ARTIFICIAL INTELLIGENCE THEORY, MODELS, AND APPLICATIONS

ARTIFICIAL INTELLIGENCE THEORY, MODELS, AND APPLICATIONS

Edited by
P. Kaliraj
T. Devi

CRC Press
Taylor & Francis Group
Boca Raton London New York

CRC Press is an imprint of the
Taylor & Francis Group, an **informa** business

AN AUERBACH BOOK

ISBN: 978-1-032-00809-7 (hbk)
ISBN: 978-1-032-10613-7 (pbk)
ISBN: 978-1-003-17586-5 (ebk)

DOI: 10.1201/9781003175865

Typeset in Times
by MPS Limited, Dehradun

Contents

Preface

The industrial revolutions Industry 4.0 and Industry 5.0 are changing the world around us. Artificial Intelligence and Machine Learning, Automation and Robotics, Big Data, Internet of Things, Augmented Reality, Virtual Reality, and Creativity are the tools of Industry 4.0. Improved collaboration is seen between smart systems and humans, which merges the critical and cognitive thinking abilities of humans with the highly accurate and fast industrial automation. The fourth and fifth industrial revolutions are affecting the roles that Indian universities and colleges prepare students for, and educational institutions are committed to help produce the workforce for this new world and the student experience to match it.

Bharathiar University has designed guidelines for Curriculum 4.0 and has prepared new syllabi for all subjects intertwining Industry 4.0 and 5.0 tools onto various disciplines such as science, social science, arts, and education. The University has identified the gap in knowledge resources, such as books, course materials, interdisciplinary curriculum, and innovative programs. To fill this gap and to prepare the future pillars of our Globe to face the Volatile, Uncertain, Complex and Ambiguous (VUCA) world, and to help the academic community, Bharathiar University has prepared guidelines for revising the syllabus, designing innovative Faculty Development Programs, establishing connectivity to the real world for students, incubating creativity and inculcating design thinking. Moreover, with the active participation of all stakeholders under the esteemed leadership of the Honorable vice-chancellor, Prof. P. Kaliraj, interdisciplinary books are being edited for Education 4.0 and 5.0.

Artificial Intelligence (AI) is a pivotal tool of Industry 4.0 in transforming the future through intelligent computational systems. AI automates repetitive learning and discovery through data. Instead of automating manual tasks, AI performs frequent, high-volume, computerized tasks reliably and without fatigue. For this type of automation, human inquiry is still essential to set up the system and ask the right questions. AI adds intelligence to existing products. Automation, conversational platforms, bots, and smart machines can be combined with large amounts of data to improve many technologies. AI is everywhere and it plays a significant role in various aspects of life. AI can be seen as a part of robotic automation, self-driving cars, healthcare and medical support, defense, online shopping, and many other technologies.

AI applications can provide personalized medicine and X-ray readings. Personal healthcare assistants can act as life coaches, reminding you to take your pills, exercise, or eat healthier. AI can analyze factory IoT data as it streams from connected equipment to forecast expected load and demand using recurrent networks, a specific type of deep learning network used with sequence data. AI provides virtual shopping capabilities that offer personalized recommendations and discuss purchase options with the consumer. Stock management and site layout technologies will also be improved with AI. In financial institutions, AI techniques can be used to identify which transactions are likely to be fraudulent, adopt fast and accurate credit scoring, and automate manually intense data management tasks.

As per the latest report of McKinsey Global Institute reports, AI is expected to create around 133 million new jobs. It shows that there is a great need for educated individuals who have expertise in this domain. And with the demand for talented engineers more than doubling in the last few years, there are limitless opportunities for professionals who want to work on the cutting edge of AI research and development. It is essential for universities and higher education institutions to offer a prescribed set of courses for a major or specialization in AI, while those with dedicated AI programs may have unique approaches to the discipline. This will create graduates who are skilled in AI and this book can aid in imparting the concepts and knowledge of AI to the graduates. This book provides a blend of the fundamentals and applications of AI with description of its fundamentals, tools, challenges, and subfields of AI. This book on AI provides relevant theory and industrial applications of AI in various domains such as healthcare, economics, education, product development, agriculture, human resource management. environment management, and marketing.

What's in the Book?

Chapter 1 entitled *"Artificial Intelligence: A Complete Insight"* describes artificial intelligence in detail from its basics to future applications and tools. This chapter provides a systematic understanding of artificial intelligence (AI) and will serve as a starting point for beginners to learn artificial intelligence irrespective of their domains.

Chapter 2 entitled *"Artificial Intelligence and Gender"* discusses gender disparity in the enterprises involved in the development of artificial intelligence-based software development. It also provides solutions to eradicate such gender bias in the AI world.

Chapter 3 entitled *"Artificial Intelligence in Environmental Management"* gives a brief overview of Artificial Intelligence (AI) potential in environmental management. The focus is to give a flavor of what AI could do in different areas, directly impacting the environment. The chapter presents a general framework for AI in environmental management, AI for cleaner air, AI for water preservation, AI for smart farming, AI for better e-waste management, and AI for climate control, i.e., smart energy optimization.

Chapter 4 entitled *"Artificial Intelligence in Medical Imaging"* elaborates the state-of-the-art AI, machine learning, and radiomics in medical imaging. It also describes the potentials and applications of using AI in medical imaging, including the challenges of AI in precision medicine.

Chapter 5 entitled *"Artificial Intelligence (AI): Improving Customer Experience (CX)"* presents the applications of artificial intelligence in improving the customer's experience from pre-purchase to purchase and then when the customer is using the product. It mainly concentrates on the applications of AI-based technology options such as chatbots and analytics in improving customer experience.

Chapter 6 entitled *"Artificial Intelligence in Radiotherapy"* describes the applications of AI in quality assurance and safety of patients during treatment using radiation. It provides insights on the ongoing technological advancements in radiation therapy and focuses on preparing researchers and students for Industry 5.0.

Chapter 7 entitled *"Artificial Intelligence in Systems Biology: Opportunities in Agriculture, Biomedicine, and Healthcare"* introduces the uses of AI in agriculture and healthcare. It describes the applications of AI in detecting the diseases in plants, provision of proper nutritional supply to plants, drug discovery, cancer cure, medical imaging, robotics, and detection of COVID-19 symptoms.

Chapter 8 entitled *"Artificial Intelligence Applications in Genetic Disease/ Syndrome Diagnosis"* shows how AI helps in the diagnosis of various diseases, such as cancer and diabetes. Diagnosing precisely and at the earliest are achieved through AI. Existing and applied AI diagnostic measures in disease and disorders diagnosis with various parameters like EEG are elaborated in this chapter.

Chapter 9 entitled *"Artificial Intelligence in Disease Diagnosis via Smartphone Applications"* discusses how AI aids disease diagnosis in the medical field using smartphone applications. The chapter identifies and evaluates the commercially available apps for promoting early diagnosis of diseases and discusses why it is safe to install available healthcare mobile applications.

Chapter 10 entitled *"Artificial Intelligence in Agriculture"* elaborates how AI helps the agricultural domain to attain supreme quality and maximum production with reduced loss. Advanced technologies in AI relieve farmers from their hard work and toil and this chapter illustrates the various AI technologies used in the field of agriculture.

Chapter 11 entitled *"Artificial Intelligence-Based Ubiquitous Smart Learning Educational Environments"* proposes a smart learning environment framework to design and implement ubiquitous smart learning. The chapter describes how this framework can be used for successful usage, coordination, and implementation of all digital resources in the learning environment.

Chapter 12 entitled *"Artificial Intelligence in Assessment and Evaluation of Program Outcomes/Program-Specific Outcomes"* describes how AI can be used in the assessment and evaluation of program outcomes and program-specific outcomes. The various machine learning models that can be used for evaluation are discussed and the chapter reiterates the role of Artificial Intelligence in the teaching–learning process.

Chapter 13 entitled *"Artificial Intelligence-Based Assistive Technology"* briefs about the significance of AI technologies in assistive technology and analyzes the different frameworks, software, and methods developed to assist differently abled people. The chapter also provides the scope of research for designers, technologists, and scientists to develop intelligent technologies to increase the capabilities of special needs people.

Chapter 14 entitled *"Machine Learning"* discusses as a subset of AI how machine learning works and the various machine learning algorithms in use. The various tools available for machine learning are also discussed and various application areas where it can be implemented are explained in detail.

Chapter 15 entitled *"Machine Learning in Human Resource Management"* shows how to apply machine learning techniques in human resource management. Moreover, the chapter explains the role of machine learning algorithms in human resource management, various applications of machine learning algorithms in human resource management, and presents some case studies.

Chapter 16 entitled *"Machine Learning Models in Product Development and Its Statistical Evaluation"* gives an idea about the role of machine learning models in product development through statistically monitoring the quality of the product and provides current emerging trends in product development to solve problems through machine learning algorithms.

Chapter 17 entitled *"Influence of Artificial Intelligence in Clinical and Genomic Diagnostics"* discusses the importance of artificial intelligence and machine learning and the influence of artificial intelligence in genomic data. Genomics is an interesting research area connected with the medical domain where DNA sequencing and modern drug discovery are significant research problems that depend on better machine intelligence.

Chapter 18 entitled *"Applications of Machine Learning in Economic Data Analysis and Policy Management"* covers machine learning (ML) in the context of economic policies and explores how economists can leverage technology advancements to make robust and effective policy decisions. The chapter also highlights the prevalent analytics and ML models and nuances of these models that warrant their prudent use in the economics and policy domain.

Chapter 19 entitled *"Industry 4.0: Machine Learning in Video Indexing"* shows how machine learning and data mining approaches can be used to provide better video indexing mechanisms to get better searchable results for users.

Chapter 20 entitled *"A Risk-Based Ensemble Classifier for Breast Cancer Diagnosis"* introduces a risk-based ensemble classifier that makes predictions by aggregating the predictions of multiple classifiers and calculating the expected risk for each class from the predictions. The experiments within this chapter are done on the Wisconsin breast cancer data set (WBCD) and the results produced reveal that the risk-based ensemble classifier outperforms the base classifiers.

Chapter 21 entitled *"Linear Algebra for Machine Learning"* brings out the relationship between linear algebra and machine learning. It introduces the basic concepts, such as eigenvalues, eigenvectors, and diagonalizable matrix of linear algebra; matrix decomposition theory, which is the foundation of data processing; Eigenvalue decomposition; singular value decomposition; and methods such as the linear dimensionality reduction method.

Chapter 22 entitled *"Identification of Lichen Plants and Butterflies Using Image Processing and Neural Networks in Cloud Computing"* provides the need to authenticate the lichen taxa's identity for the lichenologists. The proposed method of identifying lichen and butterflies is based on image processing and artificial intelligence using neural networks. It solves taxonomic problems and helps in understanding the evolution of taxa, including identification.

Chapter 23 entitled *"Artificial Neural Network for Decision Making"* provides a detailed explanation of artificial neural networks (ANNs). The chapter also provides a short discussion on the performance of ANNs for count modeling and concludes with a comparison study of ANNs with eminently used count models like zero-inflated Poisson (ZIP) and Hurdle models.

How to Use the Book

The method and purpose of using this book depend on the role that you play in an educational institution or in an industry or depend on the focus of your interest. We propose five types of roles: student, software developer, teacher, member of board of studies, and researcher.

If you are a student: Students can use the book to get a basic understanding of artificial intelligence and its tools and applications. Students belonging to any of the arts, science, and social science disciplines will find useful information from chapters on complete insight on AI, fundamentals, and applications. This book will serve as a starting point for beginners. Students will benefit from the chapters on applications of AI in *customer experience, agriculture, assistive technology, economic data analysis, healthcare, human resource management, disease diagnosis,* and *product development*

If you are a software developer: Software developers can use the book to get a basic understanding of artificial intelligence and its tools and applications. Readers with software development background will find useful information from chapters on fundamentals and applications. They will benefit from the chapters on *customer experience, agriculture, assistive technology, disease diagnosis,* and *product development*

If you are a teacher: Teachers will find that this book is useful as a text for several different university-level and college-level undergraduate and postgraduate courses. A graduate course on artificial intelligence can use this book as a primary textbook. It is important to equip the learners with a basic understanding on AI, a tool of Industry

4.0. chapter on *Artificial Intelligence: A Complete Insight* provides the fundamentals of AI. To teach the applications of AI in various sectors, say healthcare, teachers will find useful information from chapters on *disease diagnosis, medical imaging, biomedicine and healthcare, genetic disease/syndrome diagnosis, radiotherapy,* and *breast cancer diagnosis.* A course on AI for biology, too, could use the above-mentioned chapters.

If you are a member of the board of studies: Innovating the education to align with Industry 4.0 requires that the curriculum be revisited. Universities are looking for methods of incorporating Industry 4.0 tools across various disciplines of arts, science, and social science education. This book helps in incorporating AI across science, economics, and education. The book is useful while framing the syllabus for new courses that cuts across artificial intelligence and disciplines of arts or science or social science education. For example, syllabi for courses entitled artificial intelligence in science, artificial intelligence in biology, artificial intelligence in medical bio-technology, and artificial intelligence in medical physics may be framed using the chapters in this book. Industry infusion into curriculum is given much importance by involving more industry experts – R&D managers, product development managers, and technical managers as special invitees in the board of studies. Chapters given by industry experts in this book will be very helpful to infuse the application part of artificial intelligence into the curriculum.

If you are a researcher: A crucial area where innovation is required is the research work carried out by universities and institutions so that innovative, creative, and useful products and services are made available to society through translational research. This book can serve as a comprehensive reference guide for researchers in the development of experimental artificial intelligence applications. The chapters on *environmental management, improving customer experience, agriculture, economic data analysis and policy management,* and *disease diagnosis* provide researchers, scholars, and students with a list of important research questions to be addressed using AI.

*****

Acknowledgments

From Prof. P. Kaliraj:

First and foremost, I express my sincere gratitude to **Hon'ble Shri. Banwarilal Purohit,** governor of Tamil Nadu, India, who was instrumental in organizing the conference on Innovating Education in the era of Industry 4.0 during 14–15 Dec. 2019 in Ooty, which paved the way for further work in the Industry 4.0 knowledge world.

My heartfelt thanks go to Hon'ble Chief Minister of Tamil Nadu, India, and Hon'ble Minister for Higher Education, Government of Tamil Nadu. I thank Principal Secretary to Government, Higher Education Department, Government of Tamil Nadu.

I would like to express my thanks to Secretary to Governor, and Deputy Secretary to Governor, Universities Governor's Secretariat, Raj Bhavan, Chennai.

I thank my wife Dr. Vanaja Kaliraj and family members for their support and being patient.

From Prof. T. Devi:

I record my sincere thanks to **Prof. P. Kaliraj,** Hon'ble vice-chancellor of Bharathiar University, who identified the gap in the knowledge world when the professor searched for a book on Industry 4.0 and triggered the process of writing and editing books in the Industry 4.0 series. His continuous motivation during the lockdown period due to COVID-19, sensitization, and encouragement are unmatchable.

I express my profound thanks to the vice-chancellor and registrar for the administrative support. Heartfelt thanks are due to the authors of the chapters for their contributions, continuous co-operation in improvizing the chapters as and when requested, and for timely communication. I thank all the expert members who served as reviewers for providing a quality and swift review.

We wish to thank **Mr. John Wyzalek, senior acquisitions editor, Taylor & Francis/CRC Press,** who believed in the idea of this book and helped us in realizing our dream.

Special thanks are due to Mr. Todd Perry, production editor, Taylor & Francis/CRC Press, Florida, for his excellent co-ordination and Mr. Manmohan Negi, Project Manager, MPS Ltd., for his untiring and swift support.

Thanks are due to Dr. R. Rajeswari, associate professor, Department of Computer Applications for her continuous support; Sister Italia Joseph Maria and Ms. M. Lissa, project assistants, for providing earnest support.

Thanks to the faculty members Prof. M. Punithavalli, Dr. T. Amudha, Dr. J. Satheeshkumar, Dr. V. Bhuvaneswari, Dr. R. Balu, and Dr. J. Ramsingh.

Thanks to the assistant technical officers Mr. A. Elanchezian, Mr. A. Sivaraj, Mrs. B. Priyadarshini, and office staff Mr. A. Kalidas of the Department of Computer Applications of Bharathiar University, India.

Thanks are due to Mrs. K. Kowsalya, assistant registrar; Mr. R. Karthick, assistant section officer; and Mr. A. Prasanth of the office of the vice-chancellor and staff of the office of the Registrar of Bharathiar University, India.

I thank my husband Mr. D. Ravi, daughter Mrs. R. Deepiga, son Mr. R. Surya, son-in-law Mr. D. Vishnu Prakhash and grandson V. Deera and family members for their encouragement and support.

*****

Editors

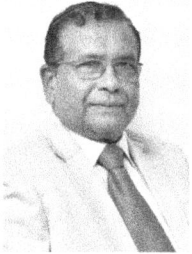

Prof. P. Kaliraj, Hon'ble vice-chancellor, Bharathiar University, a visionary and an eminent leader leading big academic teams has had more than three decades of teaching and research experience. He has held various renowned positions, such as officiating vice-chancellor of Anna University, head of the Centre for Biotechnology of Anna University, dean of faculty at A C College of Technology, and member of the syndicate for two decades at Anna University. Professor Kaliraj had research collaborations with the National Institute of Health in Maryland, USA; Glasgow University in Scotland, UK; and University of Illinois in Rockford, USA. University Grants Commission BSR Faculty Award and the Lifetime Achievement Award from the Biotechnology Research Society of India adorned the professor. **Forty-two scholars were gifted to receive the highest academic degree under his distinguished guidance**. His remarkable **patent in the area of filariasis is a boon in healthcare** and saving the lives of mankind. He is a great motivator and very good at sensitizing the faculty, scholars, and students towards achieving academic excellence and institutional global ranking. Professor Kaliraj is a recipient of the **Life Time Achievement Award and Sir J.C. Bose Memorial Award** for his outstanding contribution in higher education – research. (email: vc@buc.edu.in, pkaliraj@gmail.com)

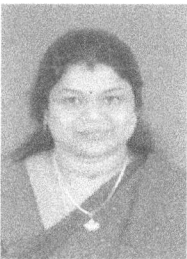

Prof. T. Devi, PhD (UK), Professor, Centre for Research and Evaluation, former dean of research, professor and head, Department of Computer Applications, Bharathiar University focuses on state-of-the-art technology that industries adopt in order to make students ready for the future world. She is a **Gold Medalist** (1981–1984) from University of Madras and a **Commonwealth Scholar** (1994–1998) for her **PhD from the University of Warwick, UK**. She has three decades of teaching and research experience from Bharathiar University, Indian Institute of Foreign Trade, New Delhi, and University of Warwick, UK. Professor Devi is good in team building and setting goals and achieving them. Her research interests include integrated data modeling and framework, meta-modeling, computer-assisted concurrent engineering, and speech processing. Professor Devi has visited the United Kingdom, Tanzania, and Singapore for academic collaborations. She has received various awards including **Commonwealth Scholarship and Best Alumni Award from PSGR Krishnammal College for Women (PSGRKCW), Proficiency award from PSG College of Technology and awards from Bharathiar University for serving for BU-NIRF, Curriculum 4.0, and Roadmap 2030 and guided 23 Ph.D. scholars**. Prof. T. Devi may be contacted at (email: tdevi@buc.edu.in, tdevi5@gmail.com)

Contributors

R. Amsaveni
Department of Information Technology
PSGR Krishnammal College for Women
Coimbatore, India

T. Amudha
Department of Computer Applications
Bharathiar University
Coimbatore, India

S. Anuradha
Operations Manager
Perpetual Systems
Coimbatore, India

M. Sakthi Asvini
Interdisciplinary Center for Water
    Research
Indian Institute of Science (IISc)
Bengaluru, India

P. Dhanalakshmi
Department of Applied Mathematics
Bharathiar University
Coimbatore, India

S. Dhivya
Department of Biotechnology
Bharathiar University
Coimbatore, India

Brijesh Kumar Gupta
IBS Software
Bengaluru, India

Hari Priya
Department of Biotechnology
Bharathiar University
Coimbatore, India

V. Kaviyarasu
Department of Statistics
Bharathiar University
Coimbatore, India

Rahul Kharat
Vice President
Zenon
Bengaluru, India

M. Krishnaveni
Department of Computer Science
Avinashilingam University for Women
Coimbatore, India

B. Malar
Department of Applied Mathematics
    and Computational Sciences
PSG College of Technology
Coimbatore, India

K. Mangayarkarasi
Department of Women Studies
Bharathiar University
Coimbatore, India

Italia Joseph Maria
Department of Computer Applications
Bharathiar University
Coimbatore, India

P. Vinayaga Moorthi
Department of Human Genetics and
   Molecular Biology
Bharathiar University
Coimbatore, India

K. Murugan
Department of Zoology
Bharathiar University
Coimbatore, India

Saradhadevi Muthukrishnan
Department of Biochemistry
Bharathiar University
Coimbatore, India

E. Kiruba Nesamalar
Department of Information Technology
Women's Christian College
Chennai, India

C. Panneerselvam
Department of Biology
University of Tabuk
Saudi Arabia

P. Ponmurugan
Department of Botany
Bharathiar University
Coimbatore, India

M. Punithavalli
Department of Computer Applications
Bharathiar University
Coimbatore, India

C. S. Rajitha
Department of Mathematics
Amrita School of Engineering
Coimbatore, India

K. M. Sakthivel
Department of Statistics
Bharathiar University
Coimbatore, India

V. Saravanan
Dean of Computer Studies
Dr. SNS Rajalakshmi College of Arts
   and Science
Coimbatore, India

J. Satheeskumar
Department of Information Technology
Bharathiar University
Coimbatore, India

R. Sathishkumar
Department of Biotechnology
Bharathiar University
Coimbatore, India

Priyadarshini Srirambalaji
Department of Applied Mathematics
   and Computational Sciences
PSG College of Technology
Coimbatore, India

P. Subashini
Department of Computer Science
Avinashilingam University for Women
Coimbatore, India

C. S. Sureka
Department of Medical Physics
Bharathiar University
Coimbatore, India

T. S. Vanitha
Department of Applied Mathematics
   and Computational Sciences

PSG College of Technology
Coimbatore, India

K. Vinaykumar Nair
BT India Pvt. Ltd.
Bengaluru, India

D. Vinotha
Department of Computer Science and
  Engineering
PRIST University
Thanjavur, India

1 Artificial Intelligence: A Complete Insight

T. Amudha

Associate Professor, Department of Computer Applications,
Bharathiar University, Coimbatore, India

CONTENTS

DOI: 10.1201/9781003175865-1

1.1   INTRODUCTION

Evolutionary changes are common in the universe, starting from the first species reported on the earth millions of years before to the species referred to as human. These evolutionary changes include physical, structural, morphological, behavioral, and mental variations. The theory of evolution also indicates a volumetric change in the brain of the species, making the species hold identical behavior from other species. The brain is an interconnected structure of millions of neurons where communication between these neurons will decide human's internal and external behavior. The sense is another significant factor that discriminates one species from the other, even every human from another human. The five senses of human beings are touch, vision, taste, hear, and smell, and the so-called sixth sense is proprioception, which means realizing self-movement and position of the body. All these senses have a strong association with the human brain.

Darwin's theory of evolution states that *"Way of successfully completing the work or the work done smartly instead of simply completing the work will play a vital role in discriminating a person from others in terms of his/her own thinking and intelligence."* Such intelligent thinking and behavior in humans are still unpredictable, whereas birds and animals exhibit their smartness through the *survival of the fittest* theory. For example, ants have their style of constructing the shortest path from their food source to nest. Human beings considered to have superior skills than ants follow the ant path construction method for deciding an efficient path to solve critical path-based problems. Similarly, humans can also widely adopt swarm intelligence to identify and optimize the solutions for numerous issues.

Figure 1.1 shows the natural, intelligent behavior of various species. However, these species are different and unique in their nature; a rare kind of intelligence can be observed in each species behavior. Many other species such as wasp, bat, cuckoo, elephant, whale, grey wolve, moth, and chicken exhibit extraordinarily intelligent characteristics. Technological developments are playing a major role in the industrial revolution, where most of the machinery has been enhanced with the support state-of-the-art technological innovations and improvements. These innovative outcomes have a stronger influence in various domains, including civil, electrical, electronics, mechanical, medical, environmental, astronomy, and other sectors. Human intelligence is more important to complete any work efficiently as well as effectively. This intelligence and intellectual thinking of human-made massive evolutionary growth by producing various devices and machinery. This ability greatly supports industries and manufacturing units for producing materials in higher volume within the stipulated time. The simplest difference between hard work and smart work is shown in Figure 1.2. Figure 1.2a

(a)

(b)

(c)

(d)

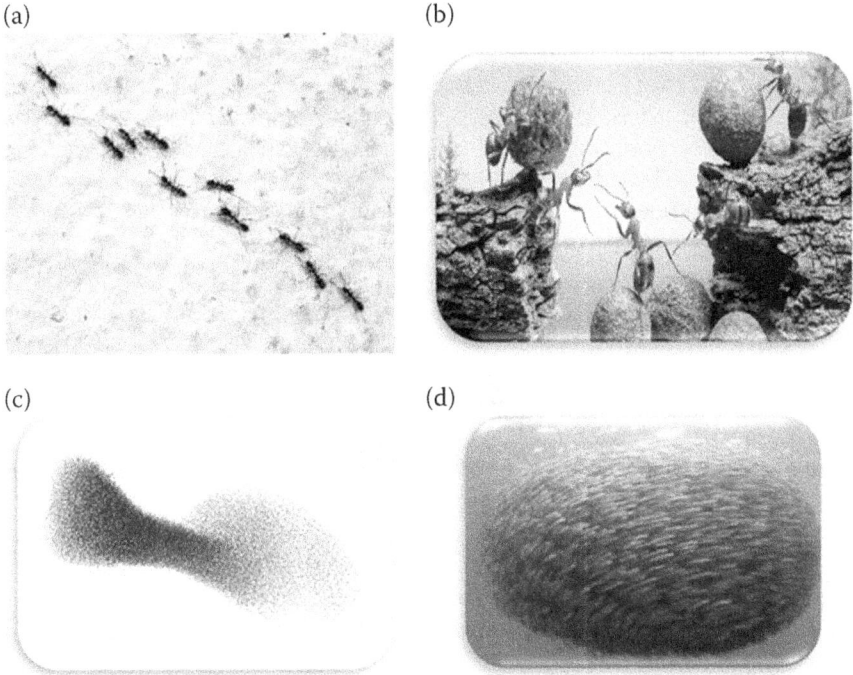

FIGURE 1.1 (a) Ant behavior, (b) smart ant behavior, (c) swarm of bees, and (d) swarm of fish.

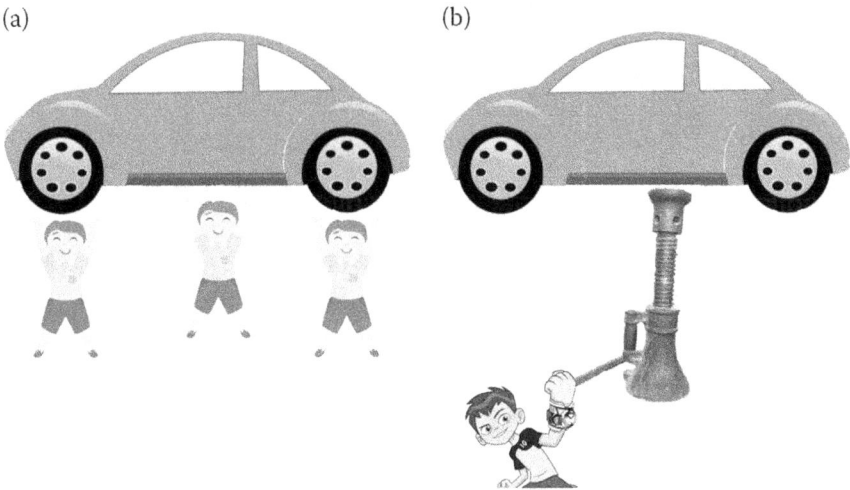

(a)

(b)

FIGURE 1.2 (a) Hard work and (b) smart work.

shows pulling up a car by a group of people whereas, in Figure 1.2b, the same work is done smartly with minimum human resources using the machine.

The latest buzzword in the industry is the *"projection and migration of industry with the support of man, machine, and automation which is referred to as INDUSTRY 4.0."* Forthcoming sections will detail artificial intelligence, which is an essential factor in Industry 4.0, its history, components, AI environment, and applicability in different domains.

1.2   ARTIFICIAL INTELLIGENCE: WHAT AND WHY?

"Intelligence" is a fascinating term that is the best fit for debate since it involves the human brain, mind, involvement, logical thinking, understanding, and applicability. The level of intelligence varies from person to person in terms of how they perceive and perform actions. In general, intelligence can be well defined as an individual's capability to do things effectively by using their own knowledge, interpretation, and insight. The term artificial intelligence (AI) was coined by John McCarthy, a Stanford University emeritus professor of computer science, and he defines it as "the science and engineering of making intelligent machines," particularly intelligent software programs. The field of AI is mostly associated with the mission of using computers to study the intelligence and associated decision-making skills of a human (Figure 1.3).

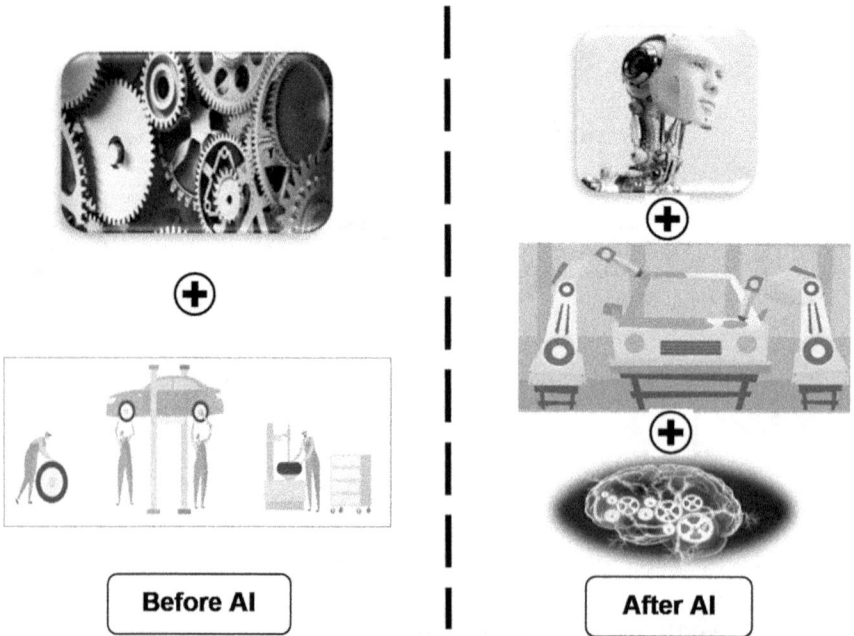

Before AI

After AI

FIGURE 1.3   Industrial scenario before and after AI.

AI is the study of agents, either softbots or robots that perceive the environment, think rationally and act accordingly like a human. In certain aspects, AI is the study to simulate the intelligence of humankind. AI aims to make machines observe and learn from people and solve problems or learn from the existing problem-solving techniques (McCarthy et al., 2006). Rather, AI is also involved in learning real-world problems which are highly challenging and finding novel solutions through experience. Researchers in AI are always instrumental in framing methods to solve highly complex problems beyond human ability and skill.

Even though humans made various innovations towards industrial and techno-logical revolutions, human resources for such material production at different manufacturing units always poses a bigger challenge due to various factors such as financial constraints, inadequate manpower, human rights, etc. Hence, there is a dire need for these industries to move towards intelligent machinery and this intelligence injected in machines made another stepping stone in the industrial revolution also referred to as *"Artificial Intelligence."* Thereby, the devices are expected to be knowledgeable about their input based on mechanical, statistical, and sensor-based inferences. In general, artificial intelligence can be defined as a *"machine with human intelligence to some extent."* Below are given a few examples of machines with a limited level of intelligence.

- Washing machines used at home have a good level of decision-making and information communication systems based on the weight of clothes, type of clothes, and the space available inside the washing drum. Even the machine can detect salt deposition in the drum.
- Intelligent televisions learn from the viewing habits and patterns of the user and can make recommendations about movies, programs, or music. The AI televisions can be operated using voice commands and connected with other smart devices at home.
- A machine used to cut the wood for pencil can accurately cut and insert the needle and segregate the qualitative pencils from the damaged ones.
- An air conditioner is one of the daily use products that have the smartness to control its cooling based on the number of persons in a room, saving power.
- Mobile phones have automatic display control using ambient light sensor technology, which helps to adjust the display's backlight for smooth visua-lization of the displayed items.
- Devices used in the agricultural sector for humidity measurement and auto-matic water flow control and irrigation support system, etc.

Arthur R. Jensen, a foremost AI researcher, has expressed that all human beings possess similar logical and rational mechanisms but differ only on certain quanti-tative parameters such as short-term memory and the ability to store and retrieve information from their long-term memory, and the speed of processing. In contrast, computers can offer massive memory space and tremendous processing speed, but the application of their capabilities is much dependent upon the rational procedures built by the programmers. It is often told that cognitive science has not completely succeeded till now in defining human capabilities. People outperforming computers always reveal the fact that the human who programmed the computers lack a clear understanding of the problem-specific and effective methodologies needed by computers.

Research in AI is always focused on the biological as well as the phenomenal aspects. The biological front is grounded on the impression that mankind is always intelligent and hence, studies in AI shall be on mimicking human psychology, behavior, and decision making. The phenomenal front is based on the study, formulation, and rational representation of the factual, worldly problems and the achievement of objectives by satisfying various real-world constraints. Both the approaches interact well and eventually work together towards progression in the field of AI.

1.3   HISTORY OF AI

Computing and intelligence are two significant words where most of us may have an identical understanding of these two words. A borderline differentiation between these two words will be helpful to have a better understanding of artificial intelligence. The word "computing" means performing any mathematical, logical, or relational operations, whereas intelligence by machine or artificial intelligence can be viewed as computing along with human intelligence. The concept of AI seems to be available since the 1940s, in various forms of intelligent computing models. The first intelligence-based computing method was introduced by the mathematician Alan Turing in 1947. He stated that more findings on machines' intelligence could be obtained by using computer programs and simulation than by using real machines. During the 1950s, most of the AI researchers have started working on computer programs rather than building machines. Turing has also discussed the circumstances to consider a machine as intelligent as a human. He strongly opined that any machine capable of mimicking and pretending as human to another human, then the machine can undoubtedly be considered as intelligent. This concept of testing machine intelligence, introduced by Alan Turing is referred to as the "Turing Test." Any machine that successfully completes the Turing test can be termed as intelligent, but an extraordinarily intelligent machine can always mimic humans even without knowing much about humans.

In 1956, John McCarthy, the researcher who actually founded the name "Artificial Intelligence" has presented his definition and views on AI in a conference at Dartmouth College, which paved the way for the beginning of the new era of AI research studies. Alan Turing had a perceptual visualization on future computing generation, which is also referred to as computing machines with thinking ability. The question challenged by Turing "Can Machine Think?" to the research community in the 1950s made a revolutionary change in the industry, which speaks on the transformation and modernization the world is now searching for in terms of Industry 4.0. Turing's concept made a strong foundation for AI, where several day-to-day applications have slowly started depending on the concept of artificial intelligence.

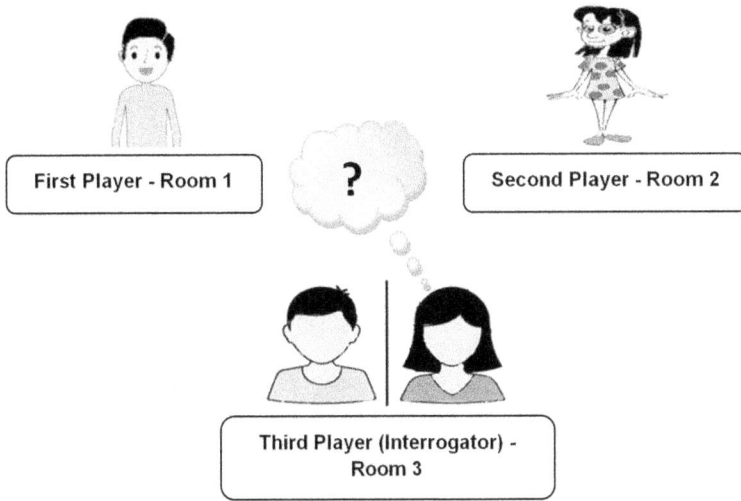

FIGURE 1.4 Party game scenario-I in turing test.

1.3.1 TURING TEST

Turing proposed his concept through the game called "party test" which is also referred to as "imitation test" (Shieber, 2004). The basic concept of this game is to find whether the participant is a human or a computer. The test scenario-I consists of three players where the first player is a "man," and the second player is a "woman," and the third player is the "interrogator" who may be either a man or a woman. The first two players will be in two different rooms and the interrogator does not know who the players are. Now, the interrogator's challenge is to find the gender of the first two players based on the written answers given by them for the questions raised by the interrogator. Another challenge will also be created by making the first player intentionally give wrong answers to the questions, which may mislead the interrogator to infer that the first player is a "woman" instead of "man." Figures 1.4 and 1.5 show the two different test scenarios of the party game.

Turing has tried to project this game with a slight change, in which he replaced one of the first two players as a computer in test scenario-II. He tried to analyze whether the machine has the ability to act like a human player by applying its own intelligence. Turing has proven through the test that; the computer has a better ability to confuse the interrogator with its intelligence, so that the interrogator has the possibility to misinterpret the first player as human instead of the computer. Machine intelligence has been proven through Alan Turing's test and widely accepted by the research community. As a result, artificial intelligence began to have a strong influence in diverse domains. Several AI-based machines and applications came into the market, providing highly accurate results and a flexible environment to the users.

Richard Karp and Steve Cook have established the NP-complete problem theories in the late 1960s. These problems are solvable, but not in a finite time and take exponential time to obtain the solution when the problem size gets increased. Such

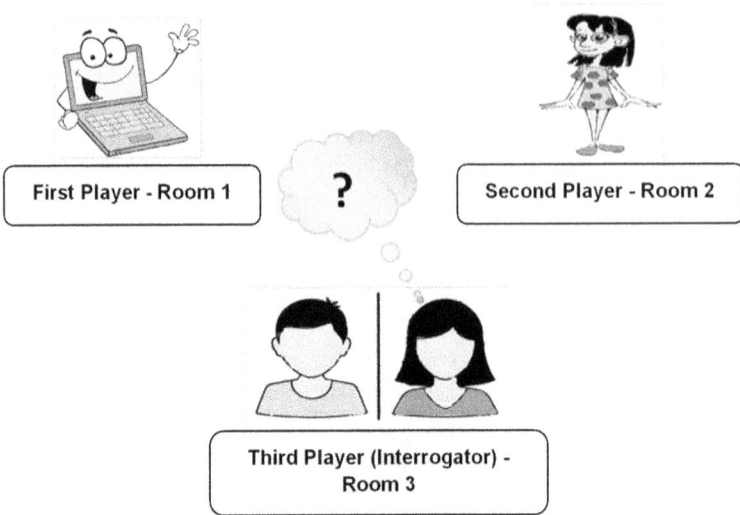

FIGURE 1.5 Party game scenario-II in turing test.

problem-solving difficulty faced in NP problem classes is termed as computational complexity. AI is expected to have capable algorithms for solving such highly computationally complex problems. However, the ultimate success in solving complex problems either by humans or by intelligent computer programs completely relies upon the specific attributes of the problems as well as the choice of suitable methods for solving the problems. It has always been a trial-and-error that could not be precisely identified by the AI research community and still remains an open challenge.

1.4 FOUNDATIONS OF AI

AI has inherited a variety of concepts, viewpoints, and practices from many other disciplines (Russell and Norvig, 2019). Learning and reasoning theories have emerged from philosophy, along with the notion that the operation of physical systems constitutes the functioning of the mind. The field of mathematics gave rise to the theory of computation, decision theory, logical reasoning, and probability. Psychology has presented investigative modes to study the human mind and systematically express the subsequent concepts. Linguistics gave the models about the structure as well as the meaning of natural languages. Above all, computer science gave the programming techniques to make AI a certainty. Likewise, various disciplines have made intellectual contributions to the fundamental theories and growth of AI.

1.4.1 LOGIC AND REASONING

Logic defines the knowledge to be possessed by the intelligent entity about the environment, the facts and proofs about the scenario in which the AI entity must perceive and act, and its objectives denoted by certain mathematical terms. The intelligent program decides the appropriate actions be performed for achieving its objectives. Logic helps to represent worldly facts, and from the facts, other facts can be deduced, and certain inferences can also be drawn. Logic is one of the key aspects of critical thinking and decision making. Analogy and creativity are the other skills highly required in AI that helps to derive logic and to make the right decisions.

1.4.2 PATTERN RECOGNITION

Any intelligent system is generally trained to observe and compare related patterns to make observations and interpretations. For e.g., an intelligent vision program to identify a human face will try to match the face with facial features such as eyes, nose, and mouth, which form a regular pattern. More complex patterns, such as natural language texts, chess positions, paintings require highly precise and improved methods than the simple pattern matching, which gave rise to several studies on AI.

1.4.3 COGNITIVE SCIENCE

Cognitive science can be well defined as the multidisciplinary study of mind and intelligence, along with neuroscience, psychology, and philosophy. Model design and building, and carrying out experiments through computational techniques is the principal strategy of AI. In the domain of cognitive sciences, psychological experiments and computational prototypes ideally go in accord. Much more research works in AI are also investigating knowledge representation, cognitive systems, and psychology.

1.4.4 HEURISTICS

A heuristic is a rule of thumb, a trial method in discovering some idea that is embedded in the code. Heuristic methods are extensively used in Artificial Intelligence for fact-finding and decision making. These functions are also used in various styles to find possible solutions in a search space, for e.g., finding the distance of the destination node from the source nodes in the given search space. Heuristic functions can make comparisons among the feasible solutions and find the best optimal solution in problem-solving. The skill to explore and exploit exponential combinations of possible solutions is of utmost importance for an AI entity or program, like moves in a chess game. Research works are continuously carried out to determine how efficiently this search could be done in various domains.

1.4.5 PHILOSOPHY

AI can be associated with philosophy in many ways, particularly because both the disciplines study mind and common sense. The mind has a strong foundation of intellectual processing and realization, which stands inherent to the real world, beyond rational understanding. Philosophy has instituted a customary practice where the human mind is perceived to be a machine predominantly operated by rational and cognitive abilities possessed within (McCarthy, 2006). It also explains the theories to establish the source of knowledge. Carl Hempel and Rudolf Carnap's philosophical concept tried to analyze the process of knowledge acquisition through experiential learning. Moreover, the association between knowledge and action is ruled by the mind and the modalities of specific associations and justifications for actions are the most needed research in AI. Thought processes, knowledge gain, and a sequence of reasonable actions play a huge role in modeling an intelligent agent that behaves rationally.

1.4.6 MATHEMATICS

Mathematical validation in the areas of computation, logic, algorithm, and probability are much needed to formulate the theories of AI. In the 9th century, mathematician Al-Khowarazmi has introduced algebra, Arabic numerals, and formal algorithms for computation. In 1847, Boole introduced formal language for making a logical inference. AI has the responsibility to explore the abilities and limits of logic and computation. Further to logic and computation, Bayes probability theory and Bayesian analysis, have served as the foundation to the uncertain reasoning approaches in AI systems. There exist certain functions that can neither be computed nor be represented by formal algorithms. Alan Turing has also expressed that there were some functions that cannot be computed by Turing machine. There is a class of problems, termed as intractable, which says that when the size of the problem instances grows, there will be an exponential increase in the time taken to solve the problems in accordance with the instance size. Problem-solving through AI should pay attention to subdividing such problems into small subproblems and solving them in a reasonable time through intelligent behavior. The decision theory, established by John Von Neumann and Oskar Morgenstern in 1944, has provided the theoretical basis for most of the intelligent agent prototypes.

1.4.7 PSYCHOLOGY

William James in the 18th century opines that the brain plays a dominant role in acquiring, holding, and processing information, attributing to cognitive psychology. Craik stated that *"If the organism carries a 'small-scale model' of external reality and of its own possible actions within its head, it is able to try out various alternatives, conclude which is the best of them, react to future situations before they arise, utilize the knowledge of past events in dealing with the present and future, and in every way to react in a much fuller, safer, and more competent manner to the emergencies which face it."* He also specified the three key aspects of an intelligent agent as follows: i. Every *stimulus* should be linked to a specific form of representation, ii. the linked *representation* should be worked out by the cognitive processes to develop more representations, and iii. the set of representations are manipulated back to a set of associated *actions*. Information processing insights have started governing the field of psychology since 1960. Later on, psychologists have believed that *"cognitive theories and computer programs work alike,"* which says that cognition consists of a well-defined transformation process operating through the information carried by the input. As per the early history of AI and cognitive science, researchers have treated Artificial Intelligence and psychology as the same discipline and it was quite common to view AI program behavior as psychological results. Nevertheless, the disparities in the methodology of AI and psychology were made clear at a later point of time, and clear-cut differences were identified between them, though they share and contribute a lot towards the development of each other.

1.4.8 LINGUISTICS

Linguistics is termed the scientific and systematic way of studying languages, making observations, testing hypotheses, and making decisions. Noam Chomsky, in his book on *Syntactic Structures,* discussed the creativity in language and showed how young children comprehend and form a sequence of words that they were never familiar with. Chomsky's theory was based on the syntactic models and he has also suggested various programmable entities. Later developments in linguistics have highlighted more of the complexities and ambiguities in language studies. Linguistics not only speaks about the structure of sentences but also about the understanding of the subject matter and context, which has more to explore concerning AI and knowledge representation. Ontology is the field that studies the categories of existential objects. Computer programs mostly deal with many types of objects and their basic properties in AI. Many early works in AI were focused on language understanding for decision making, which has naturally created a link between AI and linguistics. These two fields gave rise to certain other hybrid areas of research such as computational linguistics and natural language processing.

1.5 THE AI ENVIRONMENT

The environment of artificial intelligence consists of five major components such as machine, Human Intelligence, Machine Learning (ML) algorithms, Internet of Things (IoT), Internet Of Everything (IOE), and Data Science and Engineering as shown in Figure 1.6.

The machine is a basic as well as an implicit component in both non-AI and AI-based environment. *Intelligence* is an interesting characteristic of a human that will discriminate humans from animals and even from another human as well. Identifying the best intelligence from human brains for finding a solution to the problem plays a major role in the AI environment. This intelligence will be embedded into the machine so that the machine will act as a smart machine by carrying human intelligence, in the form of a list of instructions also referred to as program or coding. Machine *learning* is one of the efficient platforms which is used by most of the AI developers or AI programmers to produce intelligent coding. Machine learning algorithms play a major role, as they enable self-learning in AI entity from the environment and own experience. These algorithms are of much help in the

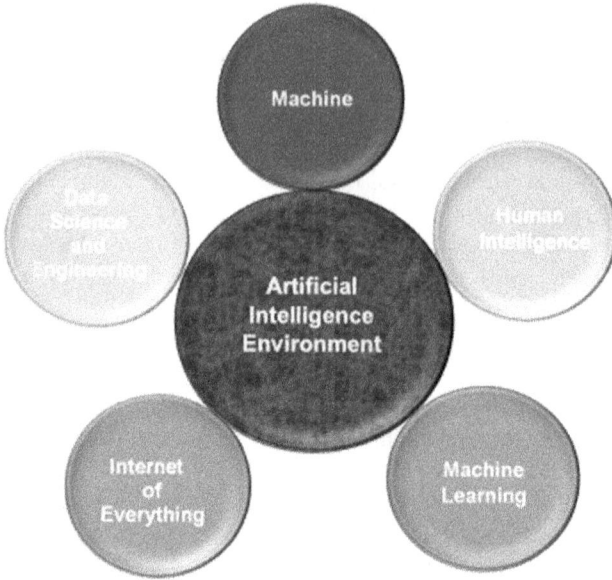

FIGURE 1.6   The AI environment.

prediction of events based on the available data and thereby forecast future trends. *Internet of Everything* and the *Internet of Things* has a very close relationship with the AI environment since most of the decision making will be depending on the real-time data produced by sensor technology. An intelligent program developed by the human in the form of coding will use the data acquired through various sensors connected to the AI environment. These data will help the machine to act intelligently so that the working environment becomes smarter. *Data Science and Engineering* is another important component in the AI environment. Data analysis plays an important role in most of the real-time applications since any decision making taken by the machine through programming majorly depend on efficient analysis of data. The integration of these components, but not limited to, will make an effective and AI environment.

1.6   APPLICATION DOMAINS OF AI

Globally, due to the immense developments and technological transformations in various sectors, the need for AI-based products and processes are on the rise even in everyday applications. Given the rapid advances in AI, it is more likely that pathology and radiology images will be analyzed by intelligent agents in the future (Whitby, 2008). AI agents in speech and text recognition are being employed for tasks like patient communication and recording of clinical notes. Figure 1.7 highlights the application domains of AI.

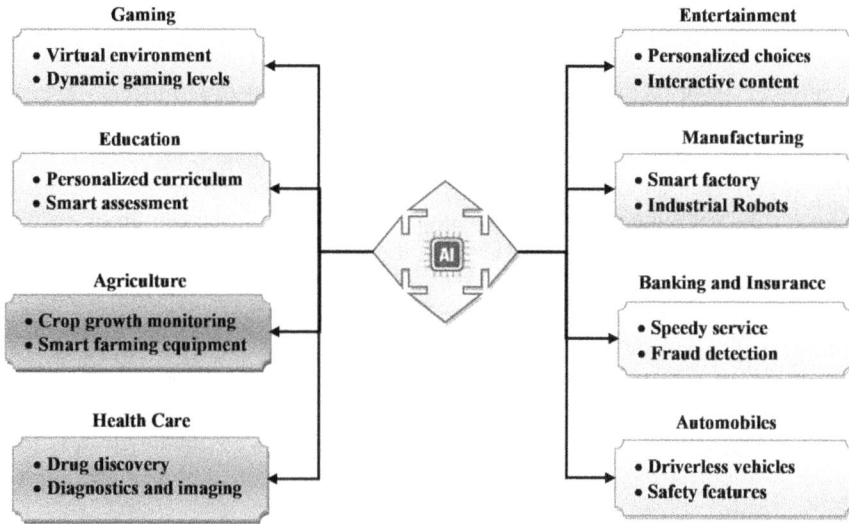

Gaming
- Virtual environment
- Dynamic gaming levels

Education
- Personalized curriculum
- Smart assessment

Agriculture
- Crop growth monitoring
- Smart farming equipment

Health Care
- Drug discovery
- Diagnostics and imaging

Entertainment
- Personalized choices
- Interactive content

Manufacturing
- Smart factory
- Industrial Robots

Banking and Insurance
- Speedy service
- Fraud detection

Automobiles
- Driverless vehicles
- Safety features

FIGURE 1.7   Application domains of AI.

1.6.1 GAMING

Artificial Intelligence in the gaming industry was dated back to the 1950s when Arthur Samuel released the Checkers game powered by AI, which successfully demonstrated the self-learning capability of computer programs. This program has given tough challenges to even professional players and could even win them on many occasions. Today, AI finds a significant place in game development, as games with AI provides a highly realistic feel and involvement to the users. Games are naturally complex and require a human mind to think in countless ways beyond imagination. Different users have different assumptions, different levels of understanding, different styles, and skills while playing games. The AI entity in gaming has to look into all these factors, train itself by taking into consideration various human perspectives, and set nearly infinite strategies to tackle the human opponents. The AI program gains knowledge and learns a lot from each and every user playing the game. It creates a huge knowledge base of reference, which gets updated with every new game played and aids in making dynamic decisions during the game. Regression algorithms and machine learning techniques go hand-in-hand in predicting the game moves of the human opponent. The gaming industry provides a risk-free virtual environment for testing the intelligence of AI applications and enables us to explore creativity without any restrictions, though challenging.

1.6.2 EDUCATION

AI has a greater potential to change the teaching-learning process, assist teachers in devising better strategies in teaching, assist students in an adaptive and improved learning experience. AI can automate the administrative responsibilities of teachers and academic institutions. Extensive research and development works are being carried out to develop intelligent educational tools, which could save teachers time by assisting them in the maintenance of student attendance, evaluation of exam papers, assessment of assignments, and other supportive activities in education. AI in education is much focussed on identifying the subject knowledge and learning capability of each and every student through investigative testing and to develop personalized and student-specific curriculum. AI can be of much help in supporting the students who struggle to cope up with the common curriculum and combined teaching-learning practices.

Personalized learning experiences are expected to overcome the major short-comings in the classic one-to-many educational models. Inclusive learning will become a reality with AI, where students from varied educational and societal backgrounds can participate in a classroom lecture and effectively engage in discussions. It is always a myth that the introduction of AI in education will lead to a replacement of teachers, but the actual fact is that teachers will be enabled through AI to perform better by providing individual attention and personalized recommendations to every student. AI can also customize the student assignments and exam question papers as well, thereby assuring a better environment for the students. Educational AI applications will facilitate students to learn in a conducive way, and the growth in this area will offer a wide range of prospective services to teachers and students.

1.6.3 HEALTHCARE

AI technology is revolutionizing the medical sector and offers multiple advantages over traditional analytics and medical decision-making practices (Yu et al., 2018). It can assist doctors and scientists in early detection and prevention of diseases, suggest personalized treatment plans for patients, unlocks various complex data sets to gain new understandings. Intelligent algorithms in AI can speed up and improve the precision in the analysis of medical data and images, which will allow physicians to gain more insights into disease diagnosis, treatment decision, and patient care. Automation of medical procedures through AI can expand healthcare access to millions of people who live in remote or underdeveloped regions where there is a shortage of trained medical as well as paramedical professionals. AI systems can also be used in taking X-rays, ultrasound, CT and MRI scanning, and many other diagnostic procedures which are in general performed by clinical support staff. AI and machine learning algorithms are capable to speed up the analysis of huge medical data, arrive at some meaningful inferences through predictions, provide early alerts about patient health conditions, recommend and support doctors in making decisions on the treatment to be given for critically ill patients. Artificial Intelligence (AI), combined with investigational technologies, is estimated to pave the way for the discovery of cost-effective, improved, and more successful drugs for various health complaints and diseases. AI will be helpful to automate and optimize the research and development in drug discovery procedures.

1.6.4   AGRICULTURE

AI-assisted technologies can support the agricultural sector in improved crop yield, pest control, soil nutrition monitoring, crop growth monitoring, and many other tasks related to agriculture. AI can help the farmers to monitor their crops without the requirement to personally supervise and observe the farm. AI is changing the traditional agricultural practices, reduce the burden of farmers, and improve crop management. AI can also be utilized to test soil nutrient availability, nutrient deficiency, and other defects in the soil. This will enable the farmers to limit the use of chemical fertilizers as per the nature of the soil and crop needs. Implementing AI can also check crop defects and diseases at an early stage, thereby improving healthy crop production and controlled pesticide usage. AI-enabled applications are highly supportive of the farmers in forecasting the weather conditions, which play a vital role in crop planning and cultivation. Weather data also assists the farmer to take the precautionary steps to protect the crops based on the predicted rainfall or drought, with the help of AI. Furthermore, AI helps farmers to selectively identify the weeds, which helps to spray chemicals only on the weeds without affecting the crops. Implementing AI in agriculture will strengthen the agricultural sector to a remarkable extent and reduce the work of farmers by providing accurate and timely guidance.

1.6.5   ENTERTAINMENT

Artificial intelligence serves as a powerful tool in the entertainment industry, bringing massive changes and thus reshaping the entertainment arena. AI along with augmented reality, data analytics, and deep learning technologies exhibit remarkable intelligence in interactive game design, innovative content production, movie design, and advertisement creation. AI has brought in an innovative style, creativity, and reality to content creation, delivery, and re-defined consumer engagement. In movie creation, AI employs massive data sets to analyze and explore the user preferences and to design scenarios, far beyond human capabilities. Various learning strategies are used by AI to learn from all possible external knowledge sources and self-experience to design interesting content. Companies use AI to monitor customer activity, assess customer behavior and to analyze customer sentiments on products, and use this analysis in improved as well as personalized service provisioning.

1.6.6   MANUFACTURING

Industry 4.0 is focused on bringing out a massive transformation in the manufacturing industry where Artificial intelligence serves as a core component in this revolutionary process. Artificial Intelligent technologies are capable of making the concept of "*Smart Factory*" a reality, which makes more productivity as well as staff empowerment. Andrew Ng, the co-founder of Google Brain and Coursera, says: "*AI can efficiently accomplish manufacturing, ensure quality control, reduce the design time, cut down materials wastage, further production recycling, and reuse, do predictive maintenance, and much more"*. Starting from materials procurement, production, warehousing to supply chain, sales, and maintenance, AI is aimed at changing the way every industry operates so far. The International Federation of Robotics has predicted that by 2025, there will be around 1.5 million industrial robots working in factories worldwide (Gonzalez et al., 2018). As more and more robots enter into the industrial shop floor along with human workers, there is a need to ensure efficient collaboration between robot and human. Advances in AI will enable robots to optimize industrial processes, handle more cognitive tasks, and make dynamic decisions based on the real-time scenario. AI algorithms play a significant role in the estimation of market demand, location and economic factors, weather patterns, consumer behavior, and much more.

1.6.7 BANKING AND INSURANCE

Artificial intelligence has gifted the banking and the insurance sector a whole new system to meet the customer demands with more convenient, smart, and safe methods to protect, spend, save, and invest their money. Artificial Intelligence will be the forthcoming trend in the banking sector as it is powered by the ability of data analytics to improve compliance, derive valuable insights, and tackle fraudulent transactions. AI can make use of the humongous data available in the insurance sector for more accurate predictions, determine trends, risks, save manpower, and ensure better information for future planning. An intelligent algorithm could realize anti-money laundering activities in no time compared to the time and effort to be spent by human resources. AI bots, digital payment consultants, and biometric fraud detection devices will reduce costs, ensure accurate and quick processing in banks, and offer highly improved quality of services to the customers. AI bots can instantly detect suspicious activities and security breaches concerning customer accounts and can alert the customers and companies well before the occurrence of fraud. Repetitive work processes can be automated, which allows human knowledge and time to be used for value-added functions, which definitely needs human expertise.

1.6.8 AUTOMOBILES

As autonomous vehicles are going to be the future, Artificial Intelligence is getting implemented in numerous ways in the design and operations of vehicles. Artificial Intelligence and machine learning have been successfully applied in the navigation of vehicles, monitoring of blind-spot, seats, mirrors, and temperature adjustment, and also in giving personalized suggestions. Various sensors controlled by AI can immediately respond to any dangerous situations by alerting the driver, applying the automated emergency braking system, or taking control of the vehicle and initiating communications to helplines. AI enables the detection of technical changes well in advance before it could affect the vehicle's performance and helps prevention of unexpected failures. Automated Guided Vehicle (AGV) is another path-breaking technology in the automobile industry, powered by AI. Without any human assistance, AGVs can identify the objects, find the optimal routes, pickup, and deliver goods to different parts of a designated location. Recently, many AI techniques are being tested and implemented in automobiles, aiming towards more effective automation and a driverless future.

1.7 AI TOOLS

Artificial Intelligence tools support the development of AI solutions for real-time, complex problems found in a variety of application domains. These tools have built-in functions and algorithms that help the user to analyze the nature of the problem, design a flexible prototype, build multiple solutions, test them and identify the best optimal solution within a very short time period. The tools can also simulate cognitive functions such as experiential learning, reasoning with logic, environmental sensing, and social intelligence like that of the human mind. Table 1.1 lists some of the successful tools in Artificial Intelligence and machine learning.

1.8 CHALLENGES IN AI

Like any technological developments, Artificial intelligence has both positive as well as negative impacts. Even though AI has a huge potential to serve mankind, there are certain challenges to be faced in real-time implementation (Harkut and Kasat, 2019). The following section discusses the major challenges of artificial intelligence in the working environment. Figure 1.8 shows the challenges of AI technology concerning various factors which include human bias, manpower, security, data genuineness, etc.

1.8.1 Loss of Self-Thinking

The intelligence of one person may make a machine to behave smart and intelligent subject to the person's knowledge who feed intelligence to the machine. It does not mean that this constrained machine intelligence will enhance the user's self-thinking ability. Instead, this kind of someone else's intelligence may lead to negative impacts as well. For instance, a machine having limited intelligence in decision making will make a human to follow it as such, though there may be better decisions that could be arrived by the human by their own intelligence.

For example, consider the scenario in which a machine having the intelligence to segregate the materials based on the color property. Assume the materials are in three different colors such as red, blue, and green and there are also other materials with a combination of the above three colors. The machine can perfectly segregate the materials with identical colors, but materials with composite colors and fading colors may be identified only through the program using color thresholding and this color thresholding is mostly static and user-defined. Sometimes, a human can do better segregation of color material than a machine that uses static intelligence. Such failure cases by intelligent machines are referred to as *false positives* and *false negatives*. Figure 1.9 shows the general representation of identical colors and degrading colors where the machine and human will be discriminated against in terms of their own intelligence.

TABLE 1.1
Tools in AI

Tool	Purpose	Website
Analyst	AI tool to analyze and organize unstructured data into a general set of rules to facilitate detailed AI and ML structures.	https://www.analyst-toolbox.com/
Tensorflow	Python-based AI library that provides diverse functionality to implement Deep Learning Models.	https://www.tensorflow.org/
ML Kit	Mobile-only SDK, which embeds machine learning technologies for face and text recognition, barcode scanning, image labeling, etc.	https://firebase.google.com/products/ml-kit
H2O	Deep learning AI platform for predictive modeling, risk analysis, insurance, advertising, healthcare, and customer intelligence.	https://www.h2o.ai/
Pytorch	An open-source AI and machine learning tool to accelerate research prototyping towards product deployment	https://pytorch.org/
DeepChem	A python-based AI tool for drug discovery, materials science, quantum chemistry, and biology.	https://www.deepchem.io/
scikit	AI tool for data pre-processing, predictive data analysis, model fitting, model selection, and evaluation	https://scikit-learn.org/stable/
DeepTox	AI tool that predicts the toxicity of chemical compounds	http://www.bioinf.jku.at/research/DeepTox/
Keras	AI tool for fast prototyping, configuring networks, and image recognition	https://keras.io/
Rainbird	AI tool for intelligent automation and decision making in finance, healthcare, insurance, and banking services	https://rainbird.ai/
AutoAI	AI tool that analyzes the dataset and discovers problem-specific data transformations, algorithms & parameter settings, builds and deploy a machine learning model	https://dataplatform.cloud.ibm.com/docs/content/wsj/analyze-data/autoai-overview.html

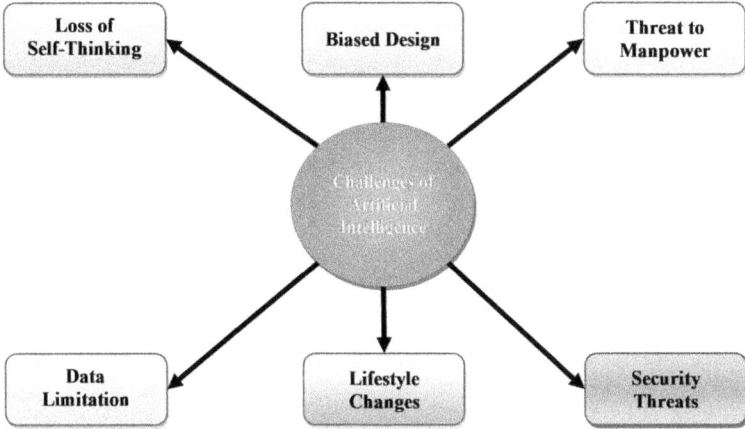

FIGURE 1.8 Challenges in AI.

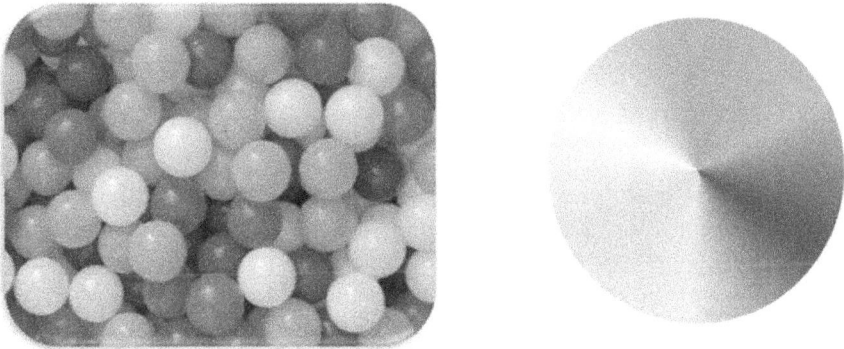

FIGURE 1.9 Representation of solid colors and composite colors.

1.8.2 BIAS IN THE DESIGN OF ARTIFICIAL INTELLIGENCE

The question *"Will it be a better model when one person's knowledge is adopted by all others?"* is a great challenge for artificial intelligence developers. The answer to this question will make us understand the influence of *"bias"* in the design of artificial intelligence. Any machine designed with human intelligence and algorithms is primarily dependent on either the knowledge of a single person or a specific group and hence, the machine intelligence will be restricted based on their limited knowledge. This intelligence can be manipulated and controlled by the developer, which may not be favorable to all scenarios. This bias in design may become a threat to society to forcibly adopt a model, though it is not a perfect fit for everyone.

1.8.3   Limitation on Data

Availability of data plays a major role in justifying the performance metrics of any AI entity. Genuineness of the data is another major challenge to the developers of artificial intelligence as well as to the AI researchers. Most of the AI-based outcomes are primarily based on existing, dynamic data being continually collected. Several data pre-processing algorithms developed by researchers are available to smooth the data before developing any intelligence model. Now the question before AI developers is *"How to find and fill up the missing data?"* In general, AI developers will use mathematical and statistical models such as interpolations, regression, and correlation methods for fitting missing values with respect to existing data. These predicted and fitted values show higher influence in artificial intelligence models. The second question is *"Will the mechanism used by AI developers for selection and rejection of data is perfect and suitable to all?"* Figure 1.10 shows two different ways to cluster the data points, a simple illustration of two possible ways to construct AI models. In the first method, lower-right data points were considered and upper-left data points were excluded whereas in the second method, upper data points were selected and lower data points were excluded. Hence, the development of AI models based on these two methods will surely give two different kinds of understanding based on the corresponding selection of data.

1.8.4   Threat to Manpower

The goal of artificial intelligence is to reduce human errors by replacing them through machine intelligence. Job opportunities will be limited due to the growth and development of human free artificial intelligence models in society. This reduction in job opportunities due to the development of AI will indirectly influence the economy, as artificial intelligence gradually reduces manpower (McCarthy, 2000). Worldwide population growth is always on the rise, and hence the development of humanless technology may pose a big threat to human survival irrespective of the country. Figure 1.9 shows the influence of robots replacing manpower in an industrial environment.

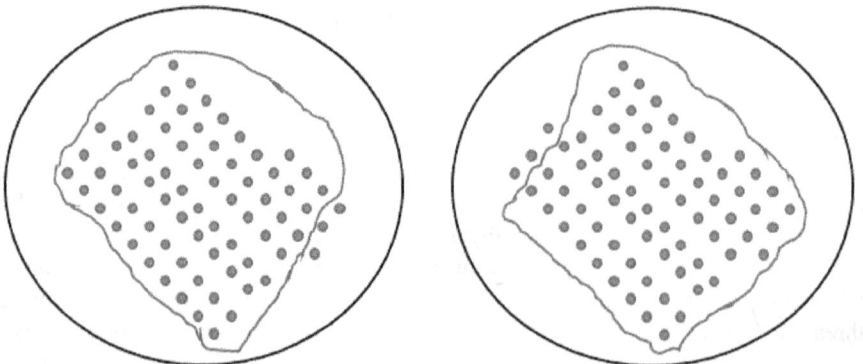

FIGURE 1.10   Two different types of clustering data to build AI model.

1.8.5 LIFESTYLE CHANGES

The current lifestyle of the human being is incomparable with the traditional life-style due to the extensive use influence of technology. Technological development is also playing its own role as one of the factors which are affecting the health of the human being. For example, most of the traditional games were replaced by technology-based games where there is no physical exercise to the human. Some AI-based games are highly interesting not only to young children but also to old age people, where unknowingly their mind and brain are affected and addicted to the games. It is another big challenge where the users undergo immense stress and struggle to come out of the virtual environment, especially the younger generation.

1.8.6 SECURITY THREATS

AI has placed its footprints all over the world in smart product development and an integrated environment. The integrated environment will help society to access AI-based products from any corner of the world but on the other side, there is always a standing threat by intruders to do unauthorized access to these AI-based products. This leads to a major threat to society, as the intruder may get access and alter the functionality of the AI products. Think about the scenario where the AI machine designed to detect and remove the "weed" in the crop field starts to remove the crop instead of weed due to security malfunctioning. Such hidden threats are always there in most of the AI-based developments.

1.9 FUTURE PROSPECTS OF AI

AI is one of the significant and powerful breakthroughs which will have a huge impact on human in all walks of life and hence it needs continuous monitoring and attention to frame standards and policies for the upcoming years. Though initial efforts in AI is highly challenging, AI is expected to master all the domains in the future. The emphasis of AI should not only be on the capability of the technologies, but also the usefulness and implementation in the respective field. AI will un-doubtedly empower the automation industry through a vast knowledge base and also infuse a high level of intelligence into the entire automation process, which will assist to prevent the associated cyber threats and contention.

AI will become integral to all processes and operations and keeps evolving and innovating with time without considerable manual intervention. For widespread adoption of AI systems, regulations and standards must be set up by the competent authorities, provision for integration must be made available, sufficient training and knowledge must be given to the user base to make them clearer about their roles and the role of AI systems. Above all, the AI system must be constantly updated and to be incorporated with day-to-day advancements in the field (Cio et al., 2020). Future developments in AI has to be more focused on bias-free, eco-friendly, non-radioactive, carbon-neutral, and energy-efficient AI environment. Figure 1.11 pre-sents the current scenario of manufacturing units, where robots assist humans in

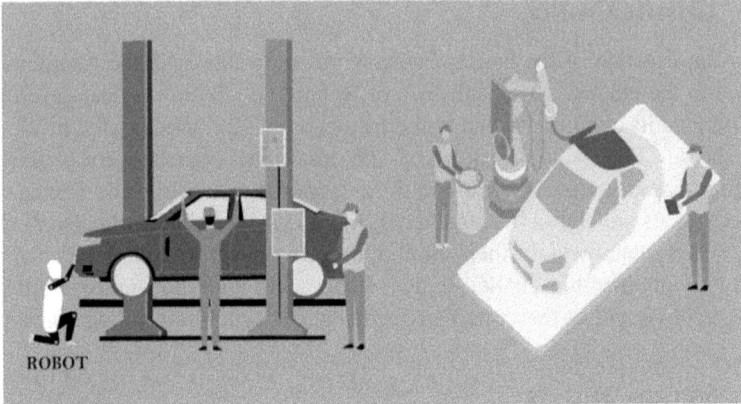

FIGURE 1.11   Present scenario of manufacturing unit.

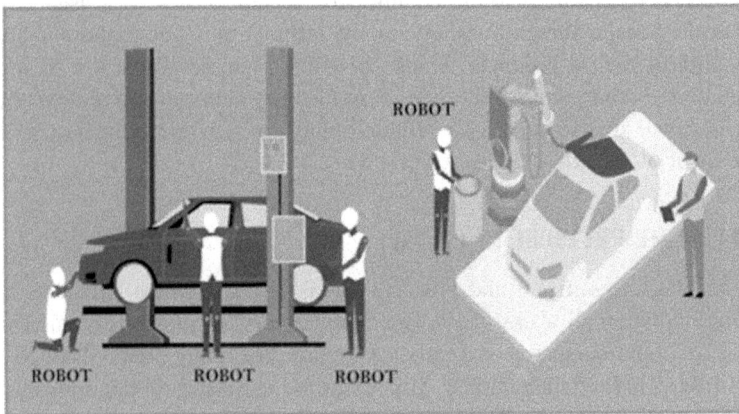

FIGURE 1.12   Future scenario of manufacturing unit.

their work. Figure 1.12 shows the future scenario, where robots carry out the entire work under human supervision.

1.9.1   APPLICABILITY

Artificial intelligence models are being developed with the available, limited data based on few assumptions. Applying and testing the AI prototype to similar applications may result in similar results and interpretation. Also, applying the same prototype for slightly varied applications may not ensure proper decision making in all cases. Hence, the development of a flexible AI model to fit global requirements will be the focus in the future for AI developers.

1.9.2 DYNAMISM IN AI MODEL

Most of the AI applications are developed for the current technologies which keep updated on an everyday basis. Hence, an artificial intelligence–based system developed with today's capability may not be suitable in the future due to the dynamic change and growth in technology (Oke, 2008). Scalability in terms of functionality with respect to the current requirements is another bigger challenge for AI designers. All the AI models developed based on the present scenario should also have the ability and adaptability to support future scenarios.

1.9.3 ECONOMIC FEASIBILITY

The cost factor involved in the development of AI models is huge and not affordable by many. Even though introducing AI in a work environment have many positive footprints, the cost involved in developing and implementing such automated environments may not be economically feasible when compared with a traditional working environment. Hence, introducing this technology in small-scale industries and its applications may not be in the position to implement the same due to the higher influence of cost factor. More works are to be done in bringing down the cost incurred in the development and maintenance of AI systems.

1.9.4 USER TRAINING

Transformation in the workplace requires the user to have preliminary knowledge as well as intense training on AI models. Training on AI technology either before launching or after launching the AI products is mandatory to the user for effective usage of the AI system. For example, intelligent word editors and text-based applications can continue the word or subsequent words when the user tries to type half of the word itself. This word predictive and suggestive system needs a minimal level of training to the user for selecting such predictive words or sentences by pressing corresponding keys. Some users do not even know how to use such word applications even though users are using the word applications in their day-to-day working environment.

1.10 SUMMARY

AI plays a highly significant and responsible role in society and of late, notable advancement has been made in this domain. AI is always a matter of interest in generating new ideas and innovative products that can adapt and maneuver the complex thought process of humans. AI has the potential to make human life comfortable and easy in several aspects. On the industrial front, AI can make wonders by incorporating intelligent bots in production, which have the power to perform tasks at an unimaginable speed with much precision as well. Many research and development works are going on worldwide to bring down the initial investment cost incurred in this industrial transformation.

This chapter has highlighted how effectively AI can be applied in various application domains such as healthcare, education, automobiles, entertainment, and so on. There is no doubt that the future is going to be AI-centric, where there will be intelligent robots all around us, carrying out a variety of automated tasks and helping mankind. On the other end, any technology is like a double-edged sword and AI is no exception to that. A time may come when smart machines will overpower the human race and will slowly make us all completely dependent on the comfort and luxury provided by artificially intelligent entities. Regulations and standards are to be framed to ensure the role of AI, invariably the intelligent machine or robot, as rightly pointed by Isaac Asimov in 1942, as given below (Barthelmess and Furbach, 2014).

- *A robot may not injure a human being or, through inaction, allow a human being to come to harm.*
- *A robot must obey the orders given to it by human beings, except where such orders would conflict with the First Law.*
- *A robot must protect its own existence as long as such protection does not conflict with the First or Second Laws.*

REFERENCES

Barthelmess U., Furbach U., 2014. Do we need Asimov's laws? *MIT Technology Review*, http://arxiv.org/abs/1405.0961, Cambridge, MA.
Cio R., Travaglioni M., Piscitelli G., Petrillo A., Felice F.D., 2020. Artificial intelligence and machine learning applications in smart production: Progress, trends, and directions. *Sustainability, 12*, 492.
Gonzalez A.G.C., Alves M.V. S., Viana G.S., Carvalho L.K., 2018. Supervisory control-based navigation architecture: A new framework for autonomous robots in Industry 4.0 environments. *IEEE Transactions on Industrial Informatics, 14*(4), 1732–1743.
Harkut D.G., Kasat K., 2019. *Artificial Intelligence - Challenges and Applications*, Intech Open Ltd, UK.
McCarthy J., 2000. Free will - Even for robots. *Journal of Experimental and Theoretical Artificial Intelligence, 12*(3), 341–352. DOI: 10.1080/09528130050111473, UK.
McCarthy J., 2006. *The Philosophy of AI and AI of Philosophy*, Stanford University Publication, Stanford, CA.
McCarthy J., Minsky M.L., Rochester N., Shannon C.E., 2006. A proposal for the Dartmouth summer research project on artificial intelligence. August 31, 1955. *AI Magazine, 27*(4), 12. DOI: https://doi.org/10.1609/aimag.v27i4.1904.
Oke S.A., 2008. A literature review on artificial intelligence. *International Journal of Information and Management Sciences, 19*, 535–570.
Russell S.J. and Norvig P., 2019. *Artificial Intelligence - A Modern Approach*, IV edition, Pearson Education, New Jersey.
Shieber S.M., 2004. *The Turing Test - Verbal Behavior as the Hallmark of Intelligence*, MIT Press, London, England.
Whitby B., 2008. *Artificial Intelligence – A Beginner's Guide*, One World Publisher, UK.
Yu K., Beam A.L., Kohane I.S., 2018. Artificial intelligence in healthcare. *Nature Biomedical Engineering, 2*, 719–731.

2 Artificial Intelligence and Gender

K. Mangayarkarasi

Assistant Professor, Department of Women's Studies,
Bharathiar University, Coimbatore, India

CONTENTS

Artificial intelligence is the most talked about technology across a wide breadth of industries. Although various expressions of artificial intelligence (machine learning, deep learning, NLP, etc.) are frequently discussed in board meetings and planning sessions, both people and media are deeply skeptical about the topic. It's quite obvious to fear the unknown. As Hollywood portrays: is the rise of machines going to wipe off mankind? Or, at the least, are they going to take over human jobs. How good or bad are they going to be? Well, the truth will unfold with time.

Like it or not, artificial intelligence is everywhere today and is growing its presence by the clock. It's impossible to live without them today, from basic

DOI: 10.1201/9781003175865-2

chatbots and virtual agents to smart home devices (IoT), industrial robots, drones, and wearables. You just think of any product or service you use daily. There's a touch of artificial intelligence in every one of them. Every business is incorporating some bits of artificial intelligence in their workflow. Because if they don't, they'll sure be left out of the game.

This article will help you understand the basics of various tools, working parts of artificial intelligence, and its ecosystem. Be it society or technology, gender bias has always been a critical issue. And artificial intelligence is no exception. We'll understand what the challenges of gender bias are and how all the issues converge. We'll also take a peek at how enterprises are dealing with artificial intelligence.

Modern artificial intelligence has its inception in the early 1950s. Since then, there is an ever-increasing demand for technologies that deal with automation, prediction, and quick data analysis. Enterprises are investing hugely in artificial intelligence and machine learning already. And the future of this technology is safe. No doubt about that.

2.1   WHAT IS ARTIFICIAL INTELLIGENCE?

Currently, we don't have a precise official definition for artificial intelligence. But, with time, different groups and organizations have come up with concepts that define artificial intelligence:

- Technology to complement human intelligence and increase our intellectual capabilities
- Thinking machines
- An intelligent computer that brings meaning to unstructured data

2.2   WHAT IS MACHINE LEARNING?

A Stanford professor and an IBM researcher, Arthur L. Samuel coined the term in 1959 when he stated: "machine learning is the field of study that gives computers the ability to learn without being explicitly programmed."

Machine learning is an intrinsic part of artificial intelligence. The technology is geared to providing solutions to problems for which they are not explicitly programmed. They are supposed to learn from instances and act as the situation demands. A large portion of techniques referred to as artificial intelligence is directly related to machine learning. There are three types of machine learning.

2.2.1   SUPERVISED LEARNING

We as humans learn from the past. Past experiences inspire our future steps. Supervised machine learning works on a similar note. It learns from large volumes of historical data and creates smart algorithms to solve similar problems in different situations. It looks for labeled data points or structured data in databases for historical problems and learns from them. The more the data, the better is the ability to provide accurate solutions.

2.2.2 Unsupervised Learning

While supervised learning looks for structured historical data, unsupervised machine learning thrives on unlabeled or unstructured data (like email messages or webpages). This technology feeds on huge amounts of unrelated data and tries to find patterns and structure within them. Naturally, this is cumbersome as there are no pre-existing pointers to assist the algorithms in comprehending the data. More and more enterprises need to process unstructured data generated by their users or customers daily in the real world.

2.2.3 Reinforcement Learning

Instead of being provided with predefined training sets, reinforcement learning agents work in a more complex and uncertain environment. It uses trial and error to come up with a solution. In other words, it learns from experience. This learning is based on a performance-based rewards system, where the agent is rewarded if it comes up with a solution. To help with this intense exercise, reinforcement learning is backed by powerful computer infrastructure. Even though the technology dates back to 1951, it was held back due to a lack of computer processing power in those days.

An interesting application of reinforcement learning today is self-driving cars.

2.3 WHAT IS DEEP LEARNING?

Deep learning is the branch of artificial intelligence that is focused on developing computer systems similar to the human brain. In this concept, machines are designed to learn using neural networks. Deep learning is geared toward developing algorithms to simulate the human brain's neural network. It tries to imitate the human brain's ability to create patterns and process data.

The building blocks of deep learning algorithms are interconnected nodes called neurons. These neurons receive inputs, perform calculations, and provide a solution for a given problem. The goal is to use computational techniques to get closer to human decision-making capabilities.

Deep learning gets its ability to solve complex issues by building several layers of abstraction. Traditional artificial intelligence was limited in its ability to learn new things without human intervention. But deep learning includes self-learning and self-teaching algorithms to interpret new and complex data.

For example, traditional artificial intelligence was competent enough to scan a zip code and an envelope's mailing address. But deep learning can comprehend from the envelope's color that it may contain a birthday card.

Deep learning finds enormous applications due to its close proximity to the human brain. Huge volumes of unstructured data are fed into the algorithms in anticipation of receiving useful patterns and insights. Deep learning offers enormous benefits by developing models using a wide breadth of data such as text, audio, video, images, etc.

Parallel computing is the backbone of deep learning. So, it naturally increases the overall performance of multiple-core computers. Faster machines and GPUs enhance the amount of training data that deep learning benefits from. The latest and greatest computers augmented with deep learning is making an impressive impact in the world of speech/image recognition and machine translation. In some areas, it's doing better than humans.

2.4   ARTIFICIAL INTELLIGENCE ENTERPRISE APPLICATIONS

Lately, artificial intelligence has become an integral component of enterprise applications. Business strategies are built to include artificial intelligence in the corporate ecosystem. With artificial intelligence's help, enterprises are focused on improving customer experiences by predicting business outcomes and accomplishing more in less time.

Artificial intelligence technologies are extensively used in financial, legal, retail, IT companies, and supply chain businesses. McKinsey Global Institute (MGI) came out with a report in 2017, which said, tech giants like Apple, IBM, Google, and Microsoft spent more than $30 billion on artificial intelligence-related technologies in 2016. Out of which, most of the budget was allocated towards R&D.

Artificial intelligence-based enterprise applications are expected to skyrocket revenue by up to $31.2 billion by the end of 2025. Enterprises are highly ambitious to gain over their competition with artificial intelligence-based enterprise applications. The applications in news headlines are online shopping, computerized billing, process management, resource planning, salesforce automation, and IT compliance. And that is not all. Enterprises are not shying away from taking bold steps. They are moving towards advanced artificial intelligence concepts to streamline corporate processes. This includes deep learning enterprise applications that are capable of working independently without human intervention. Such applications are widely being promoted as they can surpass human competence.

2.5   ARTIFICIAL INTELLIGENCE AND GENDER

We live in a gender-biased society. None of us is ignorant of that fact. So naturally, the same mindset seeps into artificial intelligence as well.

2.5.1   Artificial Intelligence Is Gender-Biased, But Why?

Artificial intelligence works with algorithms, which is nothing but opinions expressed in a programming language. And, if mostly the male-brain is developing those algorithms, the results are quite inevitably, biased.

American Psychologist Association's Center for Workforce Studies states that 76% of psychology doctorates, 53% of the psychology workforce, and 74% of career psychologists are women. The World Economic Forum made a Linkedin survey and unveiled that 78% of the talent possessing artificial intelligence skills are male. Similar research was done by Element.ai, which stated that across 23 countries, men constituted around 88% of the researchers. WIRED surveyed GOOGLE and shared its figures. Women only occupy 21% of the technical roles at GOOGLE, and only 10% of women are part of the workforce engaged in machine intelligence.

On a similar note, Facebook declared that 22% of its technical workforce is female. And only 15% of women are part of the company's artificial intelligence research team. US government figures show that women's engagement in the country's computer science bachelor programs has gone down significantly over the last three decades. So, the shortage of women among artificial intelligence researchers is not surprising.

As per the US Department of Labor, more than 94% of US administrative assistants and secretaries are women. Unsurprisingly, so is the Google maps navigation system and Siri. Currently, artificial intelligence-related projects are not taking any concrete steps to remove this bias. Instead, over the years, the issue has attracted far more controversies.

Amazon's technical team experimented with a recruiting-tool that used artificial intelligence to score candidates. But they soon realized the tool was not rating candidates in a gender-neutral way. It seemed their hiring engine didn't like women. As a result, Amazon had to scrap the artificial intelligence–recruiting program as it indiscriminately advantaged men.

The discrepancies of the physical world found their way conveniently in the world of artificial intelligence. Microsoft created Tay, a tweeting chatbot that represented a 16-year-old teenage girl. On top of that, Tay was quickly able to learn the sexist language as it's common over the Internet. Microsoft Xiaoice on Wechat, with more than 100 million users, is also a female avatar. Sophia by Hanson Robotics is perhaps the most advanced and famous human-like robot. She is the future of artificial intelligence. She is a media celebrity and the world's first robot citizen as well. While creating Erica, an advanced android human-robot, Professor Ishiguro stated that he was trying to make the most beautiful woman. Erica has a synthesized voice and displays a myriad of facial expressions. By now, it's quite clear to you that most of the world's famous artificial intelligence programs are currently female.

Both Sophia and Erica are conversation companions. Virtual assistants are mostly created with a female avatar. Maybe because of the social belief that women are better conversation companions. Meanwhile, robots that are more physically active look distinctly like a male. For example, Hermes, the disaster response robot from MIT, or Atlas, the most dynamic human-robot that demonstrates human-like agility, both have male-recognizable shape. Perhaps, stronger means male-like. Gender has a strong influence on our judgment. Search and rescue robots resemble the male form mostly because society is biased towards male human rescuers. The physical world clearly has an impact on artificial intelligence gender roles.

From Alexa and Cortana to public transport automated announcements, all have a female voice. Many teams are coming up with ideas to develop a "genderless" voice to avoid this pitfall. But still, it's unclear and directionless. What exactly is a "genderless" voice? Is that going to belong to the LGBTQ community, or is it something humans can't recognize? A lot of gray areas still need to be addressed. It's important to find an answer to develop a socially accountable artificial intelligence system.

Lil Miquela, a fictional musician on Instagram was created with artificial intelligence. Most of such visual artificial intelligence creations are female. On top of that, they are inappropriately showcased as sexually-oriented towards "white heterosexual" men. "Real" women in business have deeply expressed their unpleasantness on this matter. Why are women only exploited as artificial intelligence celebrities? Why are men not part of this game? The point is valid, but artificial intelligence doesn't seem to have an answer yet.

On the other hand, there are few areas of artificial intelligence that are unaffected by human gender. Huge tractors and vehicle movers are definitely strong but don't take up any specific gender form. Autonomous navigational drones created by DJI don't resemble any gender either.

2.5.2   LIMITED DATA FOR TRAINING

Artificial intelligence models work with input data. The larger the variety of data we provide better will be the output. If the input data is poor and misrepresents a particular group, the model's output becomes biased. The majority of artificial intelligence models are biased towards females because their input was biased towards women. Training data has to be unbiased as much as possible.

Gender bias starts during machine learning. If women don't contribute to making an artificial intelligence training dataset, there are bound to be gaps in their operations, so their results are biased.

Most of the current-day commercial artificial intelligence models are based on supervised machine learning technology. As we saw earlier, supervised learning models behave as per labeled data points. More often than not, this training data is provided by humans. Given that humans display bias, consciously or unconsciously, such biases get encoded into the artificial intelligence models. Machine learning models are built to evaluate data labels, and unwantedly, misrepresentation of particular gender stereotype seeps into the model.

The problem is historic. Before the artificial intelligence age, most of the lab research done for the benefit of the medical fraternity was performed on males. Females were excluded from such studies due to various reasons. And that is why the amount of historical data on women's health is far less than that of males. Even today, a lot of medical research continues to function the same way.

Another such problem area is facial recognition. Error rates are very high in this area for women's faces, even more for women with darker skin-tones. The reason is unsurprisingly clear. The data fed into these artificial intelligence models are limited to certain demographics.

Security applications that use facial-recognition pose a grave threat at concerts, airports, or sports events. Moreover, if artificial intelligence identifies gender as only male and female, the transgender community will feel missed out.

Speech-to-text technology also faced similar gender biases. Speech recognition is disproportionately a race and gender-biased. The algorithm gave faulty results while analyzing female speakers. This happened because the artificial intelligence models were trained to accurately analyze longer vocal cords (generally male) with low-pitch voices.

A research team at the North American Chapter of the Association for Computational Linguistics (NAACL) studied Google's speech recognition system. Even though Google was the best performer when compared to Bing, AT&T, and IBM Watson systems, it was still found to be 13% more biased towards men than women.

A question becomes obvious. Do we even need to provide gender as an input to artificial intelligence models? A lot of these smart systems identify your gender first before making suggestions. Is that process reinforcing gender stereotypes? Do we have to understand gender better to inform well? Artificial intelligence teams are beginning to take these questions seriously and focusing on ideas to eliminate bias.

2.5.3 WORKPLACE BIAS

The psychology of the job market is hugely biased. While men can apply for a job if they match 50% of the requirements, women must meet 90% of the requirements to apply for the same. There is also a grave inequality in the number of patents women file. Apart from all this, everyday workplace harassment and strange power dynamics have crept into the world of artificial intelligence. At present, technological workplaces are hugely male-dominated.

2.5.4 INDIFFERENT APPROACH TO THE "FEMALE GENIUS"

Gender roles have impacted the tech world hugely during the last three decades. In the computing industry and particularly in artificial intelligence, boys have demonstrated the talent to come up with life-changing innovative ideas while working from their garage. All the king-makers who changed the world, from Steve Jobs to Jeff Bezos, Bill Gates, to Jack Ma, all are male. Why don't we hear much about successful start-ups led by women?

An important point to ponder is that all these companies were fueled by Venture Capitalists (VC). Only 1–2% of start-ups led by women receive VC support, even though women-led start-ups have made 200% ROI. But why is that?

The answer to this question has many dimensions. Venture capitalists are mostly male-dominated. And, investors always try to find similarities while lending their trust out. In its true sense, VC funding is all about trusting the potential of the start-up founder. But research shows that while men are gauged on their potential, women founders are assisted based on their achievements.

So, the results are predictable. The more male-led start-ups receive funding, the more are the number of success stories. That is straight math. This encourages VCs to bet on even more male-led companies, while the women founders are left out of the game. It's a vicious cycle. The gender roles are boosted, causing women representation to dip further. This segment of the tech industry is massively gender-biased.

The gender-stereotype is so deep-rooted that it has become second nature. When VCs or business clients occasionally discover a rare female-led start-up founder, most of them are dumbfounded with disbelief. If students have read an artificial intelligence research paper earlier and later discover the author of the same to be a female, they feel shocked to death. In our world, female techies are highly unanticipated.

2.5.5 Artificial Intelligence-Based Harassment

A software called DeepNude takes a photo of any clothed woman and uses neural networks to create a realistic nude image of the same person. This is an awkward use of neural networks to victimize the sexuality of unwilling people. Such artificial intelligence-based harassment is pushing technology into unethical practices. Could abuse be avoided if artificial intelligence workplaces were not so biased?

2.5.6 Art Reflects Life

Popular TV shows like *Big Bang Theory,* , and movies like *Iron Man*, and *The Matrix* augment the image of the *male-dominated-genius*. Elon Musk, the Tesla icon, is often referred to as the real-life *Iron Man*. It's quite apparent to project on-screen superstars of this artificial intelligence era as males. The fictional male nerds are often projected as awkward techies who are smart and sooner or later get the novice girl. And like that is not all; these fictional male techies don't fall short of making sexist comments owing to their social awkwardness.

Science fiction is stereotyped with gender roles. From the first fiction, "Metropolis" to the recent sci-fi "Ex-Machina," female humanoids are being shown created by men in a more obedient and sexualized avatar. Be it Matrix, the Terminator, or Ultron, every sci-fi movie depicts heroes and villains as male.

2.5.7 Virtual Agents

Virtual assistants are the modern-day buzz in the customer service industry. But the issue is that digital assistants reflect the physical world stereotypes.

Think about any modern-day artificial intelligence-powered virtual assistants. Whether that digital assistant helps you maintain your grocery list or buddies up at the gym, what type of voice do you hear predominately? Research says that 67% of the popular digital assistants geared to serve others and do menial tasks are female.

In 1990, psychologists belonging to reputed speech technology companies did a study and observed that most customers prefer a female voice when reaching out to call centers for assistance. Since then, virtual assistants are built with the intent to induce a docile nature in them. They are designed and created with an enthusiastic, cheerful, and polite female voice.

Artificial intelligence implementation doesn't come cheap. Enterprises are doing everything to ensure that customers are comfortable with computerized support. Female voices are considered helpful and cordial and are therefore favored. Amazon ran a study while developing Alexa, and concluded that a female voice is far more pleasing and sympathetic. Numerous other studies in this area have come up with similar conclusions. Businesses are bound to cater to customer preferences. Women have taken the place of "assistants" in the virtual world and are serving their masters.

2.5.8 Who Will Artificial Intelligence Replace?

Media and society are highly skeptical about how artificial intelligence is going to impact the job market. This topic has attracted more attention than anything else in the tech world ever since the inception of machines that can think and learn. Artificial intelligence expert Kai Fu Lee confidently pointed out in an hour-long interview that automatic-robots will replace 40% of the world's jobs soon.

There are two important aspects to this forecast, though, which most experts fail to address. The first point is everything is not gloom and doom. Artificial intelligence is expected to create more work opportunities than it replaces. The second is that men and women are likely to be differentially affected by the artificial intelligence workforce rise.

PwC made research and revealed that women are more likely to lose their jobs by the late 2020s. The reason behind this is that women largely hold positions that are clerical based. Such tasks are at a higher risk of getting automated. PwC also points out that men will also face a bigger risk from automation in the long run. Men involved in the exclusive manual nature of work, such as manufacturing, will quickly get replaced by more capable heavy-lifting robots.

Artificial intelligence job roles require a variety of skill sets, and it's expected to disproportionately impact men and women in terms of talent. Based on research, the World Economic Forum came up with a list of artificial intelligence-related skills in which men will outnumber women. This includes machine learning, neural networks, pattern recognition, and Apache Spark. On the contrary, women are expected to outnumber men in text mining, text analytics, speech recognition, etc. These disparities need to be recognized early in any artificial intelligence project-planning phase and addressed with utmost urgency.

2.5.9 India Is No Different

Both blue and white-collar jobs face gender disparity in Indian companies. Even today, job advertisements don't shy away from specifying the preferred gender. Six out of ten jobs prefer male candidates. Women continue to be satisfied with low-quality, low-status, and low-paying jobs.

Rekha Menon, chairman and senior managing director at Accenture, India, spoke at a gender parity conference that enterprises are already strategically adopting artificial intelligence to influence decision patterns in the recruitment process.

She stressed that technology is unbiased to favor women, but it can be designed and taught to remove inherent biases against women in the system. Rekha underlined the importance of digital fluency among women if they want to ride the rising opportunity in technology.

India's female workforce has to come forward and take up the challenge themselves to rise above existing social stereotypes. Women have to micro-learn and upskill themselves to get back into the jobs for which they are outdated at present. They have to bridge this competence gap in order to be more confident while asking for their next promotion and raise.

2.5.10   STEPS ARTIFICIAL INTELLIGENCE TEAMS SHOULD TAKE TO AVOID GENDER BIAS

Gender biases are not black and white. But steps can be taken to ensure better results.

- Diverse training samples must be gathered from various backgrounds.
- Machine learning teams should check the accuracy of data coming from various demographic categories and quickly act to fix any weak areas.
- AI deployments that fail to produce fair results must be penalized. Rigorous processes have to be developed to catch any unfairness in a given model early in the lifecycle.
- A holistic approach has to be taken broadly to represent data from every gender-variants, including non-binary and transgender.

2.6   CONCLUDING THOUGHTS

Reputed American technical enterprises, including Microsoft, Google, and Amazon, came together in 2017 to lay the foundation of the partnership on artificial intelligence. Aimed at benefiting people and businesses, the Partnership has expanded to over 80 participants from 13 countries. Half of the partners function as non-profits. This is the biggest group of artificial intelligence engineers who work relentlessly to come up with guidelines and best practices in this field.

Artificial intelligence has enormous capabilities. At the same time, it has to deal with intricate challenges. The Women Leading in AI Conference 2019 presented numerous recommendations to ban tech events where panel members are all men. But no matter how much we strive to fix the gender gap, awareness is the first essential step. The Chief Scientist of AI & Machine Learning at Google Cloud, Fei-Fei Li, works to induce democracy into artificial intelligence. She strongly urges enterprises and governments to deploy artificial intelligence with diversification in mind. She reminds us that humanity as a whole is accountable for the usage of any technology, not just the tech-creator.

Artificial intelligence models are only reflecting the mindset of the people who built them. The best way to bridge this gap is to engage and diversify more women in designing and deploying artificial intelligence algorithms. It's important that the mix of people working on such tools truly reflects the society they intend to serve. Otherwise, the entire purpose of having an artificial-helping-hand fail. And the diversity should not just be limited to coding, and it has to start from the board-rooms where the discussion begins.

The artificial intelligence research community must work diligently to recruit and motivate female talent. Investors need to get rid of prejudices and support more and more female tech founders. When men and women collaborate in different areas of artificial intelligence, we'll be able to create far more efficient artificial intelligence algorithms that are free of gender bias.

Artificial intelligence is changing the world. Future opportunities and challenges can be smartly dealt with if we collaborate with female thinkers, businesswomen, scientists, academics and the like to discuss artificial intelligence's future.

REFERENCES

1. https://www.entrepreneur.com/article/326801
2. https://www.weforum.org/agenda/2019/06/this-is-why-ai-has-a-gender-problem/
3. https://towardsdatascience.com/gender-and-artificial-intelligence-5fcff34589a
4. https://www.forbes.com/sites/falonfatemi/2020/02/17/bridging-the-gender-gap-in-ai/#6777fc9a5ee8
5. https://hbr.org/2019/11/4-ways-to-address-gender-bias-in-ai
6. https://economictimes.indiatimes.com/magazines/panache/accentures-rekha-menon-on-how-ai-can-be-used-to-remove-gender-biases-at-work/articleshow/66158766.cms

3 Artificial Intelligence in Environmental Management

Rahul Kharat[1] and T. Devi[2]
[1]Vice President, Zenon, Bangalore, India
[2]Professor and Head, Department of Computer Applications, Bharathiar University, Coimbatore, India

CONTENTS

DOI: 10.1201/9781003175865-3

3.1   CURRENT WORK IN AI FOR ENVIRONMENT

Today, AI is being used in every field. We in our day to day lives are using AI extensively, without many times even realizing that there is AI algorithm guiding us to do our day-to-day task. One very common channel of AI applications is our AI-enabled smartphones. There is a very important task or rather it's a duty of every individual in this world to take care of its home, which is earth. We have got everything from earth, even the very best design applications are inspired from naturally evolved beings. This chapter will give a brief overview of AI potential in environmental management. Focus is to give a flavor of what AI could do in different areas, directly impacting environment. The graph in Figure 3.1 shows global warming projections and it shows how it is necessary to address this challenge now for future generations.

3.1.1   Organizations and Their Initiatives

Figure 3.2 gives an overview of different machine learning models and their applications across domains. Environment is shown as one of the sectors and the potential ML models mapped to the domain. Figure 3.3 depicts the organization and trends in environmental management space.

3.1.2   General Framework for AI in Environmental Management

AI initiatives in environment, or in any other industry or domain could be divided into two approaches, namely proactive and reaction. A proactive approach deals in solving for the root cause of the problem. With this approach, AI will be used to control the climate

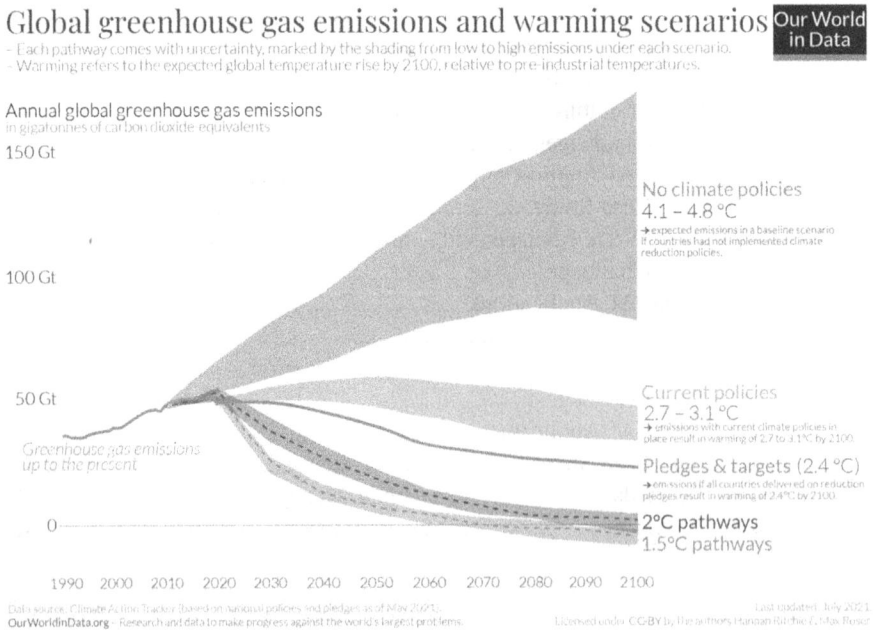

Global greenhouse gas emissions and warming scenarios

FIGURE 3.1   Global warming projections. (Hannah Ritchie and Max Roser, 2020)

Exhibit 1

Mapping usage frequency of AI capabilities to ten social impact domains identifies patterns of the relevance and applicability of AI for social good.

Lower   Higher

Usage frequency of AI capability for each domain

Capability ▼ / Domain ▶	Equality and inclusion	Education	Health and hunger	Security and justice	Info verification and validation	Crisis response	Economic empowerment	Public and social sector	Environment	Infrastructure
Deep learning on structured data										
Natural language processing[2]										
Image and video classification										
Object detection and localization										
Language understanding										
Sound detection and recognition										
Sentiment analysis										
Language translation										
Face detection										
Tracking										
Emotion recognition										
Person identification										
Optical character and handwriting recognition										
Speech-to-text										
Content generation										
Reinforcement learning										
Near-duplicate or similar detection										

Usage frequency of analytics capability for each domain

Analytics, eg, optimization, network analysis										

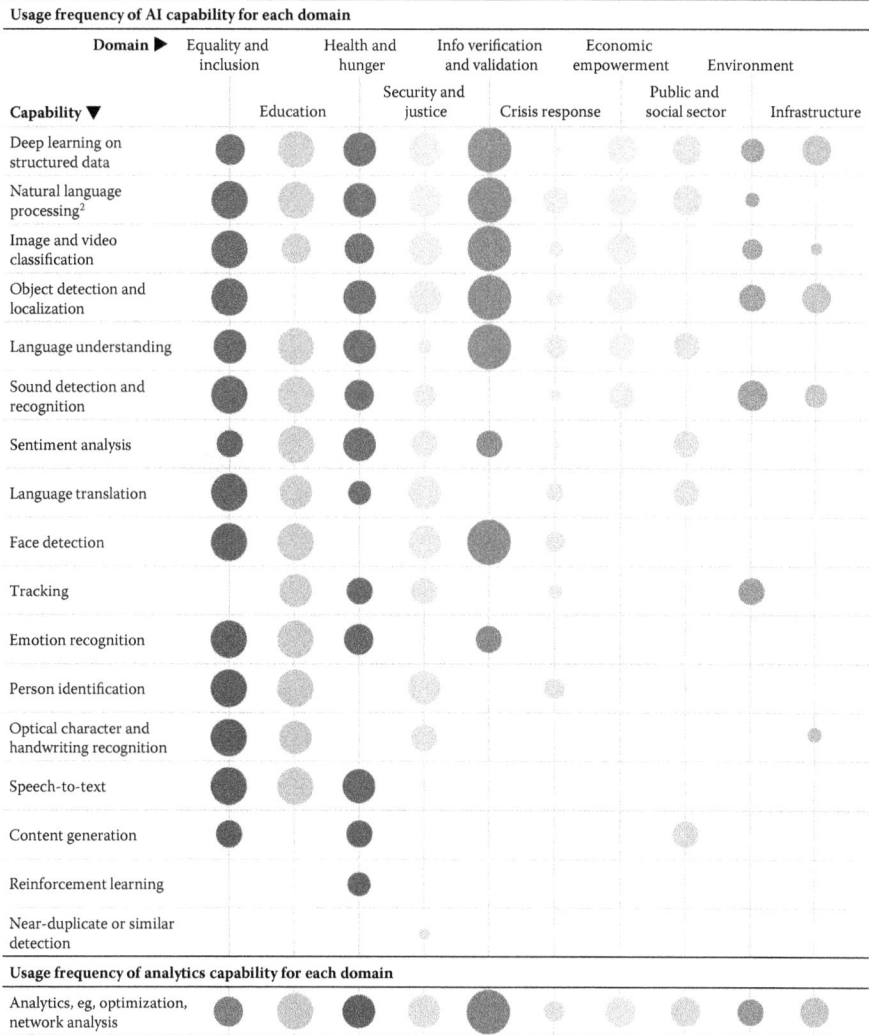

1 Log base 10 scale. Deployment frequency capped at once per hour per year to prevent skewing; capping affected only a small number of use cases.
2 Excluding sentiment analysis, speech-to-text, language understanding, and translation.
NOTE: Our library of about 160 use cases with societal impact is evolving and this heatmap should not be read as a comprehensive gauge of the potential application of AI or analytics capabilities. Usage frequency estimates the number of times that models trained using AI wouldbeused in a year to predict an outcome.

SOURCE: McKinsey Global Institute analysis

FIGURE 3.2 Machine learning models and their applications across domains. (Michael Chui, 2018)

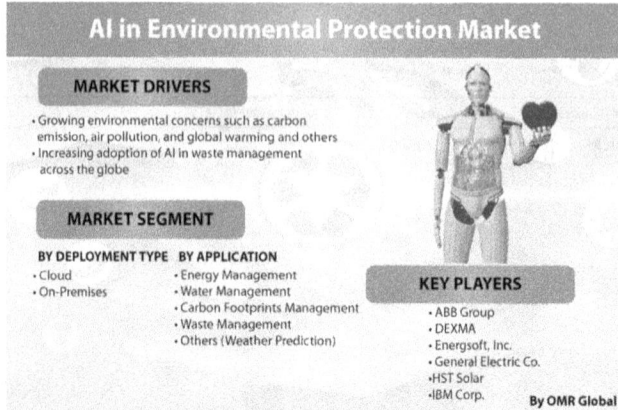

FIGURE 3.3 AI in environmental management. (OMR Global, 2019)

changes itself and try to balance the ecosystem on a whole. Reactive approach deals in solving the occurred problem such as predicting extreme weathers and disasters to prepare to deal with these problems. It can be also thought of as a risk mitigation approach.

It's also important to clearly define the boundaries of a problem when we take any of the above approach to build an AI application. Boundary is important so that the approach or a solution is not confused in defining whether it's a proactive or a reactive approach. The approaches mentioned above should be used as a guiding tool to think about the given problem and draw the right metrics for solving the right problem. Both these approaches will be studied with examples in the next sections.

Air pollution is a silent killer and is the reason for a wide range of health diseases such as respiratory difficulties, heart malfunctions and strokes. The World Health Organization (WHO) states that about 7 million premature deaths in low and middle-income countries attribute to pollution in the air. By reducing air pollution levels, countries can reduce stroke, heart disease, lung cancer, and both chronic and acute respiratory diseases including asthma. Every year around 7 million deaths are due to exposure from both outdoor and household air pollution. Keeping the pollution controlled can significantly reduce diseases and untimely deaths (Balkan Green Energy News, 2020). At the same time, it assures economic stability and protects the environment (World Health Organization, 2019). Outdoor air pollution challenges include protection of the ozone layer in the stratosphere against degradation, reducing the risk of toxic air pollutants, limiting climate change and meeting health-based standards for common air-pollutant.

3.2 AI FOR CLEANER AIR – SMART POLLUTION CONTROL

3.2.1 Current Challenges

There are many sources of air pollution such as Industrial, transportation, consumer applications, etc. Humans are working on improving the efficiency of these systems for a long-time and have come a long way. Still there exists a lot of scope, and lot of work needs to be done to improve and balance the overall ecosystem.

3.2.2 POTENTIAL AI APPLICATIONS

Very important first step is to understand the cause of the problem. Why is air polluted and what are the sources of pollution. If we eliminate or reduce the intensity of these sources, then we are attacking the root cause of a problem. One such potential application could be autonomous cars. Study shows that AI could increase the effectiveness of the autonomous vehicles to reduce the greenhouse emissions by 2–4%. The other potential application is an AI-enabled air-purifier. Such systems are often referred as smart system because of their efficiency and effectiveness in operating these systems using multiple parameters and data in real-time, which is not possible with human-defined static rules and thresholds. It's not that such rules and thresholds could not be made dynamic, but it would take a huge effort in operating and maintenance of such systems compared to data-driven continuously learning systems.

3.2.3 SAMPLE CASE STUDY

Autonomous vehicles are one of the potential applications of AI for cleaner air. One may see this application to be a luxury for humans. This application in fact has a great potential to improve effectiveness in driving and transportation. The real-time object or scenario detection and reaction systems could surpass the effectiveness of humans and will help improve the overall efficiency of the transportation eco system. This will directly impact the emissions and hence the environment. The other indirect application is connected cars which further enhances the overall efficiency and effectiveness. Though the application is still not adopted widely, but it will be one of potential applications of AI for environment and other areas.

3.3 AI FOR WATER PRESERVATION – SMART WATER MANAGEMENT

3.3.1 CURRENT CHALLENGES

Similar to air pollution, there are many similar sources of water pollution such as industrial, transportation, consumer applications, etc. Other than such sources there are indirect effect of global climate changes on controlling the quantity of hard water on earth. Humans are adopting several ways in the form of water conservation applications and water desalination applications, but all these initiatives are not enough to control water preservation and balance. These applications are merely fulfilling the current needs of humans.

3.3.2 POTENTIAL AI APPLICATIONS

Building efficient water systems and purifiers are the potential AI applications. AI could also be used to design the closed loop of water utility cycle. From source to user and then back to source keeping high the utility function of water to re-use it again and again. With all the data and information from several systems, it's possible to build the controlling mechanisms for better conservation and re-use.

The main challenges in water preservation are changing and uncertain future climate, rapidly growing population that is driving increased social and economic development, globalization, and urbanization. The world's water is increasingly becoming degraded in quality, threatening the health of people and ecosystems and increasing the cost of treatment. Some 780 million people around the globe still lack access to clean water and thousands perish daily for the lack of it. Usage of contaminated water sources is a challenge to smart water management. Globally, at least 2 billion people use a drinking water source contaminated with faeces. Contaminated water can transmit diseases such as polio, typhoid, dysentery, cholera, and diarrhoea. Water can also be contaminated by physical, chemical, biological or radiological contaminants. Examples of physical contaminants are sediment or organic material suspended in the water of lakes, rivers and streams from soil erosion. Examples of chemical contaminants include nitrogen, bleach, salts, pesticides, metals, toxins produced by bacteria, and human or animal drugs. Biological contaminants are organisms in water. They might be biological or microbial contaminants including bacteria, viruses, protozoan, and parasites. Examples of radiological contaminants include cesium, plutonium and uranium (World Health Organisation, 2019).

3.3.3 SAMPLE CASE STUDY

UN statistics suggests that about one-fifth of the population across the world, are living in water scarcity area. AI driven water management systems could be used to address this problem. Models could be used to understand the loss and distribution pattern and optimize the use and re-use of water. Necessary data collection systems will be the key to enable AI to address this problem and take the effectiveness of water management systems to its maximum potential.

AI-driven planning enables the relevant stakeholders to understand the real-time water loss and misuse, and help them design and execute comprehensive distribution networks. As research suggests applied vector regression methods AI methods can be used to forecast groundwater reserves and optimize its usage and planning.

3.4 AI FOR BETTER AGRICULTURE – SMART FARMING

3.4.1 CURRENT CHALLENGES

Due to climate changes worldwide, it has become very important to adopt modern intelligent practices in agriculture. The solution and scope is not restricted to farming alone but should be looked at the complete food supply chain. There are inefficiencies which could be addressed in the entire food supply chain using AI.

3.4.2 POTENTIAL AI APPLICATIONS

There are multifold applications possible in agricultural supply chain, right from sowing crops and monitoring farming to distribution and downstream operations. AI can be extensively utilized at multiple touchpoints to make the process overall efficient (Figure 3.4).

3.4.3 SAMPLE CASE STUDY

To approach SMART farming, the very first step is to draw down a complete picture of food value chain and find out the relevant parameters and information available at each

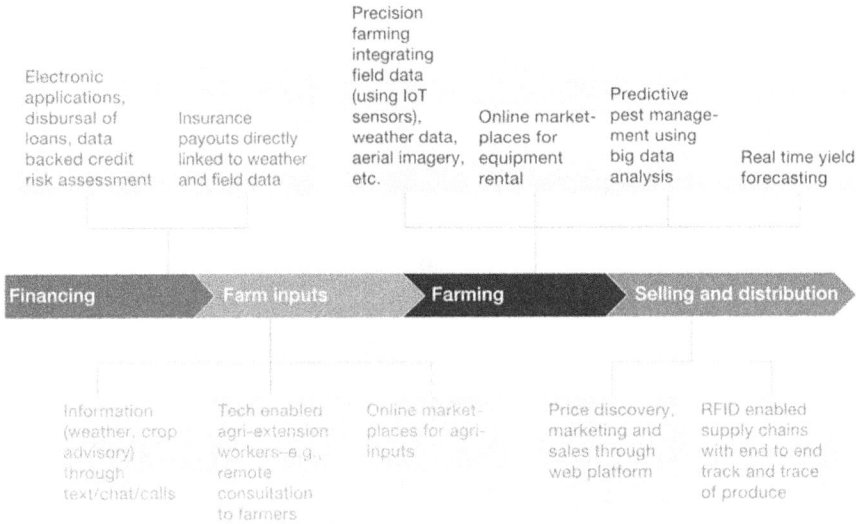

The diagram shows a process flow with four stages: Financing, Farm inputs, Farming, Selling and distribution.

Above the flow:

- **Financing:** Electronic applications, disbursal of loans, data backed credit risk assessment
- **Farm inputs:** Insurance payouts directly linked to weather and field data
- **Farming:** Precision farming integrating field data (using IoT sensors), weather data, aerial imagery, etc.
- Online market-places for equipment rental
- Predictive pest management using big data analysis
- **Selling and distribution:** Real time yield forecasting

Below the flow:

- Information (weather, crop advisory) through text/chat/calls
- Tech enabled agri-extension workers–e g., remote consultation to farmers
- Online market-places for agri-inputs
- Price discovery, marketing and sales through web platform
- RFID enabled supply chains with end to end track and trace of produce

McKinsey&Company

FIGURE 3.4 AI in agriculture. (Lutz Goedde et al., 2018)

touchpoint. This information could be further leveraged in making decision making at each touch point using machine learning models in combination domain knowledge driven systems. To give an example one point efficiency gain for a five-step process improves the overall system efficiency gain of 8–9% assuming base efficiency of 60%. This is a huge gain in terms of overall impact on the environmental ecosystem.

3.5 AI FOR BETTER E-WASTE MANAGEMENT – SMART MONITORING/CONTROL

3.5.1 Current Challenges

e-Waste is a big problem in today's digital world and it's growing at an unprecedented pace. United States and China are frontrunners in producing e-waste and other countries are not very far behind. So why is it a problem? Just to give an example, it takes approximately 500 years to decompose a plastic and almost everyone is aware of the plastic problem today. Similar e-waste carries lot of toxic material such as lead, cadmium, etc. which are harmful for the environment and needs to be handled/recycled appropriately to reduce their impact on the environment (Figure 3.5) (Forti V. et al., 2020).

3.5.2 Potential AI Applications

As we discussed in an earlier section, it's important to understand the steps involved in the current process to address the problem at each step. Let's understand the steps involved in e-waste management: Collection, Segregation, Transportation, Processing,

Global E-waste Generated by year

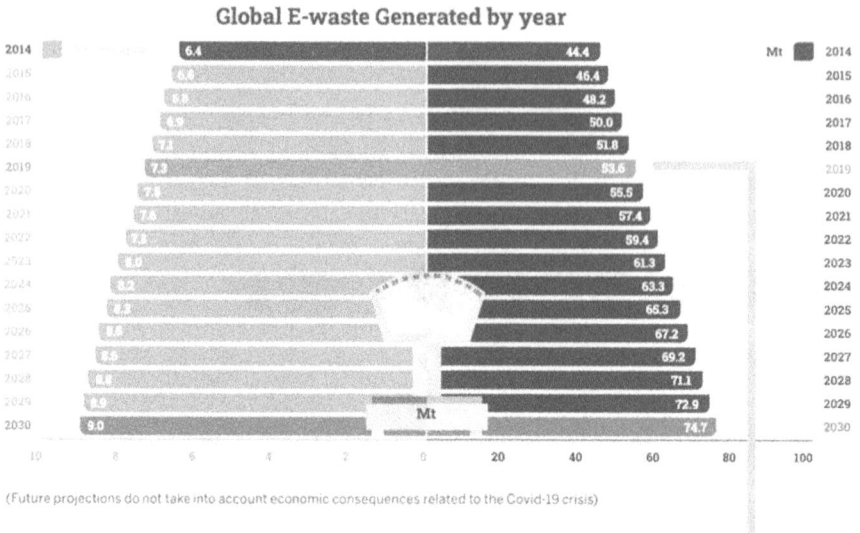

(Future projections do not take into account economic consequences related to the Covid-19 crisis)

FIGURE 3.5 Global e-waste generation (Ref: https://www.itu.int/en/ITU-D/Environment/Documents/Toolbox/GEM_2020_def.pdf). (Forti V. et al., 2020)

and Disposal/incineration. Data collected at each of the above steps could help build AI-enabled smart systems to take intelligent and effective decisions to enhance the efficiency of the overall ecosystem.

3.5.3 SAMPLE CASE STUDY

Waste classification and diversion to right disposal methodology are few of many applications of AI-driven e-waste management. Bin-E is the world's first intelligent bin that sorts waste materials. It uses a combination of sensors, image recognition and AI, and can recognize objects like glass, plastic, or paper, and compress these before placing them in containers. Refer to https://www.bine.world for more details to understand the excellent potential of AI in e-waste management.

3.6 AI FOR CLIMATE CONTROL – SMART ENERGY OPTIMIZATION

3.6.1 CURRENT CHALLENGES

One of the major impacts of climate change is the extinction of several species. Study shows that more than 20% of the species faces extinction by 2100, which is a huge problem (Renee Cho, 2018). Government and regulatory bodies over the whole world are seeing climate control as the most important concern now and in coming decades. AI is looked upon as one of the very important tools to address and mitigate this problem.

3.6.2 POTENTIAL AI APPLICATIONS

AI helps to create a flexible and autonomous electric grid enabling and enhancing the usage of renewable energy. AI has helped researchers achieve higher accuracies in identifying tropical cyclones, weather fronts and atmospheric rivers, which can lead to extreme climatic conditions and scenarios and not easy to detect by old technologies and methods. AI has helped to plan the response efficiently to keep people safe all over the world.

3.6.3 SAMPLE CASE STUDY

Hurricane Maria's winds damaged thousands of acres of rainforest, however, the only way to determine which tree species were destroyed and which withstood the hurricane at such a large scale is through the use of images. In 2017, a NASA flyover of Puerto Rico yielded very high-resolution photographs of the tree canopies. But how is it possible to tell one species from another by looking at a green mass from above over such a large area? The human eye could theoretically do it, but it would take forever to process the thousands of images (Renee Cho, 2018).

AI is the way to process these images. Refer to this excellent case study on the web for further details. There are many such case studies and applications of AI in climate control and will be seen and used as one of the most important tools in tackling this major problem of current and future decades.

3.7 RISKS AND REWARDS OF AI IN ENVIRONMENTAL MANAGEMENT

Responsible AI and AI ethics is one of the most talked about subject in recent times. It's mostly talked in context of individual privacy. Responsible AI can be extended to other applications as well. One such application is AI in environmental management. To make AI applications responsible and effective for its intended use, it's our responsibility in design the overall system with the right thresholds. AI is not about building trained machine learning models. It's very much similar to trained human resource. If we are put on a right job and integrate our skill sets well in overall system, we tend to work and perform more efficiently. If the integration and processes are not aligned to our skillsets we fail. Similarly, to make AI models to be more effective and responsible it's very important to integrate these learnings with the domain-driven knowledge models to use it effectively for recommendations, decision making, and planning. It again left to us, humans, whether we want our AI model to behave responsibly and provide more rewards over risks.

In the recent years, many applications based on artificial intelligence(AI) have been developed to monitor and control climate change (Rolnick et al., 2019). These applications help in minimizing the emissions of green house gas (GH) and in managing the disasters caused by climate changes. These applications use various techniques including causal inference, computer vision, interpretable models, natural language processing, reinforcement learning & control, time-series analysis, transfer learning, uncertainty quantification and unsupervised learning. Minimizing the emission of green house gas depends on controlling emissions in various domains such as electricity systems, transportation, buildings, industry and land use. AI can help in reducing the GHG by forecasting, scheduling and controlling emissions from energy systems such as generators. These applications make use of historical data, outputs from physical models, images and videos to forecast the generation of power. The forecasts made can be used to take appropriate measures to control the emission of GHG. Transportation systems are also responsible for emission of GHG in large amounts. AI applications have been used to reduce the transport activity, improve vehicle efficiency, provide suggestions for shifting to lower-carbon options. AI applications also help in designing energy efficiency measures for buildings and cities which will help in reducing the emissions of GHG. They can help the smart systems in buildings and cities to select and implement appropriate strategies to reduce GHG emissions. Various processes such as industrial production and logistics cause emission of GHG in large amounts. AI applications provide support in streamlining supply chains, improving production quality, predicting machine breakdowns, optimizing heating and cooling systems, and prioritizing the use of clean electricity over fossil fuels which in turn reduce global emissions. Although plants and other organisms in farms and forests consume carbon-di-oxide, they also emit methane which is one of the GHG. AI applications are used in precision agriculture to reduce the emission of GHG from soil and to improve the yield. They also help in predicting forest fire or other disasters on the farm and help in preventing them in order sustain agriculture. AI applications also help in removing carbon-di-oxide from atmosphere by enabling the plants to intake more amount of it. Many AI models have been developed to predict the changes in climate so that there are options for utilizing other sources of energy which do not cause pollution.

REFERENCES

Balkan Green Energy News, Clean Air for All – How polluted air harms human health, https://balkangreenenergynews.com/clean-air-for-all-how-polluted-air-harms-human-health/, 2020.

David Rolnick, Priya L. Donti, et al., Tackling Climate Change with Machine Learning, https://arxiv.org/pdf/1906.05433.pdf, 2019

Forti V., Baldé C.P., Kuehr R., Bel G. The Global E-waste Monitor 2020: Quantities, flows and the circular economy potential. United Nations University (UNU)/United Nations Institute for Training and Research (UNITAR) - co-hosted SCYCLE Programme, International Telecommunication Union (ITU) & International Solid Waste Association (ISWA), Bonn/Geneva/Rotterdam. ISBN Digital: 978-92-808-9114-0 ISBN Print: 978-92-808-9115-7, https://www.itu.int/en/ITU-D/Environment/Documents/Toolbox/GEM_2020_def.pdf

Hannah Ritchie and Max Roser, CO2 and Greenhouse Gas Emissions, Published online at OurWorldInData.org, 2020, https://ourworldindata.org/co2-and-other-greenhouse-gas-emissions

Lutz Goedde, Avinash Goyal, Nitika Nathani, and Chandrika Rajagopalan, Harvesting golden opportunities in Indian agriculture: From food security to farmers' income security by 2025, https://www.mckinsey.com/industries/agriculture/our-insights/harvesting-golden-opportunities-in-indian-agriculture, 2018.

Michael Chui, Martin Harrysson, James Manyika, Roger Roberts, Rita Chung, Pieter Nel, and Ashley van Heteren, Notes From The AI Frontier Applying AI For Social Good, Mckinsey & Company, 2018, 1–463.

OMR Global, AI (Artificial Intelligence) in Environmental Protection Market - Global Industry Share, Growth, Competitive Analysis and Forecast, 2019-2025, 2019.

Renee Cho, Artificial Intelligence—A Game Changer for Climate Change and the Environment, 2018, https://blogs.ei.columbia.edu/2018/06/05/artificial-intelligence-climate-environment/

World Health Organization, Drinking Water, https://www.who.int/news-room/fact-sheets/detail/drinking-water, 2019.

4 Artificial Intelligence in Medical Imaging

C. S. Sureka

Assistant Professor & Head (i/c) Department of Medical Physics, Bharathiar University, Coimbatore, India

CONTENTS

DOI: 10.1201/9781003175865-4

47

OBJECTIVES

- To understand the state-of-art of Artificial Intelligence (AI) in medical imaging.
- To explore the potentials of AI in various imaging modalities, such as Computerized Tomography (CT), Mammography, Magnetic Resonance Imaging (MRI), Medical Ultrasound, and Positon Emission Tomography (PET).
- To realize the applications and challenges in AI towards precision medicine to enhance healthcare.
- To make aware of AI's present status and future perspectives in medical imaging to develop new algorithms that can be suitable for routine clinical practice.

4.1   INTRODUCTION TO MEDICAL IMAGING

Medical imaging plays an essential role in healthcare for timely diagnosis of diseases, disease staging, management in addition to a selection of appropriate treatment, planning, delivery, and follow-up. Medical imaging originated with the remarkable discovery of X-rays by a German Physicist WC Roentgen in 1985. Within a few weeks of his discovery, X-ray technology evolved as a non-invasive imaging modality globally. From then on, there has been a series of technological innovations in the form of new or more advanced imaging modalities, viz., Radiography, Mammography, Computerized Tomography (CT), Magnetic Resonance Imaging (MRI), medical ultrasound (US), digital radiography, Positron Emission Tomography (PET), SPECT, etc. They have evolved from discoveries in physics, engineering, and technology.

The CT uses X-ray equipment and a computer system to create detailed images of all internal organs, bones, and other tissues. When the X-ray tube and detector make a rotation around the patient, the detector takes several profiles of the attenuated X-ray beam. Then, those profiles are reconstructed into 2D images for further analysis. 3D images can be obtained by spiral CT, where 3D images are obtained by acquiring a volume of data. Recently, 4D CT has been introduced to nullify the problems associated with organ movement.

Mammography is a process of examining the human breast for screening and diagnosis using low energy X-rays. It has been established to diagnose breast cancer at an early stage by detecting tumor masses or microcalcifications.

MRI works under the principle of Nuclear Magnetic Resonance (NMR) in which strong magnetic and radiofrequency fields create images of tissues. It is used to visualize morphological changes in tissues based on its ability to record changes in proton density and magnetic spin relaxation time. Medical Ultrasound, also known as ultrasonography, uses high- frequency sound waves in the megahertz frequency range. Ultrasonic images are produced when different tissues reflect these sound waves differently. The US system consists of an ultrasound transducer, which acts as both an ultrasound transmitter and receiver of echo. Doppler US scanners are used to assess blood flow in arteries and veins.

PET is a kind of radionuclide imaging modality performed in nuclear medicine departments. It uses a low amount of radioactive isotopes to produce images that can provide both anatomical and functional information. When the low level and low activity radiopharmaceuticals are injected into the body, they accumulated in the specific region of interest (normal and abnormal organs and tissues, and bones) depending upon the radioisotope. Once the organs absorb the radioactive substances, they emit radiation at variable intensity depending upon their nature (Kasban et al., 2015).

4.2 APPLYING ARTIFICIAL INTELLIGENCE (AI) IN MEDICAL IMAGING

Medical Imaging has been developed enormously in recent years due to the technological revolution globally. It starts from 2D technologies like Radiography, and Mammography moves into 3D technologies like CT, MRI, PET, Medical Ultrasound, etc., and 4D technologies as well due to the evolution of computer vision (CV) techniques. Also, conventional screen-film radiography gives qualitative information to diagnose the disease. However, digitization of Medical Imaging Technology has started to provide quantitative information on the severity of the disease, and to identify biomarkers of prognosis and treatment response. They play a major role in Oncology to differentiate benign and malignant tumor, to identify the histology of the tumor, staging, and mutations, to predict the risk of recurrence, the survival of the patient, etc.

Computer-Aided Detection (CAD) algorithms have been introduced to improve the accuracy of medical imaging, consistency in interpretation of images, image evaluation, and to decide the appropriate treatment. Even though CAD tools have a lot of potentials, they have their drawbacks to use for regular clinical practice. These limitations would be reduced with the effective usage of AI, machine learning (ML), and radiomics in association with CAD.

The term Artificial Intelligence (AI) was originally coined by an American computer and cognitive scientist, John McCarthy in 1956. It serves as a general description of the abilities and operations of computers that mimic human intelligence. AI has made enormous advancements in recent years in many areas, especially in healthcare towards precision medicine. In this section, we have given the essential concepts related to the evaluation of CAD along with the main aspects of AI applied to precision medicine (Koenigkam et al., 2019).

4.2.1   Computer-Aided Detection (CAD)

In the late 1980s, the CAD systems were involved in the processing of films in digital radiography. Later, they were used to detect pulmonary nodules on radiography and CT. Recently, they have been facilitated to diagnose other diseases like Alzheimer's disease using PET. Now, computerized auxiliary diagnostic tools have been expanded to use with all medical imaging modalities based on the developments in AI.

The CAD models have been developed by the integration of the Picture Archiving and Communication System (PACS) with the Hospital Information Systems (HIS) and Radiology Information Systems (RIS). The PACS are the foundation of filmless radiology or Digital Medical Imaging. It is a way of getting images from various medical imaging modalities (Radiography, CT, MRI, medical ultrasound, etc.) in the standard DICOM (Digital Imaging and Communication in Medicine) format, send those images to another computed system that can be accessed by Radiologists, and store them in large databases.

CAD tools are used to interpret radiological findings and for the detection of diseases at an early stage. It is aimed to enhance the consistency and accuracy of medical imaging based on the second opinion provided by the techniques associated with AI. However, the CAD systems provide information like whether there is a lesion or not, benign or malignant, etc. Hence, Content-Based Image Retrieval (CBIR) systems have been developed with plenty of potentials in medical imaging.

4.2.2   Principles of Computer-Aided Image Analysis in Medical Imaging

Digital Medical Imaging is a function of grayscale coordinates that is denoted by a matrix of either pixel (picture element with x and y coordinates) in a 2D image or voxel (volume element with x, y, and z coordinates) in a 3D image. Each pixel is identified by an integer value that can be represented by the value of the gray level. The black, white, and shades of the gray region in the image are represented by the lowest, highest, and intermediate values of gray level, respectively. Digital Medical Imaging consists of three major steps in image processing and analysis. They are: (i) image segmentation, (ii) feature extraction, and (iii) feature selection.

Segmentation is aimed to split the image into several parts to represent normal regions and abnormal anatomy. In this process, tissues and organs are separated based on their structure, using predefined regular shapes, organs are outlined, and region of interests (ROI) are marked in the image. Techniques used to segment images are generally based on grayscale levels, type of anatomical edges, threshold levels, etc. This process can be manual, semi-automatic where the user can interrupt at any step, or fully automatic.

Feature extraction is a process of calculating numerical values from the information collected from the visual format of an image. It is performed by running feature extraction algorithms called feature extractors. These algorithms execute various tasks, such as recognition of shapes and contours, classification of texture, estimation of area and volume of the region of interest, construct histograms, etc.

Followed by the extraction of features, the numerical values are represented as a feature vector. There are three types of feature extraction techniques based on the (a) grayscale, (b) texture, and (c) shape features of an image. The grayscale features extraction techniques can be performed by analyzing a histogram that describes the number of pixels or voxels along with the intensity of grayscale. But, grayscale descriptors don't provide spatial information of any image. Hence, the extraction of texture features technique is followed that can distinguish different textures of similar pixel/voxel regions. The shape feature represents the edge and geometric features of the given image.

Feature selection is an essential step to select the appropriate features of an image as per the clinical investigation. It will avoid features that are irrelevant for a given examination, redundant data, noise, and inconsistencies in the feature vector.

4.2.3   MACHINE LEARNING (ML) AND DEEP LEARNING (DL)

Most of the complex medical ontologies and classifications are represented by their underlying biologic systems simply and crudely. They do not completely describe all the factors of diseases or their causes. Besides, those classifications cannot keep pace with the medical knowledge gathered in the digital era. It limits the development of symbolic AI systems (systems that can compute and communicated using symbols) represented by CAD models.

With the advent of computer hardware, non-symbolic AI systems have been developed since mid of the 1980s. They are data-driven and work statistically. The procedures involved in the non-symbolic AI systems are termed machine learning (ML). In ML, computer systems perform a specific task independently. It means that they perform a task without direct instructions but with observational learning through big data analysis.

Generally, ML procedures are divided into supervised and unsupervised learning. In supervised learning, input data is given along with the desired output data to train the model. But, in unsupervised learning, the input data are given without any direction just to understand the inherent structure in the data. Another division of ML is conventional ML and DL.

Conventional ML involves pattern recognition based on experience gathered from previous exams as same as user intelligence. It allows the computer to learn from errors and predict outcomes. It can also classify images to identify various diseases using various tools like CAD in all imaging modalities. Artificial Neural Network (ANN) is one of the traditional ML methods developed by interconnecting nodes that consist of layers where every layer reflects the function of series of neutrons by which it represents the human nervous system.

DL algorithms have been developed to avoid the limitations of traditional ML methods, such as their dependency on segmentation and feature extraction in image processing. It is possible by integrating those processes within ANN. However, they also have their limitations, such as the need for hundreds to thousands of high-quality real images, hard to identify its logics, etc. Convolutional Neural Network (CNN) is the most commonly used system of DL algorithm in medical imaging.

Different AI and ML tools are applied in CAD, CBIR, radiomics, and Radiogenomics to analyze images in medical imaging.

4.2.4 Content-Based Image Retrieval (CBIR)

CBIR is considered an important computational tool as it has potential in medical imaging in addition to its applications in teaching and research. It is used to search for similar images based on contents matching with references case. To do so, it uses the information derived from the images, and feature vector. But, it does not search for similar images using the reports/associated texts or external annotations. The CBIR performs its function through a decision-making model experienced from similar exams. It can help radiologists to interpret the diagnosis of exams more effectively and rapidly. If there is any uncertainty in their diagnosis, they search on the internet either through a browser or an established radiology sites using appropriate keywords to confirm their diagnostic results. Likewise, it increases the confidence level of Radiologists. Hence, CBIR can be used as an effective tool in routine clinical practice.

4.2.5 Radiomics and Radiogenomics

Radiomics is considered a CAD extension with ML techniques. Radiomics can be reduced to a two-step process. In the first step, high-dimensional massive measurable data/features are extracted from tens to hundreds of Radiological exams by image processing. In the second step, these massive data are integrated into databases with patient data and clinical outcomes and shared for analysis using conventional ML. It not only shares information about the diagnosis but also provides information about the treatment, prognosis of patients, and treatment response. Based on this, "big data" of health, and methods to translate population derived radiomics signatures to a specific patient have been designed.

For example, if a patient has lung cancer, his specific texture features will be matched with the radiomics signatures of a similar exam. It will provide future knowledge about his treatment response in addition to basic information. This information will be translated to him to evaluate the prognosis of the patient. Due to the advancements in therapy, such as targeted therapy and immunotherapy mostly for cancer treatment, there is a need for a robust approach for diagnosis. Under this circumstance, radiomics has been developed to provide diagnostic image analysis in a non-invasive, fast, user-friendly, and economical manner.

Radiogenomics is a combination of radiomics and genomics (Radiogenomics = Radiomics + Genomics). It is used to find the correlation between Radiological imaging features and the gene profile of the tumor. Many studies have presented that there is a link between imaging features, gene expression profile, and mutations. They mentioned that this analysis can be used to detect various biological mechanisms in a non-invasive way with the support of mathematical and computational devices. Radiogenomics can also be used for tumor heterogeneity analysis, tumor complexity quantification, and recognition of phenotypic/genotypic sub-regions of the tumor. This information will be used to predict the tumor recurrence, resistance to the treatment, and treatment outcome. However, it will cause uncertainties/to be biased if there is no sufficient genomic data for all groups of the population.

4.3   AI IN VARIOUS MEDICAL IMAGING MODALITIES

The revolution in digital technology has made innovations in medical imaging techniques, viz., Mammography, CT, MRI, Ultrasound, PET, etc. The number of imaging studies performed and the average age of our population is increased significantly. Nowadays, the complexity and diversity of these images challenge the ability of medical imaging. Despite these changes, there is no effect on the manner radiologists interprets examinations in day-to-day clinical practice.

Generally, images are presented to the radiologist without any assistance or comment. They usually visually assess images based on their education and experience but it is subjective. Under these circumstances, AI has been demonstrated as an essential tool to recognize complex patterns and to assess images quantitatively and automatically. When AI is implemented for clinical practice as an efficient system to help radiologists, more accurate and reproducible analysis can be performed with improved patient care.

AI is capable of revolutionizing the medical industry by its enormous developments. It has the potential to impact many aspects of medical imaging starts from clinical solutions, such as improving the performance of imaging, clinical outcome, etc., to innovative applications, such as radiomics, radiogenomics, etc. With the continued development of AI algorithms, some fear that computers may replace the radiologists but it is not so.

This section discusses the importance, applications, investigations, present status, and future directions of AI in CT, Mammography, MRI, Medical Ultrasound, and Nuclear Medicine imaging modalities in a simple manner with point by point outline.

4.4   AI IN COMPUTED TOMOGRAPHY

Computed Tomography (CT) was introduced in 1972 and has been developed as an important and successful diagnostic tool in medical imaging due to rapid technological developments. The first CT machine took a long time that is about 5 min each to capture and to reconstruct images for a single scan despite poor image resolution (80 × 80 pixels). Due to the development of various generations of CT scans, the rotation speed, detector coverage, and resolution are enhanced enormously. The rotation speed of the present detector is about a quarter of a second per rotation. The detectors can cover a wide thick of the patient up to 16 cm along the patient axis. These enhancements allow the system for capturing high-resolution (up to 1024 × 1024 pixels or more) images.

Since the number of CT examinations is increasing at a rapid rate, the radiation dose received by the public is also increased significantly. It became a serious problem when it is used to scan child patients because children are very sensitive to radiation. However, CT dose has been reduced considerably due to the awareness about exposure associated health risks among the technologists and public and the efforts taken by the CT community. The most efficient way to reduce CT dose is adapting the Risk versus Benefit ratio. That is, if the benefit of taking a CT exam is higher than the associate risk, then only, this technique can be used. It should be remembered that the usage of dose reduction methods and parameters may affect the quality of the image by producing noise and image artifacts. Hence, dose reduction techniques should include provisions to treat noise and image artifacts during image reconstruction.

Based on these, various reconstructions techniques, viz., algebraic reconstruction technique (ART), and filtered back projection (FBP) technique were used in older days. Later, the iterative reconstruction (IR) algorithm was introduced and has been evolved into various advanced reconstruction algorithms (Martin and Peter, 2019; David et al., 2019).

4.4.1 CT Reconstruction Algorithms: From Concept to Clinical Necessity

In 1970, the ART algorithm (a class of IR algorithm) was developed initially to reconstruct cross-sectional images. As it has to lack computation power, another simpler algorithm namely FBP was used for more than a decade. To reduce CT dose to the child patients, more number of CT scans that can deliver low dose are acquired with FBP. But, it reduces the image quality considerably in addition to obesity. Even though FBP has the benefit of short reconstruction time, it was used in clinics to model image noise when lesser photons reach the CT detector.

Meanwhile, IR algorithms were also developed to perform high-quality CT diagnosis at low CT dose based on three basic approaches, such as (i) sonogram based, (ii) image domain-based, and (iii) fully iterative algorithms. In parallel to IR algorithm development, low-cost computational tools like programmable graphics processing units (GPUs) were also developed for fast CT reconstruction. In combination with these developments, many advanced reconstruction algorithms were developed in the medical industry and introduced in clinics by various vendors.

A few of them are Iterative Reconstruction in Image Space (IRIS), Adaptive Statistical Iterative Reconstruction (ASIR), Sinogram Affirmed Iterative Reconstruction (SAFIRE), iDose4, Veo, ASIR-V, AIDR3D, etc. Recently, a model-based IR algorithm namely Forward projected model-based Iterative Reconstruction Solution (FIRST) was introduced for clinical CT imaging. It can reduce the CT dose up to 76% with the same image quality. Later, many investigators verified the efficiency of the IR algorithm on image quality and CT dose at different body regions. They found that the IR algorithm reduces the radiation dose of chest CT, CT angiography of the heart, coronary CT angiography, and abdominal CT exams considerably without compromising the image quality.

4.4.2 Importance of AI-Based Detection in CT

Current medical imaging practice is confronted with two major challenges:

1. The number of CT examinations is increased rapidly every year. But, there is not much change in the number of radiologists and the frequency of urgent pathologic conditions.
2. The time from admission to initiation of surgery is a major factor to determine the survival of patients. Unfortunately, the identification of real urgent cases in routine clinical practice is presently not satisfactory since the present system either misleading or missing prioritization.

One possible solution to address these challenges is to use DL algorithms in clinical practice. These algorithms can be used to detect abnormalities after the acquisition of the raw data and to highlight special and urgent studies in the worklist. They would be used to assist radiologists to detect visual abnormalities and to minimize both false-positive and false-negative cases. They may also reduce the time to therapy and to report case completion. The feasibility of the DL approach in CT has recently been demonstrated in detecting intracranial hemorrhage, acute ischemia, metastatic brain tumors, and to determine tissue types in abdominal regions.

4.4.3 PRESENT AND FUTURE DEVELOPMENTS

Currently, the speed of introducing IR related algorithms into clinical practice for CT examination has been reduced. However, technical developments to reduce CT dose is still an important area of interest. Another possibility of reducing CT dose is by acquiring a lesser number of images. But, the CT dose remains the same in all the slices. This approach is known as sparse-sampling CT. The advantage of the sparse-sampling approach is higher SNR by removing the electronic readout noise. This advantage deposits just half of the CT dose when compared to the present technology but its raw data are undersampled. Therefore, it necessitates a complete IR algorithm to reconstruct cross-section images from these data.

Based on these, many investigators recommended various IR solutions that would be implemented clinically soon. However, its implementation highly depends on the availability of hardware like advanced X-ray tubes and its relevant technological advancements. A few of their advancements are:

1. Confirmed the usage of CT to measure BMD (Bone Mineral Density) quantitatively with the support of a sparse sampling technique and an IR algorithm together.
2. Incorporation of former knowledge into the image formation and reconstruction process of the IR algorithm. For example,
   a. In the case of follow-up in Oncology, many patients may undergo a series of studies of the same examination. There should be common anatomical information in between the scans. This information can be shared and used in an IR algorithm to improve the diagnosis as well as by reducing the CT dose.
   b. Integration of prior understanding regarding orthopedic implants (shape and material composition of the implant) into the reconstruction process. It will reduce metal artifacts and improves image quality.

3. Introduction of a novel dual-energy CT (DECT) technology with IR. It can reduce artifacts and enhance contrast when compared to conventional CT.
4. Introduction of another novel photon-counting CT (PCCT) technology (also known as spectral CT technology) with an IR algorithm. It consists of (i) multi-energetic information rather than single energy information, (ii) additional detector to improve spatial resolution of images, (iii) complex software setting depending on the configuration of the detector and hardware. Therefore, PCCT technology should use the power of IR algorithms to integrate the PCCT data into a clinical model.
5. Introduction of a new phase-contrast and dark-field CT technology with tailored IR algorithms. Phase-contrast and dark-field CT can provide higher soft-tissue contrast and structural information respectively.
6. Evaluation to apply the emerging AI to enhance CT image reconstruction by various approaches, viz., optimizing IR algorithms, training convolutional neural networks, etc.

4.5   AI IN MAMMOGRAPHY

In mammography, 10–30% of breast cancers can be missed due to dense parenchyma obscuring lesions, poor positioning, perception error, interpretation error, etc. Also, inter-reader variability to detect breast cancer and recall rates that are caused by false negatives became a serious issue.

Based on this, investigators have developed CAD for mammography and described its basic rationales, approaches, and limitations during the 1970s. They have proved that CAD tools can improve the sensitivity of cancer detection, and characterize clusters of microcalcifications as benign or malignant. They have also analyzed various aspects of the size, density, and morphology of individual microcalcifications and pattern of clustering. However, the effectiveness of CAD became a challengeable one by recent large-scale clinical trials as it has failed to improve the diagnostic performance of radiologists. Due to the high rate of false-positive cases, radiologists need to analyze more number of false-positive marks of CAD which leads to disappointment and necessitates unnecessary additional tests for confirmation. Also, important information may be lost because of the incorporation of human-designed descriptors in the traditional CAD (Carl and Maryellen, 1994).

Recently, AI-based CAD incorporates mammographic features as a descriptor. Due to the advantage of using self-learned descriptors rather than human-designed descriptors, AI can be developed to achieve a similar performance of Radiologists. Hence, mammographic detection and characterization tasks can be performed better than unaided radiologists if the radiologists are supplied with sufficient information and support by AI (McKinney et al., 2020; Geras et al., 2019).

4.5.1   LIMITATIONS OF HUMAN OBSERVERS

The human observers of mammographic image analysis are limited even when simple targets are detected on uniform backgrounds because of the noise in the image. If the image contract is very low, the internal noise observed in the eye-brain system is also low. Under this situation, the information observed about the size and exact location of the target may not sufficient to diagnose the disease. But, the eye-brain system performs the diagnosis at a high level due to the low internal noise. It can be further improved by varying the viewing distance, adjusting the magnification factor of the image, and using computer algorithms.

However, the majority of the diseases are represented in the complex background of normal anatomy. It causes structured noise due to the superimposing of normal structures. This is the reason for the failure of human observers to accurately diagnosis diseases at an early stage. Such superimposing can confuse the computer algorithms also which leads to false-positive (interpret normal structures as abnormal structures) detections. Also, normal breast anatomy is varied from patient to patient. Because of these variations and complexity, radiologists may interpret abnormal structures as normal structures (false negative). Another important limitation of the human observer is the oversight of abnormalities in the computer-aided diagnostic techniques. It also increases the false-negative interpretations even in high-quality mammography. These false detections affect the performance of mammography.

Based on these, it has been recommended to train the radiologists' at least to a basic level, encourage interpretation of a single mammographic exam by two radiologists, and develop an approach to review the images by both human and computer observers.

4.5.2 COMPUTER VISION (CV) AND AI

Computer-based image analysis is possible if the images are represented in an appropriate digital format. Most of the examinations have already been upgraded to acquire digital data either directly or indirectly. Digitization of mammogram requires images with high spatial resolution, high contrast, and sensitivity. Researchers confirmed that pixels of size 50 μm with 12-bit quantization may be enough to represent the mammographic details.

Image processing is the first step in CV based detection algorithms followed by the image acquisition in digital format. Image processing enhances the SNR (Signal to Noise Ratio) of the image by suppressing unwanted details. Potential targets of interest are identified from the processed images. Then, features of potential targets of interest are extracted from the image which serves as the basis for further detection. Here, detection is performed based on the characterization of abnormalities. It is important to note that feature extraction plays a vital role in the CV.

CV techniques can provide reproducible data and consistency in performance. In CV, the decision related to detection and characterizations has been performed indirectly unlike the Radiologists approach. Usually, Radiologists consider the physical appearance of the image.

To determine the final output, the details of the mathematical pattern are extracted from the individual feature by the radiologists. If this pattern is simple, it can be analyzed straightforwardly using simple algorithms. To analyze complex patterns accurately and in reproducible ways, AI techniques have been developed by mathematical and physical scientists. These techniques include expert rule-based systems and discriminant analysis methods along with artificial neural networks.

4.5.3   Detection of Microcalcifications and Breast Masses

Microcalcifications are considered to be an ideal target in mammography algorithms to detect abnormalities present in the breast. Because they are visible in images, their structure is different from normal anatomical structures, and they are clinically relevant for diagnosis. Many investigators study microcalcifications in CAD. They used different approaches in their detection algorithm at the image-processing stage, feature analysis, and decision-making stage.

For example, a subtraction-image approach is an important approach used at the image-processing stage of an algorithm. Here, the original digital mammogram is spatially filtered twice, i.e. one time to enhance microcalcifications and another time to suppress them. Then, these digital images are subtracted to improve the SNR of the microcalcifications and to suppress the soft tissue present in the breast. Following image subtraction, the pixel value of the image is analyzed to detect microcalcifications. If the pixel value at a particular place reaches the threshold pixel value of microcalcifications, it can represent its presence in the image. Usually, the threshold value is routinely updated based on the results obtained from true positive exams to improve the sensitivity for detection. Further, a few more features and criteria (Ex. Mathematical morphology, new clustering filters, artificial neural networks, etc.) of the threshold images are used to avoid the possibility of false-positive detection of microcalcifications and to detect true clusters of microcalcifications.

Detection of breast masses is more difficult than microcalcification detection because breast masses are suppressed and hidden by normal tissues in the image. This is due to the similar appearance of breast masses and normal breast parenchyma tissues in mammography. Therefore, investigators discussed various approaches to detect breast masses. They used the asymmetry between the left and right breast to detect subtle masses. Such asymmetry can be enhanced using multiple subtraction images at the image processing stage. Feature extraction is another approach used for morphologic filtering, to determine the size and shape of lesions and their distance from the breast border. Template matching, detection of stellate abnormalities in the breast, and multi-resolution image processing approaches are used to identify breast masses in their initial stage. Likewise, these approaches play a major role to reduce the number of false-positive detections. They are also used to classify clusters of microcalcifications or breast masses as benign or malignant. Despite many approaches to classify benign and malignant lesions, there is a possibility for misclassification. It can be rectified by improvement in computer algorithms in association with human observers.

4.5.4   Present Status and Future Directions

At present, there are many approaches and techniques like CNN-based CAD that have been developed to detect mammographic abnormalities and they improved the performance of radiologists as well. However, they require various parameters, such as filter characteristics, threshold levels, etc., to make decisions. Therefore, no simple complex theory approach can be used for better performance. This approach must be evaluated by comparing the testing case against an actual case. But, the outcome of this evaluation strongly depends on the type of clinical case. Hence, the present approaches do not report the sensitivity, specificity, and other characteristics of computer performance.

Based on these, investigators proposed that a standard set of images would be developed as a reference database and the same would be shared among all the investigators to compare their results in a meaningful manner. Until this development, any CAD approach can only be evaluated against the human observer. Recently, investigators have reported that AI can be used to combine individual image features into correct mammographic diagnoses and shown the ability of neural networks better than the radiologist's outcome. They also proved the advantage of the neural network over radiologist's performance for patient management as well.

In the future, the on-going large scale efforts in CAD-based mammography will advance the present technology. It will be in the form of either continuous up-gradation of the present approach or introduction of new and novel techniques. Importance will also be given to time management and efficiency to complete the desired task as simple as possible. Hopefully, other obstacles to implement CAD techniques in mammography for routine clinical practice will also be removed in time. Once it is achieved, radiologists and patients will be benefited from the re-volution of digital technology.

4.6 AI IN MAGNETIC RESONANCE IMAGING (MRI)

MRI is a leading image modality for the assessment of musculoskeletal (MSK) disorders which offers high-resolution images with good soft-tissue contrast. Generally, MRI image acquisition is a slow process due to the high sampling requirements. The increase in data acquisition time causes image artifacts due to patient movement, patient discomfort, low patient output, and increases the cost of MRI imaging. These limitations necessitate the development of faster MRI imaging methods that explore the potential of AI. AI applications have led to innovations in MRI image classification, segmentation, super-resolution, and reconstruction.

4.6.1 DEVELOPMENTS OF AI IN MRI

1. The complexity of modern multi-parametric MRI has increasingly challenged interpretations of its images. ML has emerged as a powerful tool in personalized predictions of clinical outcome, in breaking down broad diagnostic categories into more detailed and precise subtypes, estimating cancer molecular characteristics in a non-invasive manner, contribute to the field of precision medicine, to introduce more specific diagnostic and predictive biomarkers of clinical outcome, and to select better treatment to patients.

2. The performance of a DL approach called the SMORE algorithm was demonstrated to improve the visualization of brain white matter lesions, to improve the visualization of scarring in cardiac left ventricular remodeling after myocardial infarction, on multi-view images of the tongue, and to improve performance in parcellation of the brain ventricular system.

3. The localization and quantification of subcutaneous adipose tissue (SAT) and visceral adipose tissue (VAT) were explored in MRI with the support of ML technology.

4. A convolutional neural network was proposed to perform segmentation using MRI images with synthetically introduced intensity inhomogeneity as data augmentation. It will simplify the segmentation process during image processing.

5. A method of contrast harmonization, called Deep Harmony, which uses a U-Net-based DL architecture, was proposed to produce images with high contrast and also to improve volume correspondence significantly.

6. Since DL methods are limited by the number of training samples, a wider denoising neural network to MR images was applied using a small sample size. The excellence of denoising performance of deep-learning methods is due to (i) the increased capacity and flexibility for exploiting image characteristics as it uses CNNs algorithm with very deep architecture, and (ii) choosing smaller intervals rather than the whole interval.

7. Radiomics and DL algorithms were used to differentiate metastatic lesions in the spine that originated from primary lung cancer.

8. A novel dual-domain convolutional neural network framework was proposed to improve structural information of routine 3T images. With this well-trained model, it can synthesize high-quality 7T-like images from input 3T images.

9. An ML analysis along with MRI-derived texture analysis (TA) features was evaluated to assess the presence of placenta accreta spectrum (PAS) in patients with placenta previa (PP). It can provide information about the histological abnormalities behind the PAS in patients with PP thus helping in differentiating positive from negative cases.

10. An efficient Bayesian diffeomorphic registration framework in a band-limited space was developed to quantifying image registration uncertainty based on a low-dimensional representation of geometric deformations.

11. Infant brain MRI analysis is a tedious task as it has many inherent challenges such as inhomogeneous tissue appearance across the image, considerable image intensity variability across the first year of life, and a low signal to noise setting. However, convolutional networks have shown success in infant brain MRI analysis specifically infant brain tissue segmentation at the isointense stage and presymptomatic disease prediction in neurodevelopmental disorders. This is possible because of the ability of the DL algorithm to learn non-linear, complex relationships in variable, heterogeneous input data.

12. Neuroanatomical volume and shape asymmetries have been considered as potential preclinical imaging biomarkers to predict Mild Cognitive

Impairment (MCI) and Alzheimer's disease dementia. A DL framework utilizing Siamese neural networks is used to harness the discriminative power of whole-brain volumetric asymmetry.

4.6.2 FUTURE DIRECTIONS

1. The SMORE algorithm should be evaluated using MR images instead of the natural images, require improvement in its resolution, and should address motion artifacts.
2. The speed of ML methods used for SAT and VAT quantification needs to be increased even though the quantification process is fast. Then, multicentre data should be collected to train the AI algorithm of all regions.
3. The fetal MRI slices that are heavily affected by motion artifacts are hard to manage during the segmentation process. Generating those slices would be an interesting area for future work.
4. The Deep Harmony architecture should be trained with non-representative data in addition to representative data using transfer learning. Even though it requires a high sample size, it will improve segmentation performance.
5. A combination of traditional MR image denoising methods and deep- learning methods would be investigated in the future to improve MRI performance.
6. The spine lesion segmentation method and DCE analysis methods performed with radiomics should be improved with a large case number and validated to apply for all related studies to investigate its clinical value for diagnosis and prognosis.
7. Even though dual-domain convolutional neural networks have multiple advantages in MRI image processing, it requires further investigation on functional information and disease diagnosis of synthesized images to evaluate image synthesis comprehensively.
8. The ML analysis along with MRI-derived texture analysis (TA) features should be further investigated on a larger cohort to validate this new diagnostic approach in the clinical practice.
9. Most of the present studies focus on classifying a single disease versus controls. However, the ability of a diagnostic system to discriminate between multiple psychiatric disorders is much more useful in a clinical setting. Hence, there is a need to assess the efficacy of ML models for differential diagnosis. Also, integrating rs-fMRI with diffusion-weighted MRI can yield even better neuron phenotypes of disease, and it is another challenging study in the future.
10. The novel Bayesian model for registration uncertainty quantification requires further investigation to completely assess the model uncertainty, and for extending its application to real clinical settings, e.g., real-time image-guided navigation system for neurosurgery.
11. The open challenges exist in convolution DL algorithm to analyze infant brain image, such as low data size restrictions, class imbalance problems, and lack of interpretability of the resulting DL solutions need to be addressed in the future.

12. It is proposed to apply a Siamese framework to different asymmetric features, such as shapes, voxel intensities, and cortical thickness, to seek other promising biomarkers associated with Alzheimer's disease. Also, more related works are recommended to verify the connection between biomarkers in MRIs and clinical diagnosis associated with Alzheimer's disease pathological features.

4.7   AI IN MEDICAL ULTRASOUND(US)

US imaging has been recognized as one of the most important imaging modality for many specialties. It is most commonly used in prenatal screening because of its high safety, low cost, non-invasiveness, user-friendly and real-time display. It has many advantages over Radiography, CT, and MRI. They are, the US does not use ionizing and non-ionizing radiation, and strong magnetic field, it is portable as it is compact, high accessibility, and economic. Therefore, US imaging allows point-of-care imaging at the bedside, during emergencies, in rural clinics, and developing countries. US imaging is applied to many specialties, viz. echocardiography, obstetrics and gynecology, intravascular US, etc.

Despite all these benefits and advantage, it has its challenges include (i) low image quality caused by noise and image artifacts, (ii) its performance highly depends on the operator and experience of the radiologists, and (iii) high variation in inter and intra- operator observation across different institutes. For example, the sensitivity of the US to detect malformations during the prenatal stage is varied from 27.5% to 96% among different diagnostic centers. This information implies that there is a necessity for advancements in US image analysis to make US diagnosis a more accurate, objective, and intelligent technology.

DL is considered to be a state-of-the-art approach to perform image analysis tasks automatically in the US. It can directly process and automatically represent raw data into higher-level features by combining the raw data with lower-level features. DL is successfully applied to many research domains such as CV, natural language processing (NLP), and speech recognition in addition to US image analysis. Recently, DL is demonstrated in various tasks of the US, such as image classification, segmentation, detection, registration, biometric measurements, and quality assessment as well as the 3D US, and image-guided interventions and therapy. However, there is a challenge to get more number of samples to train the model to achieve excellent learning performance.

This section discusses the basic information about the ultrasound imaging process, the role of AI and DL methods to execute these processes, architectures of DL algorithm in US imaging, benefits of DL in the US, and its potential future trends and directions (Shengfeng et al., 2019).

4.7.1   DL ARCHITECTURES

DL architectures are categorized into three main classes. They are:

1. Deep discriminative models or Supervised deep networks. These models are commonly used for the classification, segmentation, and detection of anatomical structures in US images. Examples of Supervised deep model are Convolutional Neural networks (CNNs) and Recurrent Neural Networks (RNNs).
   a. CNN's are a class of discriminative deep architecture with many modules. Every module consists of a convolutional layer and a pooling layer.
      i. The convolutional layer is used to detect local features at different positions in the input feature maps. As it performs its function through convolution operations on input images, it is termed as a convolutional layer. It involves three hyper-parameters, such as depth (number of filters), stride (control the filter), and padding (to remove the cause of dimensional reduction).
      ii. The pooling layer is used to subsample the output of the convolutional layer to reduce its data range.

   a. RNNs can model sequence data like US video sequences because of the structural characteristics of the network. However, it has not been implemented as it is hard to train the RNN to capture long-term dependencies. To date, RNNs have mostly applied in text or speech- recognition domains, but they are less applied in US image analysis.

2. Unsupervised deep networks or deep generative models
   These models are used to generate data samples by sampling from the networks. There are three basic approaches in medical US analysis. They are, (i) Auto- Encoder (AE), (ii) Restricted Boltzmann's Machines (RBM), and (iii) Deep Belief Networks (DBN).
   a. AE is a nonlinear feature-extraction approach. It is used for effective encoding of the raw data in hidden layers and representation learning. It consists of at least three layers: (1) an input layer to represent the original input features, (2) hidden layers to represent transformed information, and (3) an output layer to match the input layer to activate hidden layers.
   b. RBM is a single layer, undirected graphical model. It consists of a visible layer and a hidden layer that are connected symmetrically like in AE. Therefore, RBM is an AE but it is rarely used alone since there is no connectivity among units within the same layer.
   c. DBN is made up of a visible layer and many hidden layers. It can perform generalization because its layers are pre-trained using unlabeled data. Finally, it requires a fine-tuning step to practice a specific task as it is an unsupervised process.

3. Hybrid deep networks: These networks use the components of the generative and discriminative model together.

4.7.2   APPLICATIONS OF DL IN MEDICAL US IMAGE ANALYSIS

DL applications play a major role in (1) image classification, (2) detection of objects of interest, and (3) segmentation of various anatomical structures, and also (4) in 3D US imaging technology.

1. Image classification: Image classification is the identification of certain anatomical or pathological features to differentiate normal and abnormal structures in US images. Since computers cannot reproduce all the information required to interpret the images, the automatic classification of regions of interest became a developing technology in CAD systems. DL is applied to classify various following anatomical features as below.
   a. Traditional ML approaches can classify breast tumors or mass lesions using handcrafted and heuristic lesion-extracted features. However, DL can extract object features from US images automatically and directly. Example of such adaptive models are Adaptive Deconvolutional Networks (ADNs), CNN, stacked denoising auto-encoder (SDAE), GoogLeNet, etc.
   b. The US is an advanced imaging modality for the diagnosis and follow-up of thyroid nodules because of its real-time and non-invasive nature. It became an alternative tool to excisional biopsy methods and fine-needle aspiration (FNA) biopsy. A combination of high-level image features collected from CNNs and low-level image features from conventional hand-design are used here.
   c. Fetal abdominal circumference (AC) measurement, location of the fetal heart, and classification of the cardiac view should be performed very accurately. If not, it may cause inaccurate fetal weight estimation and increase the risk of misdiagnosis. Therefore, there is great importance to ensure the quality of fetal US imaging. This can be executed with the support of the DL models include fetal US image quality assessment (FUIQA) scheme, fully convolutional neural network (FCN), and a trained CNN model.

2. Detection: It is essential to detect objects of interest viz., anatomical objects, tumors, nodules, etc., on US images or US video sequences followed by classification. It plays a major role in object segmentation, for differentiation of benign and malignant tumors, and localization of anatomical objects. In this aspect, various DL models are applied to enhance the performance of the US as below.
   a. A combination of US, DBN DL model, and digital pathology is executed successfully for the detection and grading of prostate cancer. Another DL model namely Single-Shot MultiBox Detector (SSD) showed improved performance in terms of precision and recall to detect breast lesions.
   b. With the support of transferred deep models, the detection of fetal standard views and the fetal abdominal views were accomplished by radiologists in 2D US images. Likewise, a transferred RNN based deep model has also been applied for the same in US videos.

c. A deep residual recurrent neural network (RRN) was proposed to automatically recognize cardiac cycle phases. Similarly, a fully convolutional regression network was presented for the detection of measurement points in the heart.

3. Segmentation: The segmentation of anatomical structures and lesions is an essential step to analyzing clinical parameters (Ex. shape, volume, etc.) quantitatively in addition to detection and classification. However, there is a challenge to perform segmentation accurately due to the low contrast between the objects of interest and background in US images. Also, the available manual segmentation methods are tedious, individual dependent, and time-consuming. Therefore, it is essential to develop advanced automatic segmentation methods using DL models.

a. Various ML methods such as active contours and deformable templates have been widely used to successfully segment the left ventricle (LV) in Echocardiography. However, they need prior knowledge about LV shape and appearance. Recently, a dynamic CNN based method was proposed to gather multi-scale information, segment LV, fine-tuning for fetal LV segmentation, and to separate the connection area between the LV and LA (left atrium).

b. Boundary incompleteness is a big challenge for automatic segmentation of many anatomical structures (e.g., prostate, breast, kidney, fetus, etc.) in medical US images. Various DL methods (Ex. FCN segmentation network, ResNet-based deep framework, etc.) are presented to perform this task accurately and fast.

4. 3D US analysis: The present DL methods are applied only on 2D US due to various limitations to implement it on 3D US. A few of the challenges are (1) Training a DL network on a large scale for real clinical application may be computationally expensive due to the requirement for more memory and computational process, and (2) Requirement for more training samples. Therefore, various models have been proposed to address these challenges. Few of them are:

a. FCN based two-step algorithm for the measurement of endometrium thickness in a fully automatic manner.

b. Deep Learned Snake (DLS) segmentation model to detect and segment the endometrium from 3D trans-vaginal US volumes.

c. Hough-CNN to perform the detection and segmentation of brain regions.

d. 3D CNN to detect needle voxels in 3D US volumes.

e. Combination RNN and 3D FCN for segmentation of many objects simultaneously.

4.7.3 FUTURE PERSPECTIVES

Even though DL methods have been updated continuously in various aspects of US imaging, there is still a requirement for improvement to overcome its challenges.

Such improvement depends on the number of sample datasets used for training. Presently, the available public datasets are limited. To address this issue, intra-modality and inter-modality cross dataset learning, also known as transfer learning is recommended.

Transfer learning is a method of transferring the knowledge learned from the source task into the target task to improve learning performance. The effectiveness of any transfer method for a given target task depends on the source task, and how it is related to the target.

There are two main ideas to use transfer learning while handling small sample datasets. They are, (i) by directly using a pre-trained network as a feature extractor, and (ii) fine-tuning the small datasets by fixing the weights in parts of the network. However, the pre-trained network also requires a large training sample for good generalization. Therefore, a specially designed small network may be used as smaller-scale training datasets.

It is recommended to develop domain-specific DL models to perform a specific task to improve the performance of US imaging with less computation complexity. However, it is not recommended to train the models using natural images. Because, natural images consist of low contrast, texture-rich, and single-channel data. Generally, multiple imaging modalities (Ex. US, MRI, CT, etc.) are used to diagnose a single disease. Under this situation, cross-modal transfer learning is recommended. It is difficult to collect large samples from a single site (hospital). But, it is possible to collect large samples from multiple different US machines. With this data, cross-machine transfer learning of the US modality can be performed.

Further, future studies should address the issues associated with the present transfer learning algorithms as well. A few of the issues are (1) negative transfer, (2) heterogeneous features between target tasks and source, and (3) lack of generalization across different tasks. The negative transfer may be avoided by various strategies that include (i) recognition and rejection of unwanted source knowledge, (ii) selection of suitable source tasks from a group of source tasks, and (iii) modeling the similarity among the suitable source tasks. Heterogeneous features may be handled by mapping.

Even though 3D US imaging is an essential modality in medical imaging, there are many challenges associated with the DL model in 3D US and they should be addressed in the future. It is emphasized that more innovative 3D DL algorithms need to be established to perform various tasks and to improve the performance of 3D US imaging with the support of computer experts and radiologists to implement it for routine clinical practice.

4.8   AI IN NUCLEAR MEDICINE IMAGING

Nuclear Medicine (NM) imaging is used to collect functional information of organs and tissues in addition to structural information, and for molecular profiling by detecting radiation coming from the region of interest after a radiopharmaceutical is injected into the patient.

Positron Emission Tomography (PET) and Single Photon Emission Computed Tomography (SPECT) are two important and rapidly growing NM imaging modalities. They provide macroscopic information on molecular processes and altered cellular biology in several diseases, especially in cancer. This information is very important to understand the phenotypes of an individual tumor, behavior of tumor during invasion and metastasis, the interaction of tumor cell with their environment, and predict the tumor response to therapy.

The initial diagnosis of tumor disease and its molecular profiling are performed commonly by an invasive method namely biopsy. Then, non-invasive imaging, such as CT, MRI, PET, and SPECT need to be performed to know the staging of the tumor and to monitor the disease to plan the treatment. These modalities provide digitized images which are analyzed using mathematical algorithms.

It is accepted that many of the image features, such as proliferation, hypoxia, necrosis, angiogenesis, tumor genotype, and intra-tumor heterogeneity are not visible to the nuclear medicine physician or radiologists. Therefore, there is an increasing interest to develop algorithms with AI methods. The field of medical imaging that investigates the creation and application of these algorithms, termed radiomics has also been developed rapidly (Ian et al., 2019; d'Amico et al., 2020).

4.8.1 DEFINE A RADIOMIC DIAGNOSTIC ALGORITHM

The group of features that appropriately classify the radiological data in radiomics are termed as radiomic signature. The workflow of the radiomic diagnostic algorithm to define a radiomic signature consists of five major sequential steps. They are:

1. Identification of a group of patients to be studied: A large group of patients should be selected. To get the required number of patients, a small inhomogeneity in the group is acceptable. But, it should be noted that the increased number of variables selected due to heterogeneity will affect the result. There is a possibility for hundreds of features that will complicate the process. Hence, it is recommended to perform multi-institutional studies during the image standardization process.

2. Image acquisition: Image acquisition is one of the most difficult processes in nuclear medicine imaging because it has highly variable acquisition parameters. It should be performed in a reproducible and standardized manner. Initiations have been taken to standardize image acquisition nationally and internationally. The usage of the point-spread function, the reduction in voxel size, usage of narrow Gaussian post-filtering, and radiomic methods can minimize feature variations.

3. Definition of lesion contours (segmentation): Different segmentation methods are possible depending upon the Standardized Uptake Value (SUV), percentage of tracer accumulation compared with the point of maximum signal intensity, and the ratio between the signal of an organ and standard. However, none of these methods have yet been validated clinically. Recently, a method has been proposed to evaluate data on physiologically different regions of the tumor against the radiomic data extracted from these regions.

4. Features extraction: Data extraction features are divided into semantic and non-semantic features. Semantic feature deals with the data, such as diameter, volume, and shape of the tumor. Non-semantic features deal with the data extracted from the mathematical elaboration of the image. Data extraction features can also be classified according to their mode of definition mode as the first order, and second-order variable. First-order variables deal with the signal values of the tumor voxels but not about their spatial characteristics. However, second-order variables depend on the spatial distribution of the signal which is termed texture analysis. The texture is defined as a regular repetition of patterns or elements with the characteristics of brightness, color, size, and shape. Finally, various data sets can be calculated by analyzing the tumor based on their fractal features. It means that the datasets are selected if they are non-redundant, stable, and relevant ones. Then, the stability of the data is assessed by evaluating the consistency of the data in tests that are repeated at different times or by comparing the data extracted from different methods of tumor segmentation.

5. Model building and clinical validation: Once the suitable data is identified, an algorithm is defined to process the data to collect a response to any clinical question. Generally, the research population is divided into two groups: a training group to build a model, and a testing group to validate the model clinically. It is well known that each of these steps shows specific problems in the field of nuclear medicine.

4.8.2 Applications of AI in Nuclear Medicine

Nuclear medicine based imaging workflow can be divided into 4 major steps: (1) planning, (2) image acquisition, (3) interpretation, and (4) reporting in addition to admission and payment. This section gives an insight into AI that how it is applied in that step to improves, accelerates, or automates the process.

1. Planning: Before performing an examination, the planned procedure should be verified. Such an important process can be executed effectively with the support of AI systems as below:
   a. The feasibility of predicting no-shows in the medical imaging departments are demonstrated using simple ML algorithms and logistic regression.
   b. ML algorithms can be used to search patient-related information to prepare and plan the examination easily.

2. Scanning: Modern scanner technology has already started to use ML. For example,
   a. Attenuation maps and scatters correction is being performed for PET and SPECT imaging. A modified U-Net (special convolutional network architecture) is demonstrated to generate the attenuation maps for whole-body PET/ MRI.
   b. A deep residual CNN is used to improve the image resolution and noise property of PET scanners with large pixelated crystals.

    c. CNN's are used to improve timing resolution by 20–23% compared with conventional discrimination methods.

    d. AI-based methods are used to predict drug-target interactions (DTI) quickly. Therefore, the cost and time to develop radiotracers are reduced drastically.

3. Interpretation

    a. AI assistants working in the background can alert the radiologists to check the missing findings. It can also be used to detect recurring secondary findings.

    b. DL algorithms have already been demonstrated to detect Alzheimer's disease and mild cognitive impairment.

    c. A combination of threshold-based detection and ML-based classification has been addressed to evaluate 18F-NaF PET/CT scans for bone metastases in prostate cancer patients.

    d. ML algorithms are used in 18F-FDG PET to estimate the arterial input function to quantify regional cerebral metabolic rate for glucose.

    e. AI systems can support the interpreter in the process of classification and differential diagnosis.

4. Reporting

    a. ANN-based models have been proposed to predict later skeletal metastasis in 18F-FDG PET/CT with improved sensitivity and specificity.

    b. Radiomics features from 18F-FDG PET/CT and ML models have been demonstrated to predict local disease control with therapy.

    c. AI-based models have been evaluated to predict coronary artery disease and its associated risk.

    d. The AI-based automatic image annotations have the potential to search and find similar cases that can be useful in real clinical scenarios.

4.8.3 FUTURE SCENARIOS

Many investigators have explored the possible clinical applications of radiomics. AI-supported segmentation of head and neck tumors can be applied to plan the radiotherapy and to differentiate tumor from surrounding normal tissues accurately. In 18F-FDG PET investigation, fractal-based algorithms can be used to distinguish malignant lesions and non-aggressive nodules from the images of pulmonary solitary nodules.

The application of radiomics in FDG PET to investigate lung, esophageal tumors, and sarcomas has shown an appreciable outcome. However, it should be validated to implement clinically. Nowadays, the process of standardizing image acquisition and reconstruction in PET appears to be a challenging task. Since these processes having many potential clinical advantages, their present challenges must be sorted out with the advancement of AI in the future.

The involvement of AI in medical imaging will influence the Nuclear Medicine practice and research through the development of AI-assisted CT and MR applications in SPECT/CT, PET/CT, and PET/MR hybrid imaging. However, it is important to note that human supervision is strongly recommended as an additional or mandatory option even though AI-based systems can provide excellent results.

4.9 SALIENT FEATURES OF AI IN MEDICAL IMAGING

After the invention of digital computers in the 1940s, the term AI (AI) has been developed enormously for applications in various areas of science and technology. This section discusses the various characteristics of AI to develop strategies to explore the potential of AI in medical imaging (James et al., 2018; Lia et al., 2019).

4.9.1 OPPORTUNITIES AND APPLICATIONS

The development of AI has the following opportunities in medical imaging:

1. Integration of systems and Information Technologies (IT) in medicine.
2. Standardization of medical procedures and their digital formats.
3. Establish a categorical model to handle the various research and clinical developments and applications of AI.
4. Establish reference datasets of confirmed cases to check and evaluate AI programs.
5. Establish criteria to standardize and optimize protocols correspond to medical imaging to use them for AI applications. '
6. Establish a common lexicon to describe and report AI applications.
7. Aggregate material from multiple institutions to analyze medical images.
8. Develop standards and robust methods to ensure the quality of shared images and integrity of imaging data.
9. Establish reference datasets (like "ImageNet") in all applications to record the demographic variation among the patient population.
10. Establish image sharing networks at the national and international level by connecting healthcare professions into networks to share their digital information.
11. Develop training models using images labeled by experienced radiologists, and histopathological experts for manpower development, and to help general radiologists and trainees to gain confidence and competence.
12. Establish infrastructure to frame standards.

All of these opportunities facilitate the following applications and benefits:

1. Optimization of workflow and value in healthcare.
2. Teleradiology and telemedicine to provide primary healthcare and diagnostics in remote areas in an economic way.
3. Improved diagnostic accuracy because of the AI-enabled CAD with two achieving human-level performance.
4. Day to day clinical issues will be reduced by (1) optimizing worklists to prioritize cases, (2) alerting radiologists and physicians about the patients

who require urgent treatment, (3) analysis of cases in high-volume applications to avoid observer fatigue, (4) extracting additional information from images that are not visible to the naked eye, and (5) improving the quality of reconstructed images.

5. Help radiologists to achieve diagnostic excellence and to enhance patient healthcare through precision medicine.
6. Tumor recurrence, resistance to the treatment, and treatment outcome can be precisely predicted by radiogenomics.
7. Increased workload since the time required to collect images is shorter than before.

4.9.2 CHALLENGES

Even though AI has many opportunities and applications, it also has its challenges. They may be either circumstantial challenges or intrinsic challenges. Circumstantial challenges are related to human behavior in society. Intrinsic challenges are related to the limitations in science and technology.

A few of the circumstantial challenges are:

1. It is well known that medical images are varied patient to patient and population to population. If the number of available images for a specific application is limited, training the AI system will be a challenging task. It may create a risk of "overfitting" the data and prevent its usage in various areas.
2. The numbers of Radiologists who are expertise in radiology AI methods are limited.
3. The introduction of AI technology into clinical practice will be expensive as it includes the cost of expert salary, hardware, and software.
4. There are many legal and regulatory issues to judge who the owner of the data is, who is responsible if the machine makes a mistake, and who has the right to use the results.

A few of the intrinsic challenges are:

1. The complexity of the data
   a. Low resolution and contrast, high noise, and artifacts in the image affect the image acquisition process.
   b. Analysis of different models among multiple centers and modalities would be a challenging task.
   c. Need for curated data to train the machine- learning algorithms.

2. The complexity of the targets of interest
   a. The targets of interest in medical images, such as bones, soft tissue organs, lesions, implants, etc., show complexity in their nature and shape. Such complexity can't be easily represented by a mathematical model.
   b. The objects of interest show both intra-subject variability caused by movements associated with the respiratory activity, bowel activity, etc.,

and inter-subject variability caused by pathological and biological modifications. These changes also induce complexity and uncertainty when
designing a model.

c. Similar objects of interest can show variation in their shape and intensity
due to difference in time points.

3. Complex validation

a. The assessment of the absolute accuracy of diagnostic images is a tedious
task in most of the applications due to a lack of ground truth. However,
ground truth can be provided by manual analysis by a clinical expert (for
example, manual delineation in image segmentation and manual annotation of corresponding anatomical landmarks in image registration). But,
such manual analysis is also subjected to intra- and inter-observer
variability.

b. Validation of results mainly depends on how best the source of truth is
established.

c. Like accuracy, other parameters of any imaging modality, viz., robustness,
consistency, precision, etc., also creates complexity during validation.

d. In most cases, the gold standard of interpretation is also degraded due to
the shortage of pathologic proof.

4.9.3 PITFALLS

The obstacles to the successful implementation of AI in clinical practice are:

1. AI programs require a few thousands of exams for training. Unfortunately,
xenophobia at institutions and other owner's interests limit access to data
among institutions.
2. Failure to collect training models to produce trained manpower.
3. The risk of overfitting as indicated previously.
4. The tolerance limit to use AI programs in imaging at individual and population levels is unknown.
5. Failure to realize that AI programs are not common for patients of different
ages and cultural groups.
6. Complexity in considering the variation in organ size and occurrence of
diseases among the population.
7. Failure to incorporate the immunity power of the individuals.
8. Failure to consider the errors introduced when transferring an AI program
from one protocol to another.
9. Lack of expertise to reduce the inherent challenges of AI programs.

4.9.4 GUIDELINES FOR SUCCESS

The important guidelines for successful implementation of AI programs are:

1. Create opportunities through discussions.

2. Generate value in the outcome of healthcare, increase diagnostic accuracy, trigger the effort to reduce the time taken by the radiologists to complete a task, and quick display of results.
3. Develop AI programs that are suitable for various data acquisition protocols and to work in a heterogeneous group of patients.
4. Understand the circumstantial challenges completely to implement an AI program successfully.
5. Bring new ideas and business processes to minimize its cost for making advanced technologies available to a wider group of populations who are deprived of healthcare.

4.9.5   REGULATORY AND ETHICAL ISSUES

The ethical issues associated with the applications of AI programs in medical imaging can be categorized into three categories. They are (1) Data ethics, (2) Algorithm ethics, and (3) Practice ethics.

Data Ethics:

1. It is necessary to protect the patient data according to the existing directives and legislation of the patient's country.
2. Data privacy and data confidentiality are inter-linked issues however these terms are not interchangeable.
   a. Data privacy indicates the rights of owners on their medical data and results.
   b. Data confidentiality means that maintain privacy by a person who is responsible for the data.

3. AI algorithms will be biased against the individual patient, geographic variations, gender, socioeconomic background, culture, immunity of individuals, the occurrence of disease, lack of genetic studies among the population, etc. Hence, all the users and developers of the AI system should be aware of this bias and verify that corresponding variations are provided in the database to avoid unintended bias.

Algorithm Ethics:

1. The progress, path, and limitation of every algorithm should be clear for the users.
2. The Radiologist would approve the AI tools based on the approval given by the regulatory authorities, and standards of healthcare. The regulatory approval should be obtained from the US Food and Drug Administration (FDA) or analog organization to validate the AI tools, their procedures, and applications.

Practice Ethics:

1. There should be a policy to promote the developments in AI and protect the rights of every Radiologist as well.

2. The policy should allow the users to realize their mistakes in social media like Facebook and learn from them.
3. The reason to use AI tools should be verifiable and transparent.
4. Practice policies should incorporate the effects of a so-called collective brain on human behavior.
5. It is difficult to predict the malfunction of AI tools and hence they should be bound by ethical principles. Moreover, Radiologists are responsible to validate the AI associated things to do now and in the future.

REFERENCES

Carl J.V. and Maryellen L.G. (1994), 'Computer Vision and Artificial Intelligence in Mammography', *American Journal of Roentgenology*, 162, 699–708.

d'Amico A., Borys D., and Gorczewska I. (2020), 'Radiomics and Artificial Intelligence for PET Imaging Analysis', *Nuclear Medicine Review*, 23(1), 36–39.

David J.W., Tobias H., Thomas J.W., Daniel T.B., and Bram S. (2019), 'Evaluation of an AI-Based Detection Software for Acute Findings in Abdominal Computed Tomography Scans Toward an Automated Work List Prioritization of Routine CT Examinations', *Investigative Radiology*, 54(1), 55–60.

Geras K.J., Mann R.M., and Moy L., (2019), 'Artificial Intelligence for Mammography and Digital Breast Tomosynthesis: Current Concepts and Future Perspectives', *Radiology*, 293(2), 246–259.

Ian R.D., Amanda J.B., and Neil V. (2019), 'Improving PET Imaging Acquisition and Analysis with Machine Learning: A Narrative Review with Focus on Alzheimer's disease and Oncology', *Molecular Imaging*, 18, 1–11.

James H.T., Xiang L., Quanzheng L., Cinthia C., Synho D., Keith D., and James B. (2018), 'Artificial Intelligence and Machine Learning in Radiology: Opportunities, Challenges, Pitfalls, and Criteria for Success', *Journal of the American College of Radiology*, 15, 504–508.

Kasban H., El-Bendary M.A.M., and Salama D.H. (2015), 'A Comparative Study of Medical Imaging Techniques', *International Journal of Information Science and Intelligent System*, 4(2), 37–58.

Koenigkam S.M., Raniery Ferreira J.J., Tadao Wad D., et al. (2019), 'Artificial Intelligence, Machine Learning, Computer-Aided Diagnosis, and Radiomics: Advances in Imaging Towards to Precision Medicine', *Radiologia Brasileira*, 52(6), 387–396.

Lia M., Silvia D., and Loredana C. (2019), 'Artificial Intelligence in Medical Imaging: From Theory to Clinical Practice', USA: CRC Taylor & Francis Group.

Martin J.W. and Peter B.N. (2019), 'The Evolution of Image Reconstruction for CT - From Filtered Back Projection to Artificial Intelligence', *European Radiology*, 29, 2185–2195.

McKinney S.M., Sieniek M., Godbole V., et al. (2020), 'International Evaluation of an AI System for Breast Cancer Screening', *Nature*, 577(2), 89–114.

Shengfeng L., Yi W., Xin Y., Baiying L., Li L., Shawn Xiang L., Dong N., and Tianfu W. (2019), 'Deep Learning in Medical Ultrasound Analysis: A Review', *Engineering*, 5, 261–275.

5 Artificial Intelligence (AI)

Improving Customer Experience (CX)

K. Vinaykumar Nair
BT India Pvt. Ltd., RMZ Millenia, Bangalore, India

CONTENTS

OBJECTIVE

This chapter provides high-level insight into the customer journey when the customer decides to go for purchase and how AI can be used to improve the customer experience starting from the pre-purchase phase to purchase and then when the customer is using the product. This chapter tries to map the whole customer journey and how AI can be used across the customer journey.

DOI: 10.1201/9781003175865-5

5.1 INTRODUCTION TO ARTIFICIAL INTELLIGENCE (AI)

5.1.1 WHAT IS AI? – THE BASICS

AI or artificial intelligence is a branch of computer science that allows machines to learn constantly from the environment to gain knowledge and develop cognitive (human-like) skills. AI allows machines to learn, keep learning and adapt to new inputs and based on what has been learnt to make better decisions. The goal of AI is for machines to learn from the environment so that it takes actions based on past learnings, thereby maximizing the chances of achieving its goals.

One of the most common examples of AI is the maps application which we use on our mobile phones, it gives the prediction about how much time it's going to take to reach from location A to location B. It also provides the details about the best possible route to reach the destination with minimum time. All this is possible only because of AI being used by the maps which constantly learns from the various sources about the traffic patterns regularly which allows it to predict the duration and the best possible route from location A to location B.

Another example of AI is autonomous cars. A fully autonomous car can drive on its own, it can drive the same way as a human driver, make the same decision that a human driver will take depends on the road and other external factors. How is it able to achieve this? The car is fed with all the data on how to behave under certain conditions (road condition, weather, etc.), the car senses the environment using the sensors, and based on the inputs from the sensors the car behaves in the manner in which it is programmed. The car also learns from its environment and improves its behavior.

Let's take another example which we see very often, the voice assistants – the voice assistants constantly hear what is being said and pick up the commands which activate them, for example – Alexa or "OK Google," then whatever question you ask or commands you give, it acts upon it. Voice assistants use NLP or natural language processing to understand what you said. The language is then converted to text and it either actions the command or searches the Internet or database to find the matching response to your query. This is again converted to speech and played back to you.

These are some of the commonly seen examples where AI is used. One of the other Interesting fields where AI is used heavily is the area of customer experience or the digital customer experience. We will discuss more the use of AI in the area of customer experience and how AI helps in providing a better customer experience (CX).

5.2 CUSTOMER EXPERIENCE (CX) AND THE USE OF AI

Customer experience is the experience which the customer of the product has with the organization during the course of their relationship. Customers can start interacting with the organization the moment they start the search for a particular product. The search can be an online search or a search in the physical store. For the customer, the whole journey from trying to search for the product to making the purchase decision to buying, using, and getting support throughout the life of the product is what makes the whole customer experience.

Customers like to stick to organizations that make things easy for them. They prefer the ease of dealing with the organizations. Organizations that make the whole process from deciding to buy to using and in-life support easy for the customers are the ones who are more successful, but this is not an easy task as it may sound. But there is help available, AI has been very successful in creating an excellent customer experience. In this chapter, we will discuss the various aspects of AI and how it can help create an excellent Customer Experience (CX) for the whole customer journey.

5.2.1 CUSTOMER JOURNEY

Before we discuss AI, let's try to understand the customer journey. We did touch upon this at the beginning of this section, and the customer journey is the process that starts when the customer begins the search of the product to satisfy the need and continues until the product's end-of-life.

Figure 5.1 will explain the customer journey. The customer journey has five key steps starting from awareness of the need and the product, which can satisfy the need to considering suitable options, making the purchase decision, using the product, and remaining loyal to the organization or switching to another alternative. Let us discuss these stages in a bit more detail:

i. Awareness/Need Identification – In any customer journey, the starting point is the "Need Identification" by the customer and the awareness about the possible options to satisfy that need. There should be a need to buy a certain product to meet a certain requirement. For example: I need a laptop, or I need a mobile phone, etc.

ii. Consideration/Searching Suitable Options – Once the need is established, the next step in the journey is to search for suitable options. Usually, there is

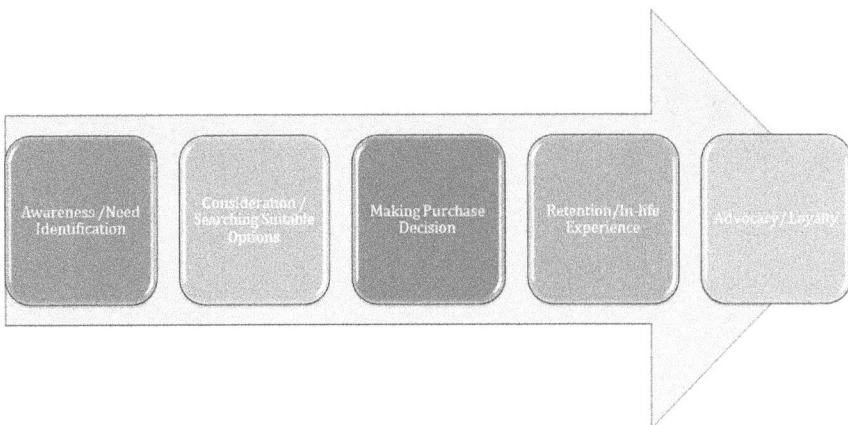

FIGURE 5.1 Typical customer journey.

more than one option to satisfy the need. There can be multiple products or offerings which the customer can go for based on price, features, color, size, etc. At this stage, the customer explores all possible options which can satisfy its needs.

iii. Making Purchase Decision – Based on the review of the suitable options the customer makes a purchase decision to buy a particular product.

iv. Retention/In-life Installation – Once the successful purchase has been made, at this stage customer starts to use the product. At this stage, the customer is using the product regularly and will approach the organization only if needed. For example, if there is any problem with the product or if the customer wants some more information about the product/feature or if there is a renewal of the maintenance contract, etc.

v. Loyalty – If the organization can demonstrate excellent customer experience throughout the journey, it can create customer loyalty meaning that customer is likely to stick to the organization and also promote the product or the organization to other potential customers.

5.2.2 CUSTOMER TOUCHPOINTS

During this whole customer journey, the customer has interacted with the organization at multiple points, also known as "Touchpoints." These are the touchpoint which the organization needs to focus on, giving excellent customer experience at these touchpoints is what makes the organization successful. There are two types of touchpoints: physical touchpoints and digital touchpoints (Figure 5.2).

i. Physical Touchpoint – These are touchpoints in which the customer experiences the organization or brand in the physical world. For example, walking

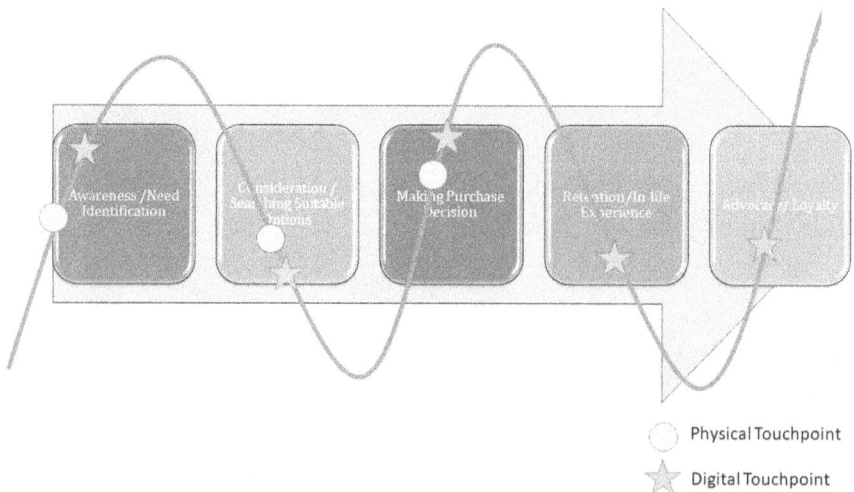

○ Physical Touchpoint

★ Digital Touchpoint

FIGURE 5.2 Customer journey mapped to touchpoints.

into the physical store and experience (touching, using) the product or getting to see and experience the product at a marketing event, etc.

ii. Digital Touchpoint – These are the online touchpoints that try to interact with the customer in the digital world. Examples are the organization website, Twitter handle, Facebook page, etc.

5.2.3   CUSTOMER JOURNEY MAPPING AND TOUCHPOINTS

During the whole customer journey, the customer interacts with the organization using either the physical touchpoint or digital touchpoint. Let's try to understand these touchpoints across the customer journey.

i. Awareness/Need Identification – Customers most likely know what they want to achieve and which organization/brands/products may be able to offer them solutions using their product. This can happen both online as well as offline. Online by engaging the customers on social media channels, company website, etc., and offline via physical stores, newspaper advertisements, etc.

ii. Consideration/Searching suitable options – Customers prefer organizations/brands whose product information is available readily. It can be via physical touchpoints or via digital touchpoints. Physical via visiting the organization/brands' store and digital via the organization/brands' website, Twitter handle, social media page, etc.

iii. Making purchase decision – Making a purchase decision again can be made via a physical touchpoint or via a digital touchpoint. Purchase in the store or online.

iv. Retention/In-life experience – The experience which the customer gets once the product is delivered and installed and also when the customer faces any problem with the product makes a huge difference in customer experience. Customers prefer organizations/brands which are easily accessible, especially in a crisis situation. Customers expect ease in dealing with the organization/brand wheatear it's the ease to contact the organization/brand for any problems or faster resolution to their problems. Most of the time, customers will reach out to organizations/brands using digital touchpoints.

v. Advocacy/Loyalty – Based on the experience which the customer gets across, the touchpoints defines brand loyalty, and brand loyalty can be seen when the customer starts recommending the product not just to the friends and family but also on the Internet where the customer starts engaging on the social media channels and starts recommending the brand/organization to others.

5.3   CUSTOMER EXPECTATIONS FROM CX

Let's now focus our attention on the changes in consumer behavior as that will articulate the expectations which the customer has from the organization/brands across the customer journey. Today's customer is a digital customer who has the power of connectivity and information is at the fingertips. The customer can search for information whenever they want and are clear about what they expect from the organization/brands.

There have been many studies conducted from time to time, trying to understand the changes in customer behavior. One of the most recent ones is the recent study done by BT (BT Telecommunications Plc) and Cisco called Autonomous Customer 2020 (A study on changes in the customer expectations when it comes to customer experience). The study has the following key findings (BT, 2020a and 2020b) (Figure 5.3):

i. The majority of the customers still prefer a phone call to reach out to the organization/brand. Yes, many people may have thought that the phone is dead and people prefer texting to a phone call. That's not true; majority of the respondents said they would still prefer a phone call.

ii. Email is the next preferred channel. The good old email is still a preferred channel for communication. After voice, it's still the most reliable channel.

iii. The customer wants choices of other channels like WhatsApp, Facebook Messenger, etc. Customers just don't want to stick to traditional channels. Popular digital channels are what the customers may use based on requirements.

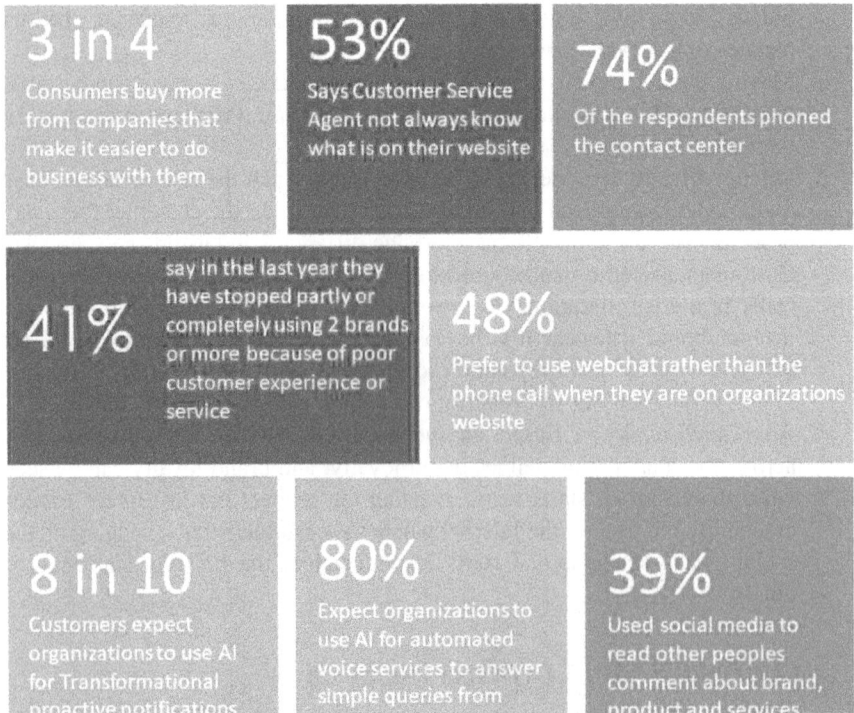

FIGURE 5.3 Autonomous customer 2020.

Source: The Digital Customer 2020-BT Telecommunications Plc/Cisco.

iv. Social media is less preferred for customer complaints but is preferred for general communications and promotions. Customers usually review the ratings and feedback of the organization/brand/product on social media before making a purchase decision.
v. Customers are open to the use of AI in the customer experience, customers want ease and security and are open to the use of AI if that makes things easy and secure for them.

In summary, customers reward organization/brand which makes things easy for them. Customers want the interactions to be simple, personalized, and continuous. Today's customer is digital and does most of the research themselves. A great customer experience means that brands/organization needs to focus on all aspects of the customer journey and not just one interaction when the customer calls the contact center.

Today's digital customer prefers to use a variety of channels, though voice remains the preferred means, the customers want to use different channels based on convenience. Customers may want to start with a messaging app (WhatsApp, Facebook messenger, or even an SMS) for less important communication but want to shift to a voice channel if there is something complex or more serious.

Customers don't want to repeat the same conversation which they completed on the messaging channels once they want to talk to the agent, the agent should be aware of the conversation which the customer had on the messaging channel and should be able to deal with the complex issue straightaway for which the human agent has been involved.

If the organization/brand is unable to provide a great experience in every part of the customer journey, customers are less likely to remain loyal to the organization/brand. As per the recent survey done by Adobe – Digital Trends 2020, organizations are putting maximum emphasis on customer experience (Adobe, 2020a and 2020b). Most companies surveyed consider CX as the most exciting business opportunities.

Customers are willing to explore new technologies like AI if that makes life easy and secure for them. All these are easier said than done. It's important to have the right technology supported by AI or another technological advancement to create a seamless customer experience.

In the next section, we will discuss more about the customer journey and how AI can help create a seamless customer experience across various physical and digital touchpoints to help organizations and their customers provide a superior customer experience.

5.4   CUSTOMER JOURNEYS AND THE USE OF ARTIFICIAL INTELLIGENCE

Let's now try to understand how AI can help organizations/brands improve customer experience across the customer journey.

5.4.1 NEED IDENTIFICATION/AWARENESS CREATION

This is about creating awareness of the products, clearly communicating with the potential customers about the product, what it can do and how it's better than other products in the market in satisfying a certain need.

The use of AI to create awareness is more relevant for a digital touchpoint. AI can help awareness creation in many ways:

i. Targeting the right customers – using AI the organization/brand can target the product to the right customers. AI can be used to identify who is interacting or searching for their products on the internet and can be targeted.

ii. Target messaging – AI can also be used to tailor the messaging around a product or a brand. Using AI, organizations can understand the needs of the customer better based on the internet search, location, age, device, etc., and can provide custom messaging addressing the needs of the customer.

iii. Online support – AI can also help answer potential customer's queries regarding the product. This online support to answer customer queries can be automated using Chatbots. Chatbots are software programs that have the capability to understand the text written by the customer and respond to the question with an appropriate response. The behavior of a chatbot is very similar to a human agent and it has the intelligence to respond to most of the common queries from the customer.

iv. Targeted Advertising – When the customer is visiting the organization's website, by analyzing thousands of data points, past interactions, past purchases, etc., AI can push relevant advertisements which will help improve conversion rates and improve customer experience.

v. Personalized Content creation – AI can understand the customer's behavior on the organizations' website, capture the whole information across multiple data points, and then can draft a personalized and relevant email. A personalized email is far more impactful than a general email. AI can achieve this by analyzing multiple data points about a customer and send relevant information to the customer improving conversion rates.

vi. Churn reduction – AI can provide details about customers who are not engaging with the organization and are likely to churn. Organizations need to work with these customers giving them attention and trying to resolve their outstanding issues which will help retain these customers.

vii. Intelligent customer Insights – AI can help you provide detailed insight into customer behavior, buying patterns, likes, and dislikes and this data can be used to enhance the customer experience.

5.4.1.1 Use of Social Media in Awareness Creation

Social media is best suited for organization/brand awareness. Combined with AI it can help promote the brand/product to the right audience. Some of the key points to show how social media can be leveraged are as follows:

    i. Social media can help increase the website traffic – By targeting customers based on age, region, previous browsing history, etc., the right ads can be pushed to customers prompting them to visit the company website.

    ii. Building Conversations – Social media is a great tool to build positive conversations with existing and new potential customers. AI can be used to respond to general queries or comments on social media.

    iii. Managing customer reviews – A bot can search for the right keywords, for example, a brand/product name on the internet or popular social media platforms and send an alert to the helpdesk to take suitable action regarding the same. This helps the organization manage feedback on social media.

Most customers do search social media for feedback about a particular product. Organizations need to manage social media carefully and deal with negative feedback immediately.

5.4.2 Consideration/Searching Suitable Options

Once the customer has decided to make a purchase the next step is to deep dive into the organizations' products they would like to consider. This can happen via two different touchpoints, either by visiting the physical store or trying to find information online. More than 80% of the sales happen using physical stores, not online as we think.

When the customer reaches the physical store, the expectation is that the customer gets the same experience which they may have got from the organization/brand online. AI can be used in the digitization of instore experience and personalized experiences to the customer. AI can bridge the gap between the online experience and in-store experience. An AI-powered app which the in-store sales representative can request the customer to download for best offers and discounts can seamlessly provide a similar experience for both in-store and online. As soon as the app is download, based on the mobile number which the customer may have provided when searching a product online, the app can start showing the preferred product based on customers' choices. The app can also tell the customer in which rack/floor that particular product is available so that customers don't have to search for that product in the whole store. The app can help the customer navigate the store at ease just like the customer can navigate the online store. Merging the online and in-store experience is what will delight the customer and create a superior customer experience.

In case of retail merchandise, organizations can install "Smart Mirrors" which allows customers to wear the merchandise virtually, it can also show various color options, and this is the same experience customer gets online. Smart Mirrors scan the body shape using cameras and sensors and suggest the customer best suiting clothes and all this without actually getting into the traditional trial room. This significantly reduces the wait times to make a purchase and significantly enhances the customer experience.

Organization/brands can also deploy an Interactive control panel in the trial rooms using which the customer can request the next size/color if they want to try the selected merchandise.

If the customer wants a different size or color, the store can check if the inventory is available and if not, the store can check if it's available in any other stores and using AI can predict how long will it take for that particular item to arrive at the store from another one where it's available. If the customer prefers to get the same delivered at the home address then an Integrated AI can predict the delivery timelines which even the customer can track on the app.

If the customer decides to make the online purchase without visiting a physical store the customer is likely to search the product online first to understand the reviews from other customers, the ratings given by other customers significantly influence the decision making.

If the customer decides to make the purchase online the en customer is likely to visit the organization/brand's website. The website needs to be intuitive and engaging enough for the customer to get all the relevant information. If the website has all the usual details about the product and is arranged in a manner that is easy for the customer to consume, the customer will self-serve themselves and will go ahead with the purchase but customers prefer support to be available readily, in case if needed. Usually, the easiest way to offer help on the website is by using a FAQ. Today's customers want everything quickly and FAQ is usually too long and time-consuming to go through. The quicker option is Chatbots on the organization's webpage. Chatbots come in many flavors and the most sophisticated are AI-powered intelligent programs that can understand the question from the customers and provide an appropriate response. There are different types of Chatbots, as shown in Figure 5.4.

a. Rule or menu-based Chatbots, are the basic types of Chatbots and will throw the options which the customer has to click to get a reply and move to the next step as shown in Figure 5.5. Rule-based chatbots are fine for limited and simple operations.
b. Keyword Recognition Chatbots are more sophisticated and try to understand the keyword in the sentence customer has submitted. For example, if the

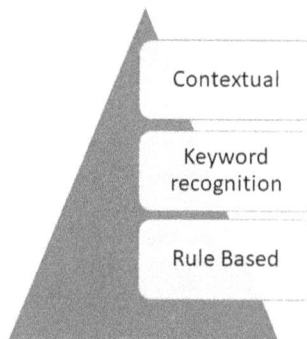

FIGURE 5.4 Chatbot types.

Hi

Hey! Got any queries related to
your Tata Sky connection?

Reply 1 for **Packs**

Reply 2 for **Bill & Recharge**

Reply 3 for **Technical**

Reply 4 for **Account**

Reply 5 for **Get Connection**

Reply 6 for **New Buy**

3

Not able to view after recharge,
reply **REFRESH**

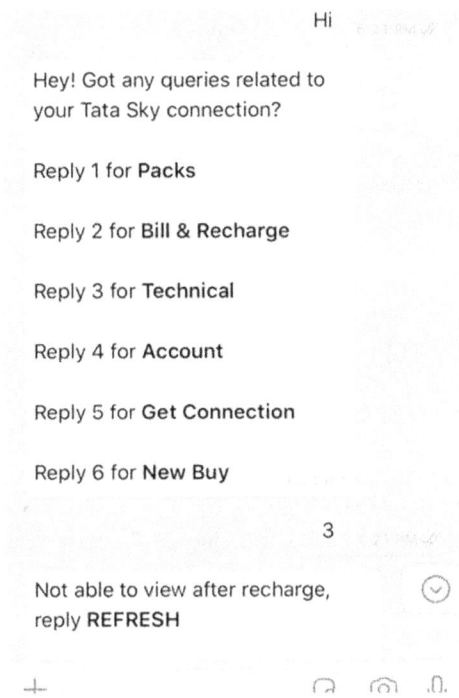

FIGURE 5.5   Example of rule-based chatbot.

customer says "I have to reset my password," the Chatbot will pick up the
keywords "reset" and "password" and provide an appropriate response.
c. Contextual Chatbots are AI-driven chatbots and try to understand the whole
text as a human would do. They can answer a completely different question
on the fly still retaining the original intent of the customer. These chatbots use
NLP (Natural language processing) to understand the question and respond
accordingly.

Organizations/brands must deploy the right chatbots based on the complexity of the
business. Organizations need to offer a great experience on the company website as
it influences the buying decisions.

5.4.3   PURCHASE DECISION

Once the customer has decided to go with a particular organization/brand based on
superior customer experience, the whole purchase process has to be made smooth
for the customer. At this stage of the organization, one cannot afford to go wrong.
Whether the purchase is being made online or in the store, AI can help. If the
customer is new and has visited the store or online for pre-purchase analysis, the
organization/brands should have most of the details of the customer already.

When the purchase is made either in-store or online, to create a great customer experience the customer should be able to get all the details of the purchase on email and the app (if the customer has downloaded the app during pre-purchase stages). The email should also provide details about the delivery status (mainly in case of online purchases or big size items from the store, for example, a TV or washing machine), the status of the installation, an email with the user manual, and guidance on where to reach out for help. Some brands mainly in the high-value technology space also invite the customer to join user forums which is a good idea as to its best if the new users of the product can get help from the existing users. It also helps the brands in keeping the customers engaged and motivates them to buy more and increase customer advocacy.

By this time the organization/brands should have all the information about the customer, purchase history, preferences, likes, and dislikes, etc. Using AI-based tools, the organization/brand can keep track of the purchase behavior of the customer. AI can also help suggest new products based on the purchase history which will help sell more to the existing customers. Customers can be kept updated on similar products, enhancements, and new launches. Customers are kept engaged and this helps in improving brand loyalty.

AI can also prompt the organizations the details of the customers who are completely disengaged, this helps organizations/brands to reach out to such customers proactively to understand if they have any issue with the product.

5.4.4 RETENTION/IN-LIFE SUPPORT

This is one of the most complex and expensive challenges which the organization/brands face. In-Life support of the product. This is a make or break phase where an inferior experience will lead to the customer moving to alternate options. Organizations are well aware that it is always cheaper to keep the customer than to acquire a new one.

At this stage, the customer is already using the product and will reach out to the organization/brand only when the customer needs more information about the product, want to buy something more, or if there is an issue with the existing product. Depending on the case the customer may choose a particular channel. Irrespective of the channel chosen by the customer, organizations need to recognize the customer. The first time the customer reaches out to the helpdesk and if the organization doesn't recognize the customer, that's the biggest letdown. It is for organizations to ensure that they have the details of all their customers and are greeted in a personalized manner. Whether it's the BoT response or the human agent responding, customers like if they are greeted in a personalized manner, especially the customers who are the existing users of the organization's products. AI can help the organizations collate all the data and provide personalized and meaningful information about the customer which will help not only in creating a better customer experience but also chances of selling more products.

Customers like the ease of use and secure transitions, if the customers are greeted with personalized messages then the organization/brand has made a good initial impression. When the customer reaches out to organizations, organizations need to ensure that customers feel secure. If the customer is not getting the feeling that the transaction or interaction is secure, it's for the organization to lose. How do organizations do this? It is for the organization to invest in new technologies to provide a safer and secure environment for its customers.

How do organizations recognize genuine customers and fraudsters? How can organizations give customers the confidence that the transaction is safe and secure? AI can help in providing security of the transaction to the customers. In text-based communications AI can looks for patterns that can alert the organization about the fraud. In a voice-based transaction, AI can provide security with ease by using technologies like Voice Biometrics. Voice biometrics technology stores the unique attributes of a person's voice. The next time the person calls, the attributes of the callers' voice is compared with the one which is stored. If the voice is matched the call is considered verified. Technologies like AI-driven voice biometrics allow easy and secure access, free up human resources in the support center as they don't have to spend time verifying the callers/customers.

AI-driven speech biometrics is becoming very popular in the banking and financial industry. Some of the leading global banks have incorporated this technology and provide ease of access to their customers. Voice biometrics can also be used as two- factor authentication besides a telephone PIN or a mobile-based OTP for added security.

Customers can reach out to the organization via multiple channels, traditional channels like voice are still popular but the newer generations may prefer new channels like a Facebook messenger or WhatsApp. It is for organizations to ensure that they support their customers not only the traditional channels but also new-age digital channels. Figure 5.6 shows the most popular channels used by organizations to provide customer service.

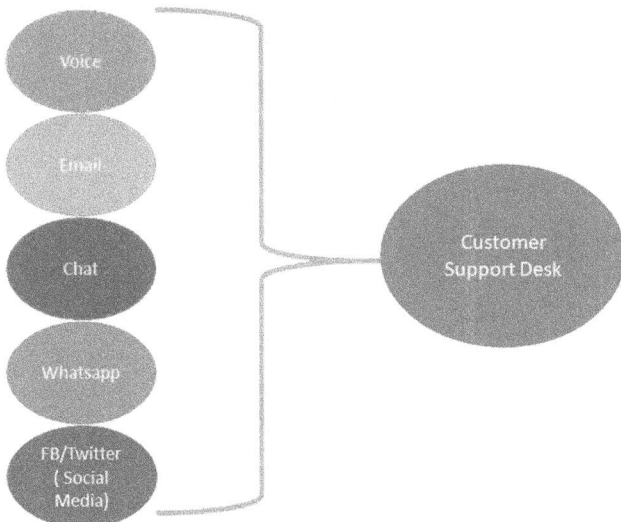

FIGURE 5.6 Commonly used channels for customer interaction.

Customers can use any channel based on their preferences and organizations need to support the majority of the commonly used channels. The choice of the channel by the customers to reach out to the organization is driven the urgency. For example, if it's about renewing the AMC (annual maintenance contract), the customer may prefer an email or webchat but if there is a breakdown or the product has certain issues customer may prefer a voice call to the organization's support desk.

Organizations need to provide excellent customer service at reduced costs, to support multiple channels organization/brands needn't necessarily hire additional agents in their customer service desks as AI can help improve the efficiency of the support desk by incorporating technologies like chatbots which can help answer all the less complex queries from the customer. Chatbots are AI-driven and can open a new ticket, update the customer on the status of an existing ticket and all the other less complex and repetitive tasks can be handled by chatbots. Organizations should also give the option of escalating the call to a human agent so that if the customer feels that they are not getting the right responses from the chatbot the call can be escalated to a human agent to deal with complex issues.

A chatbot that is for text-based chats originating from either the company website, company's app, or on the digital channels (WhatsApp, Facebook messenger, etc.) can be upgraded to a voicebot and can take on voice calls as well. A voicebot can understand the customer's voice and respond in voice. Figure 5.7 explains how voicebots work.

A voicebot converts the voice into text and queries the chatbot engine in text and gets a response in text format which is again converted into speech and played to the caller. The text to speech (TTS) and speech to text is done using the TTS/STT engines.

Upgrading the chatbots with voice functionality will further reduce the number of calls reaching the agent desk as the routine calls can be handled by the voicebots. This will reduce the wait times and improve customer experience. Organizations deploying voicebots should give the option of escalating the call to a human agent if the caller wishes to do so.

When the call does hit the human agents, there are AI tools that help the agents to respond to the call efficiently. For example, agent assist is an AI-enabled program

Cloud Contact next generation digital channels and bot framework

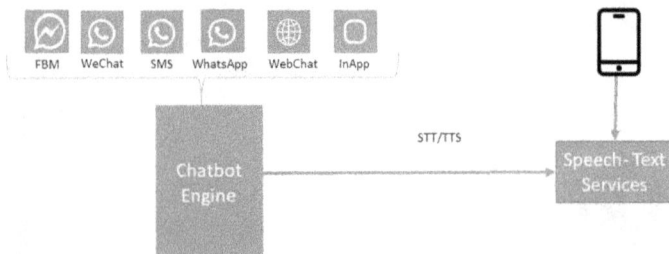

FIGURE 5.7 Voicebot high-level diagram.

that can help the agent respond efficiently based on the context of the call. AI-enabled agent assist helps the customer helpdesk agents to provide better responses to their customers. This also helps lessen the monitoring requirement from the contact center supervisor, improves the accuracy of the response, and also create employee satisfaction as agent's effort is reduced to respond to a complex problem.

AI can also help the agents make better decisions. Let's take the example of a travel desk agent where the customer reaches out to the agent and want to book a group tour. There are four families coming from three different countries and have different arrival and departure needs. It is very difficult for a human agent to plan this trip and book the hotels and tickets and there are multiple variables and the whole planning can take a lot of agents' precious time. If the agent is assisted by an AI-based tool the whole planning can be done in a few seconds and the AI system can recommend the best possible flight and hotel options.

AI can also help understand human emotions online and can advise the agent according to the caller's emotions. Using speech analytics, AI can suggest some responses to the agent in real time by understanding the customer's intent much before the agent can understand it and pop up a message on the agent's deck suggesting the next best action.

Post interaction with the customer, AI can also help in text and speech analytics and suggest guidance to sales and marketing to improve sales. AI is fast in looking for data points across all the customer interactions and suggests improvements in the processes, staffing levels to improve customer satisfaction and bring efficiencies.

5.4.5 LOYALTY

Whatever the organization is trying to do by improving the customer experience to achieve brand loyalty, to try and give customers an experience which customer is thrilled and sticks to the brand.

A positively engaged customer is more likely to remain with the organization. Organizations need to keep the customer engaged and AI can be of great help by doing the following:

i. Proactive engagement with customers – with AI, organizations can send the customers the details of their new products, features, events, etc. to remain connected to the customers.
ii. Personalized Messaging – AI systems can help create personalized messages based on past purchase history, likes, and dislikes. This can be clubbed with offers and discounts for loyal customers.
iii. Brand Loyalty Program – AI can also help in creating customer loyalty programs, whenever a customer buys a product, likes a comment or promotion on social media, shares a products video on social media, make a favorable comment, the AI system can track all these positive behaviors and reward such behavior by offering more loyalty points or discounts for such customers.
iv. Keeping a check on pricing – AI can help organizations keep a check on pricing as pricing is one of the most important criteria in the customers'

minds. Organizations need to keep a check on the pricing of their products in comparison to alternatives and adjust the pricing from time to time. AI can help organizations compare the pricing across all possible alternatives and make suitable recommendations.

It is important to note that a loyal customer will not only buy more from the organization but also promote the products on all platforms including social media platforms.

A disengaged customer is also an opportunity for the organization and AI can help identify such customers who had a less positive experience with the organization. It can also suggest corrective actions. Organizations need to identify the disengaged customer and engage with them early on to improve their experience with the organization and prevent churn.

5.5 CONCLUSION

Across the customer journey, AI has a role to play to provide an excellent customer experience. Figure 5.8 summarizes the technology options which can be used.

During the awareness phases, organizations/brands need to use AI to target the right customers, provide as much information as they can on the organizations' website, get insights into customer preferences based on time spent on the website, and manage social media interactions with customers.

During the consideration phase organization can provide an excellent and personalized online and in-store experience. Instore experience can be digitized using AI to match the same with the online experience. Organization/brands can also incentivize customers to download their app which can provide a superior in-store and online experience.

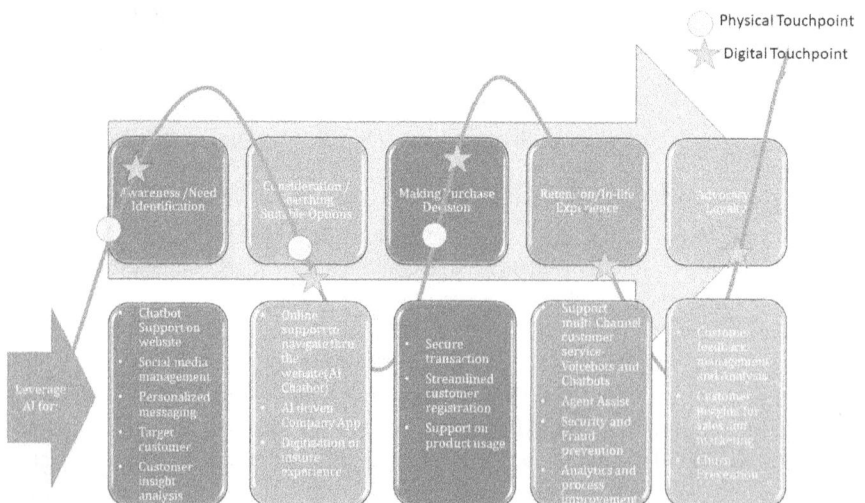

FIGURE 5.8 AI use across customer journey to improve customer experience.

During the purchase phase, the organization can enable AI to provide secure transactions, registering the customers on the company's CRM (Customer Relationship Management) systems which can be fed with intelligent data about customers based on purchase history and engagement with the organization. CRM can also help organizations to send product details like product brochures, manuals, etc. Using AI, customers can be encouraged to engage with the organization both online and offline.

During the retention phase, AI can be leveraged for smarter customer interactions using automation by incorporating chatbots, voicebots, and also enabling the new-age digital channels to support the customer. AI can also be used to enable agents (Customer Support representatives) to serve the customers better by providing real-time assistance and suggesting next best actions. AI can also suggest process improvement to serve the customers better and also analyze the interactions (text and voice) to provide insights into customer pain points and marketing insights.

During the loyalty phases, AI can detect customer's interaction with the organization, keep a check on the purchase history, and suggest new launches and products to the customer based on personalized preferences. AI can also help identify disengaged customers, the pain areas of these customers and suggest corrective actions to engage them better.

In summary, AI can be very useful across the customer journey. Organizations need to implement AI across customer journeys in a manner that its fully integrated end to end to understand the end to end customer experience better. Any siloes across the journey may not be able to provide the full benefits of AI.

5.6   FUTURE OF AI

5.6.1   Future of AI in Customer Experience

AI is being used extensively by organizations for improving the customer experience. The future will see further usage of AI in this area:

i. Pre-emptive Care – More devices will be connected over the internet and sending the health checks to a centralized AI system, which will either resolve the problem or raise the alarms for human intervention. This means lower downtime of devices.

ii. Voice-based virtual agents – though it's in the initial stages now and we don't see much voice-based virtual agents this seems highly likely that AI-based virtual agent which can behave exactly like human agents take the customer experience to the next level.

iii. Video-based contact center – we haven't seen massive adoption of video-based contact centers but with 5G connectivity around the corner, we can expect video-based contact centers for specific sectors like Banking and Healthcare. These video contact centers will have the security aspects taken care of by AI-based systems.

iv. 24 × 7 Support – with AI-based chatbots, voicebots, virtual agents, etc., customers will get 24 × 7 support even for complex issues.

5.6.2   FUTURE OF AI ACROSS VERTICALS

There is probably no industry untouched by AI. As we go to the future the use is AI in everyday life is likely to increase. Let's take the example of a few industries and how AI may bring in the transformation:

   i. Healthcare – AI can look into multiple data points across millions of patients and help physicians prescribe drugs that can provide better results. AI and robotics may be able to take a blood sample from patients, evaluate the results, and prescribe medicines.
   ii. Manufacturing – AI will bring more robotics to manufacturing. Humans may be doing more skilled jobs and all the repetitive jobs will be done by AI-powered robots.
   iii. Transport – Increase in the number of autonomous vehicles on the road.
   iv. Education – Online education with AI-powered facial recognition to understand if students can understand the concepts, getting bored, not interested, etc.
   v. Security – You will see more and more governments deploying technologies like facial recognition to make their countries secure.

REFERENCES

Adobe, 2020a, Experience Index 2020 Digital Trends.
Adobe, 2020b, https://www.adobe.com/content/dam/www/us/en/offer/digital-trends-2020/digital-trends-2020-full-report.pdf [accessed 17 April 2020].
BT Telecommunications Plc (BT), 2020a, The Autonomous Customer.
BT, 2020b, https://www.globalservices.bt.com/content/dam/globalservices/images/downloads/whitepapers/The-Autonomous-Customer-30012020-final.pdf [accessed 15 April 2020].

6 Artificial Intelligence in Radiotherapy

C. S. Sureka

Assistant Professor & Head (i/c), Department of Medical Physics, Bharathiar University, Coimbatore, India

CONTENTS

OBJECTIVES

1. Learn the importance of artificial intelligence (AI) in radiotherapy (RT) to make it a boon to society.
2. Understand various aspects of AI in RT and aware of the threats associated with it.
3. Explore the potential of AI and radiomics during treatment delivery, dosimetry, quality assurance, radiation biology, and safety.
4. Create awareness of the ongoing technological advancements in RT among radiation oncologists, medical physicists, and other radiation professionals.
5. Encourage researchers and students to focus on an appropriate, safe, economic, and efficient mode of RT to enhance the clinical outcome and prepare them for Industry 5.0 as well.

6.1   INTRODUCTION

Radiotherapy (RT) is considered to be an effective modality to treat 48.3% of the cancer patients with all types of cancer using RT alone or in combination with surgery or chemotherapy. Even though it is a life-saving technology, it is not accessible to all people who are in different geographical regions, below the poverty line, etc. The field of RT has been developed enormously over a century. It uses ionizing radiations such as photons (X and gamma rays), electrons, protons, etc. to kill tumor cells by protecting surrounding normal structures. It is broadly classified into (i) external beam radiotherapy (EBRT) or teletherapy, where the source of radiation is located a specific distance from the patient, and (ii) brachytherapy, where the radioactive substance is kept close to the patient inside the tumor.

EBRT has witnessed continuous developments by the introduction of various techniques starts from telecobalt machine, and conventional medical linear accelerator-based treatment into 3D conformal RT, Intensity Modulated Radiotherapy (IMRT), Volumetric Modulated Arc Therapy (VMAT), Image-Guided Radiotherapy (IGRT), Stereotactic Radiosurgery (SRS), Stereotactic Radiotherapy (SRT), Stereotactic Body Radiotherapy (SBRT), Cyberknife based treatment, proton therapy, etc. In brachytherapy, various techniques are depending upon the location of the tumor-like intracavitary, intraluminal, interstitial, intraoperative, intravascular, and surface mold. Also, radiation dosimetry that deals with the quantification of radiation using various detectors, radiation biology that describes the biological effects of radiation, quality assurance procedures that ensure the RT procedures, and radiation safety have welcomed enormous advancements.

With the advent of RT, executing an appropriate technology with limited time, budget, and high clinical outcomes would be a challenging task for radiation oncologists and medical physicists. Artificial intelligence (AI) is evolving as the most popular technology in academics, medical institutions, and industry in this digital era of the fourth industrial revolution. Therefore, the future of RT should be the introduction of AI into clinical practice and hence this chapter discusses the importance and developments of AI at various processes of RT based on the information collected from articles published by researchers.

6.2 IMPORTANCE OF ARTIFICIAL INTELLIGENCE (AI) IN RADIOTHERAPY

AI systems can assist and enhance the competence of RT workflow through the developments in ML algorithms. Generally, the RT workflow consists of many steps, as given in Figure 6.1.

Immobilization: Desired immobilization devices are designed to avoid the movement of patients during the treatment. Image acquisition: The most commonly used modality for image acquisition is CT since the algorithms for dose calculation require electronic density data. Even though MRI has excellent features for soft tissue imaging, it is not possible to transfer CT data to MRI and PET CT data to PET MRI due to electron density dependency of CT to correct attenuation. To provide a suitable solution to this problem, various methods like learning methods, sparse coding methods, atlas methods, etc., have been developed to utilize the data acquired from MRI to make a CT. This is termed synthetic CT or sCT. Out of these methods for sCT, a type of AI method namely deep embedding convolutional neural network (DECNN) can produce images of higher resolution with lesser artifacts in a lesser time and more efficiently. Hence, AI-based methods have high potential in the future to generate sCT from MRI data with limited electron density information to generate a treatment plan. The sCT can also be applied in the image segmentation process with lesser error because sCT data can be fused accurately and easily with MRI data.

Image segmentation: Image segmentation and contouring is an important step in RT planning. But, it is a time-consuming process and depends on the expertise of the radiation oncologist and medical physicist. Based on this, auto segmentation algorithms have been developed to increase the speed of the process and to reduce inter-expert variability. There are many algorithms and approaches available for auto segmentation. Originally, they applied to contour OAR that can be identified by tissue density. Then, auto-contouring methods were merged with atlas to contour normal tissues three-dimensionally. Recently, AI-based ML and DL methods like deep dilated convolutional neural networks (DDCNN) are in widespread use to perform many tasks. Researchers confirmed that DL methods have performed better than manual contouring with auto segmentation for the esophagus and spinal cord by consuming 79% of the lesser time and reducing Intra and inter-observer changeability. Still, it requires further improvements to make it suitable for all cases.

To measure the segmentation accuracy and consistency of an algorithm, the Dice similarity coefficient (DSC) was used. Even though, DDCNN can contour many

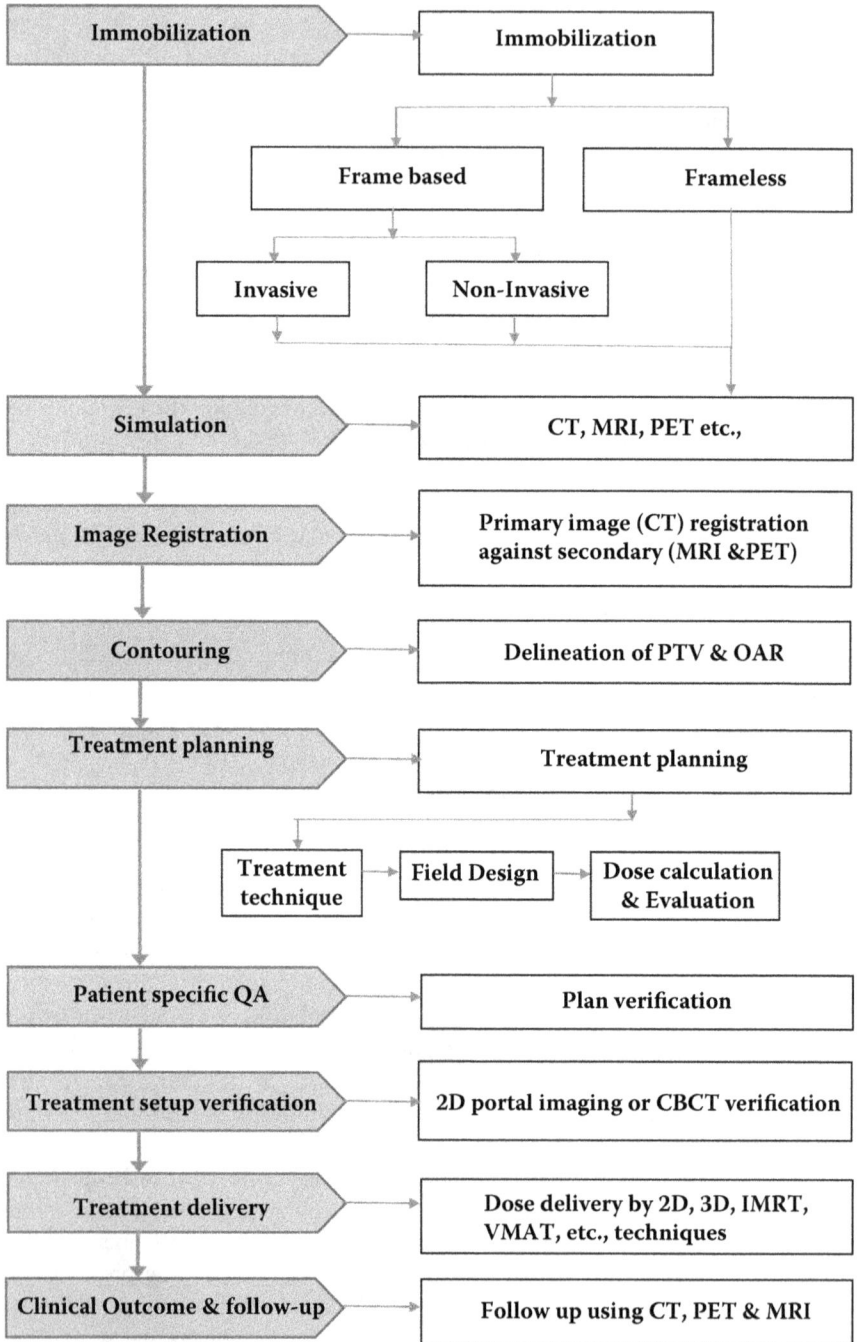

FIGURE 6.1   Radiotherapy workflow.

organs such as CTV, bladder, left and right femoral heads, colon and intestine with high DSC value and low test time, it shows high uncertainties while segmenting structures like submandibular glands, optic chiasm, etc. Due to the continuous research activities on AI-based tools like CNN, the auto segmentation quality will be improved in the future by incorporating more number of high quality and less variable data as input to train the algorithms. Also, the anatomical knowledge and experience of the users are necessary to monitor the outcome of the algorithm. Despite many developments in AI, technology can only assist the users in the contouring process of RT.

Image registration: The next step of RT workflow is to spatially align multiple images of the same scene acquired at different viewpoints and times concerning an image. This process is termed *image registration.* It uses a mathematical transformation to align an image with the reference image. Even though, there are many registration methods available commercially, rigid techniques and intensity-based methods are commonly used in RT. Based on a survey, researchers confirmed that DL-based image registration techniques will make the image registration process more user-friendly and easier than the earlier one.

Treatment planning: It is a tedious process of optimizing dosimetric objectives using computer-based algorithms before delivering radiation to patients. It is a time-consuming and laborious step that involves a trial and error concept. AI technology has been progressed to get more efficient and rapid planning process as given below:

1. Voxel-based dose prediction and dose mimicking methods were used to plan head and neck RT.
2. ML methods and multi-patient atlas selection were applied to calculate dose distributions per voxel to generate automated RT planning.
3. AI-based methods have been applied with maximum accuracy in the shortest time because of their rapid auto segmentation and image registration process to make it suitable for adaptive RT planning.
4. Knowledge-based ML algorithms have been used to generate a dose-volume histogram (DVH) of a given plan with a provision to perform inverse planning in less time.
5. AI algorithms can include patient-specific parameters such as sex, age, geographical variations, genetic makeup, etc., in addition to the ability of conventional algorithms.
6. Another development of AI in RT is personalizing the dose delivery to a patient by incorporating dosimetric, clinical, and biological information of the patient and accessing the treatment outcome. It will enhance tumor control and minimize the toxicity of the treatment.
7. In the future, AI technology can select the patient who can be benefited from RT or exclude the unsuitable patient by measuring the radio-sensitivity of the tumor based on radio genomic assays like PORTOS.

RT dose optimization is a part of the treatment planning procedure where AI-based approaches have incorporated hundreds of prior plans of multiple diseases to improve the efficiency and reproducibility of a plan. Records show that this approach can save approximately 80% of the time and can be applied in multiple clinical conditions that include SBRT planning, DVH data analysis, etc. However, AI-based planning is not completely automated now as it needs expert's supervision to ensure the treatment plan.

Beam delivery methods: While delivering the planned dose throughout the full course of treatment, complications associated with patient movement and biological movement of the tumor and internal organs within a fraction and in between fractions became a challengeable task. However, AI-based techniques can decrease the uncertainty related to patient motion. Researchers have demonstrated a soft-robot actuator to treat head and neck cancers without any immobilization device that uses a position-sensitive soft robot to consider the movement of a patient. The uncertainty that arises due to internal tumor motion can also be tracked with the support of AI. There is a time lag in conventional techniques that is caused by a delay in recording the movement and correcting it. This time lag can be avoided by AI-based tumor tracking systems where various breathing patterns and breathing cycles of many patients are incorporated. Intra and inter-fraction fuzzy deep learning (IIFDL) algorithms have been developed to predict intra- and inter-fractional variation by incorporating breath pattern data with lesser computation time in the order of 1 to 2 ms.

Quality assurance (QA): Generally, advanced RT QA workflow requires a complete evaluation of the treatment plan of every patient without expecting any result. Now a day, AI-based techniques have been implemented to predict the passing rate of the advanced QA procedures, to predict error in image-guided modalities, and to assess the performance of Linac. Although AI algorithms have been applied for preventive maintenance of machine data, they may help to avoid technical failures and reduce machine downtime. Therefore, they can enhance the work efficiency of the department and worker's satisfaction even though they add additional cost for the algorithm. However, additional quality assurance procedures for the inherent AI-based algorithms and processes should also be performed periodically.

Clinical decision support and prediction of treatment outcome: It has been evolved as another area of interest to apply the power of AI with the principle of using the available treatment and outcome-based data and models to give efficient and timely recommendations and directions. A few of its benefits are: (1) to assist radiation oncologists to inform their decision to the patient about his/her treatment modality, schedule, basic dosimetric information, etc., (2) integrate dosimetric data with diagnostic imaging, genomic, and other medical data to build an outcome-based model, and (3) radiomics data will be used in the future to predict the risks associated with the treatment before initiating it. However, its accuracy and scope are limited because of the lack of outcome data of curative treatments, data sharing among institutions, and standardized processes. Therefore, many approaches such as OncoSpace, EuroCAT, MAASTRO, LAMBDA-RAD, and models such as ontologies, HL7-FHIR, etc., are in the process of getting acceptance (Reid et al., 2018).

6.3   AI TOOLS FOR AUTOMATED TREATMENT PLANNING (ATP)

As discussed in the previous section, many AI algorithms have been progressed to improve the efficiency of the treatment planning system (TPS), for ATP, and for optimizing the dosimetry. In addition to the automatic nature of ATP systems, ATP can also reduce treatment planning time, error, and enhance the plan's consistency and efficiency. This section discusses the most commonly used AI tools for ATP, AI applications and advancements in ATP, AI challenges and research guidance in ATP, and collaboration and regulations to implement AI in clinics (Chunhao et al., 2019).

6.3.1   PRESENT ATP TECHNIQUES

Based on the effect of RT workflow in clinical practice, the present ATP techniques are classified into three categories. They are (1) Auto Rule Implementation and Reasoning (ARIR), (2) simulation of previous knowledge into clinics, and (3) Multi-Criteria Optimization (MCO).

Generally, basic TPS parameters are implemented based on the guidelines and rules of individual institutions and expertise of the medical physicists which are simple adjustments. But, the reasoning of the TPS process needs more knowledge and complexity too but that can be simulated by binary logics like "if-then." Therefore, the ARIR technique can be used to reduce the need for manpower involvement to generate a plan most commonly while performing repeated procedures. Vendors of various TPS have brought ARIR based solutions for scripting functions based on the input given by the user. These special functions can enable users to develop automatic programs as per their clinical need and research includes beam setup, dose calculation, DVH optimization, etc. Many researchers have been analyzing the automation capability of the ARIR technique in IMRT and VMAT treatment planning developed by various vendors. Recently, the ARIR technique has also been used with ML algorithms in the case of pelvis and breast TPS.

An approach of simulating previous knowledge of similar good cases can naturally enhance the efficiency of manual planning. That is, parameters in earlier cases such as beam alignment, and DVH components are inserted into the treatment planning procedure or considered as reference parameters to decide for a present case. Based on this, scientists have introduced statistical models to find important features from previous high-quality cases using knowledge and clinical decision. When using those features as input, those models can improve the efficiency of the treatment planning. This approach is called knowledge-based planning (KBP). Many analyses have been performed with DVH based KBP as they improve the quality of the plan. Recently, Varian has developed the DVH-based KBP as Rapidplan in Eclipse TPS. However, its usage is limited due to deficiency of spatial data, and the complexity in dealing with rare OARs and targets.

In the case of inverse planning optimization using DVH, a cost function is generally determined to reduce the problem in the planning process. This function represents the data collected from all regions of interest as a single dosimetrically weighted total of the penalty. Then, the compromise between the OARs and targets are marked by a coefficient of dosimetric criterion. If the preference of the user is modified in terms of its dosimetric parameters while evaluating the plan, then the original plan needs to be optimized once again which limits the usage of DVH-based approach. However, its alternative approach would be a time-consuming one. Therefore, MCO was introduced in the inverse planning procedure that will generate multiple model plans at a time for evaluation. Here, each plan is optimized as per a single DVH parameter for maximum sparing of normal structures without compromising the dose to the target. If the user modifies the dose distribution, the corresponding plan will be generated immediately without optimizing the plan once again. The MCO based approach is available in RayStation TPS and Eclipse TPS.

6.3.2 AI APPLICATIONS, ADVANCEMENTS, AND RESEARCH GUIDANCE IN ATP

ATP along with a potential AI tool will be an efficient and effective system in the future with less manpower. A few of the AI applications in ATP are as follows:

1. AI tools can be instrumental to perform all reasoning logics and manual procedures in RT by incorporating the complete anatomical details of the patient.
2. AI can decide the RT parameters such as dose prescription, beam delivery, etc. instead of a medical physicist.
3. The implementation of AI in routine clinical practice will reduce the number of manpower and hence the saved manpower can be utilized to perform other tasks that require human involvement.

A few of the AI advancements in ATP are as follows:

1. KBP approach in ATP was developed very long back. Recently, researchers demonstrated its clinical applicability in IMRT to treat prostate cancer using two different algorithms namely weighted K-nearest neighbor and multi-nomial logistic regression algorithm and it is confirmed that both of them perform well.
2. Researchers confirmed that the KBP approach with the support vector regression model is more suitable for rectum and bladder DVH prediction than the RapidPlan model.
3. When the 3D dose distribution of a plan is predicted accurately, it will improve the quality and efficiency of manual TPS and can simplify the decision-making process. Also, it can be utilized to make the ATP workflow completely automatic without plan optimization. Researchers developed AI-based models such as the ANN-based dose model and U-net to predict the 3D dose distribution in advanced modalities (SBRT, IMRT, etc.) accurately. Fully convolutional neural network-based models such as DoseNet, DenseNet, and ResNet were also introduced to predict 3D dose distribution with lesser network redundancy.
4. U-net models were introduced to perform the image segmentation process by maintaining the original dimension of the image that can avoid the feature

extraction process and reduce the need for data interpretation while performing the KBP process.

5. The success of 3D dose distribution prediction is converting its parameters into a real treatment plan to make it a deliverable plan. Researchers proposed various frameworks such as KBP workflow and ResNet-based framework for auto planning to generate an actual plan.

A few of the research guides for effective implementation of AI in ATP are as follows:

1. As discussed in the previous chapter, the developments in deep CNN-based algorithms are potential research areas for AI-based applications in medical imaging. In parallel to this research, investigation to improve the efficiency and accuracy of 3D dose prediction is a potential area of focus in the future. Therefore, DVH-based plan optimization may be replaced by a plan generation algorithm through image reconstruction when the predicted 3D dose data is considered as reference data.

2. Another interesting area of research is predicting the RT plan parameters directly to generate plans automatically. It may be possible by using CNN-based algorithms to predict the dose parameters like 2D fluence data and convert them into equivalent images.

3. More focus on the decision-making approach may enable the researchers to implement the fully automatic ATP workflow into routine clinical practice without human involvement.

4. Human reasoning approaches can be simulated by implementing reinforcement learning from an easy case with a lesser number of cases and extend the same to the complete ATP workflow on large scale.

5. AI-based Generative Adversarial Network (GAN) algorithms have already been implemented for diagnosis, image segmentation and to predict 3D dose distribution in RT. GAN can be investigated in the future to model the treatment planning decision-making process.

6.3.3 AI CHALLENGES IN ATP

The major problem with the current RT planning process is its complexity since each step of its plan generation needs to be assessed after the dose calculation process is completed. Therefore, the ATP workflow modeling became expensive on simulation aspects when compared to other applications. However, its computational cost and complexity can be reduced when the decision-making processes are simplified by incorporating basic rules in ATP workflow. This is also possible by integrating the basic rules followed in the manual treatment planning process such as clinical preference, institutional guidance, etc., using simple logics (e.g., If-else), related variables, or physical concepts like the effect of built up regions. Also, these challenges can be nullified by the team efforts of oncology personnel and researchers.

ATP applications became a challengeable task because of limited data set caused by lesser patient involvement, variation in data acquisition, heterogeneous imaging data, insufficient infrastructure, etc. It triggers the need for separating each data set into three subsets namely test data, validation data, and training data. The test data set is used to test the performance of the model that was trained using validation and training data sets. However, this three-part data method may also critical when we use it for highly complex AI methods. Also, the KBP-approach-based ATP algorithms shows low performance in more complex and advanced cases due to overfitting and simulation error associated with small sample size.

Such issues associated with limited sample size can be handled by various approaches such as transfer learning, data augmentation, and the addition of features into model learning. The transfer learning approach creates a model algorithm using small data sets to adjust a model that was trained by big data sets from a different application. The data augmentation approach increases the number of data sets by adding a modified form of its original data. In the third approach, a model learning that incorporated the features selected from previous cases is considered as representative statistics where extra operations can be included to remove overfitting. Unfortunately, this approach can be successfully executed by users with sufficient computational skill to handle AI algorithms. Hence, this area requires further research towards the development and adaptation of new methods to tackle the issues related to small data size.

To introduce the AI-based ATP techniques into regular clinical applications, it is essential to validate them in terms of their efficiency and quality. Despite that, medical physicists should play a major role to follow the RT workflow to ensure the quality and safety of a plan. To validate and generalize the AI techniques successfully, they require more number of patients in each group of disease, data types, imaging modalities, RT plan, clinical results, etc. It can be achieved in the future through collaboration among institutions by making guidelines for the RT plan generation.

Professional associations, committees, and vendors have already made efforts over the last decade to strengthen research on RT big data analysis by expecting more number of plans that are generated based on recent guidelines. Also, the number of recent plans can be increased by using the current ATP techniques in clinics that will enable future research activities. Since every step of the RT workflow needs manpower involvement to ensure its safety and accuracy, open-access software can be used to demonstrate the suitability of the novel AI techniques in ATP. When it is validated for clinical implementation, a suitable platform with vendor-specific parameters for automation needs to be incorporated. Under this situation, issues associated with intellectual property rights (IPR), data security, and quality assurance procedure development may be handled carefully by developing an industry model- academy collaboration to bring a new paradigm in RT treatment planning.

6.4   AI IN INTENSITY MODULATED RADIOTHERAPY (IMRT)

ANNs have been developed to overcome the challenges associated with image classification using CNNs and image segmentation using dilated CNNs (DCNNs). These AI-based models were originally established to perform non-medical activities like credit card fraud detection, label products, etc. Recently, these models have been used to solve the issues related to IMRT H&D treatment planning processes such as auto segmentation, dose estimation, ATP, decision making, and outcome prediction. This section deals with AI applications in various steps of IMRT for H&N cases (Georgios et al., 2011; Vasant et al., 2018).

6.4.1   AI FOR IMRT DOSE ESTIMATION

H&N IMRT planning requires experienced medical physicists to plan the treatment and it is a time-consuming process as well. They should have enough knowledge about the general 3D dose distribution/volumetric dose of any case as it is an important part of the workflow. Because it can estimate the dose received by the patients so that guides to correct the treatment plan. Presently, there are four techniques to estimate the 3D dose distribution in IMRT for H&N cases. They are:

1. Deformation-atlas dose estimation: Generally, automatic H&N treatment planning models use the data collected from previous cases to estimate the 3D dose distribution for new cases. One possible way to accomplish it is by reconstructing images and gathering volumetric information of target and OARs. However, AI-based techniques reduce the volume of information from the input subset and use alternative structured data. For example, the regression forests model is supported with density prediction among the various features to choose the most suitable plan among the past plans from the plan library. Therefore, the prior dose will be selected for the new case. Among various models available for dose estimation, the atlas-based models are the first ML-based model that can support medical physicists to generate a new plan using previous plan data. It has three sub-processes: (a) reducing the number of image data and contour data into the input data sets, (b) relating those input data sets to a matching patient by the model, and (c) adjust the dose distribution of the matched previous case suitable for the new case through image registration. Hence, the accuracy of this model depends on the errors encountered in each process.
2. Probabilistic-atlas dose estimation: Generally, ATP converts the dose estimated/voxel into a full-fledged dose distribution of a given IMRT plan. Atlas-based regression forest (ARF) model can simulate the correlation between the 3D dose distribution per unit voxel and image features of a given case such as the geometry of the patient, shape of the region of interest, and appearance of the image. Another model was developed to choose the most appropriate ARF model to plan a new case based on the number of image features used. If less number of image features are used to plan a new plan then that ARF model will be considered as the best one. It was aimed to simulate an expert's view on images of a new plan, choose a similar case from the library of cases, and reproduce the dose distribution of the selected plan into the new plan.
3. Fully connected neural network-based dose estimation: Researchers found an alternative to the previous atlas-based models by directly estimating the dose by studying a series of classified features using ANNs. This model can help in

IMRT planning using a semi-unstructured technique. Even though they are multipurpose, suitable for most of the planning processes, easily trainable, their performance is affected by overfitting and more memory requirement.

4. CNN-based dose estimation: CNN-based dose estimation technique has been demonstrated as a substitute for the fully connected ANN technique to estimate the dose distribution volumetrically. Generally, there are two types of CNN models: Tiramisu models and DCNNs. Tiramisu models (e.g., U-net) use a convolution approach for down-sampling during the encoding process to study the series of features and then a de-convolution approach for up-sampling during the decoding process to restore the input data. DCNN models use a convolution approach to reduce the number of features during the encoding process and in turn, enlarge the field of coverage. However, they are complex, not easily trainable, and need advanced hardware facilities.

6.4.2 AI FOR IMRT PLANNING SUPPORT

To reproduce dosimetry, to provide planning support, and to reduce the issues in ATP, many AI-based algorithms have been developed. Out of which, a few of them are discussed here in the following two aspects.

1. Reproducing dosimetry: Many models have been proposed to reproduce the dosimetric aspects of a planning process in IMRT. In one of the models, an additional program constructed on a commercial TPS to select the suitable planning parameters from the plan library and generate an efficient plan. It contains three parts that include a commercial TPS, a library of previous plans, and a separate module for optimization by reproducing the routine dosimetric concepts.
2. Optimization of planning parameters in TPS: Few more models have been developed that use a separate algorithm to find relevant objective specific parameters to decrease workload by ATP. One such technique is the optimization of control parameters such as the threshold dose of various organs and geometry of the beam. Many researchers confirmed that a similar plan can be generated by using DVH as the main function for optimization. These approaches can perform many planning processes automatically.

6.4.3 AI FOR MODELING IMRT OUTCOME AND PLAN DELIVERABILITY

As discussed earlier, many AI-based models are available to analyze the modeling efficiency of TCP, NTCP, and deliverability of a plan. Those models that predict the treatment outcome have a high potential to support decision making, to select a treatment method, and to optimize a plan as well. A few of the AI-based models that are used to model the treatment outcome and deliverability of a plan on three aspects are as follows:

1. Model for TCP prediction in IMRT: The present radiobiological models that are used for TCP prediction are rigid as they have many mathematical

structures so that AI-based models are preferred to overcome the shortcomings. Generally, TCP is formatted with a Gompertzian function that corresponds to TCP parameters and dose that includes TCD50 and the slope of the TCP curve. It gives a rough idea about the radiosensitivity of different types of tumors. When non-dosimetric parameters are integrated into these multivariable models, estimation of possible interactions would be a challengeable task. Therefore, many genomic biomarkers have been demonstrated recently to estimate the RT response but they are not yet used for H&N cases. So that the combined effect of ML models and genomic profiling may explain new interaction among the characteristics of the tumor, dosimetry, and tumor microenvironment with the patient. For example, a combination of the Cox-Proportional Hazard (CoxPH) model with a Kaplan-Meier (KM) model. Also, radiomics will play a major role to design models for TCP prediction that is discussed here in the later section.

2. Model for NTCP prediction in IMRT: Due to the toxicity of IMRT of H&N, the patient may get mucositis (ulceration and inflammation in the mucous membrane) that results in acute pain, dysphagia, and finally spoils the quality of patient's life. If the patient gets mucositis during the treatment, it may break the conventional treatment which compromises the normal tissue complication that can be achieved by IMRT generally. Therefore, researchers developed ML-based models using forest classifiers with the capability of accurately predicting the mucositis by analyzing the spatial dose distribution, dose-volume, and examination data of the IMRT treatment.

Similarly, IMRT of H&N can also cause xerostomia (dry mouth caused by a malfunction in the salivary gland) and increases the acidity of the surrounding region, and in turn affect the quality of the patient's life. To predict the xerostomia and its related toxicity, researchers have recently developed ML-based models using a multivariate logistic regression approach with input variables derived from dosimetric and clinical data like mean OAR dose. It is also demonstrated that non-dosimetric variables such as age, education, economical condition, and tumor stage can also estimate the IMRT treatment-induced xerostomia.

1. Model for Quality assurance in IMRT: Generally, H&N planning in IMRT is complex when compared to other cases that increases the chances of failure in patient-specific QA. It may be one of the reasons to postpone the treatment and increases the clinical burden. Based on these, researchers developed many ML-based models to estimate the failure rate of IMRT patient-specific QA for H&B cases. A few of them are as follows:
   a. A virtual algorithm for IMRT QA that utilizes cross-institutionally evaluated generalized additive methodology to estimate the passing rate of QA procedures. This approach uses a series of features designed by experts to measure the deviation between the planned and delivered systems and then predict the failure rate using ML-based algorithms. The study results showed that the failure rate of IMRT H&N QA procedures is

higher than in other cases. However, this algorithm also shows high institutional dependency.

b. A CNN-based model to estimate the failure rate of IMRT QA from the dose distribution of the plan without any special features. Since its performance is not better than the previous model, a combination CNN model and the previous model with expert-designed features can improve its predictive accuracy. However, a CNN-based algorithm can perform inter-institutional analysis well.

c. Another ML-based algorithm that uses SVMs can predict what are the N&N cases require re-planning. However, all these algorithms are under the developmental stage. If it is implemented successfully, it can enhance treatment efficacy and clinical outcome.

6.4.4 AI FOR AUTO-SEGMENTATION OF OAR IN IMRT

Segmentation of OARs and targets by manual processes affect the IMRT delivery due to high uncertainty and inconsistency in contouring associated with a broad margin. Generally, NTCP-based models depend on OAR segmentation and hence its accuracy highly depends on the contouring precision. To reduce those issues associated with manual contouring, models for auto segmentation have been introduced. The two forms of auto segmentation models are as follows:

1. Atlas-based auto segmentation (ABAS): ABAS models create new contour sets to choose a similar patient using a library of model atlas of prior images and contours by image registration process despite many variations. Following this, voxels that are anatomically similar in both of the CT images are registered deformably. Then, the prior contours are transferred onto the new plan using that deformation vector. Even though ABAS has been implemented clinically, it is affected by image artifacts, noise, and low tissue contrast. However, it can be further improved by enhancing the accuracy of the image registration process.
2. Auto segmentation using CNN: Many of the approaches of CNN-based image segmentation models have solved the issues associated with IMRT H&N segmentation. They have a good learning environment since they receive feedback from more images, however it is under the developmental stage.

6.4.5 FUTURE DIRECTIONS

1. The developments of AI in the IMRT planning process lead to many developments as discussed earlier. Since most of the models were developed independently, the organization of these models altogether to perform multiple tasks would be a potential area in the future. For example, a model that performs contouring, dosimetry, and plan optimization can efficiently model plan prediction, plan deliverability, and patient outcomes.

2. Since the AI-based models need a large number of good quality data, collaboration among institutions should be developed to enhance the performance of those algorithms. Therefore, distributed learning practice is recommended to face challenges associated with data aggregation among institutions.
3. Most of the AI-based models are under the developmental stage. Therefore, extended educational and training activities along with clinical professionals are recommended.
4. Efficient AI-based algorithms may be developed to train users to understand the mechanisms behind the decision-making process of various algorithms.
5. It is well accepted that AI will make the future of IMRT bright by providing economic and high-quality patient care.

6.5 AI IN BRACHYTHERAPY

AI techniques have not been studied much in brachytherapy. Recently, ANN-based models have been demonstrated in image-guided brachytherapy to correct dose modification at OARs during the gynecological treatment. It was aimed to change the final brachytherapy plan to correct anatomical changes on OARs and variation in applicator position by keeping the same dose distribution. In this study, treatment plans of 30 cervical cancer patients, each received around 50 Gy dose over 5 weeks in teletherapy and suitable for intracavitary brachytherapy were chosen. ANN methods were used to estimate the variation in DVH during the treatment and help the professional to generate a good plan.

Generally, it is a completed process and very difficult to solve by conventional analytical approaches as it is an inverse issue in the brachytherapy plan. Also, the problem characteristics are such a way that the data size is high and there is no prior data and knowledge that relates the variation in organ position and dose. Hence, analytical methods cannot solve it so that ANN-based models were used to solve the inverse issue. Here, a network of radial basis functions (RBF) and multilayer perceptron (MLP) was validated to confirm their ability to predict an outcome (Ramin et al., 2017).

6.6 AI IN RADIOTHERAPY QUALITY ASSURANCE

The recent developments in AI techniques result in many promising steps in the quality assurance (QA) of RT. Generally, treatment plan assessment and QA include contouring OARs and targets, field collimation and arrangement, dose uniformity inside the target, and sparing of normal tissues. But, these procedures became complex due to advancements in radiation technology and also a challenging task in institutions having limited staff since they are reviewed manually using checklists and charts. Also, the manual review may lead to errors that necessitate the implementation of AI methods to automate its processes, reduce complexities using simple rules, and include provision for individualized assessment. Therefore, the quality of the plan, treatment planning time, advanced dosimetry, safety procedures, and the development of new QA procedures will be improved (Alan et al., 2019).

6.6.1 DEVELOPMENTS IN ML TOWARDS QUALITY ASSURANCE

Various aspects of RT QA procedures were developed to identify the best algorithm to perform all the QA procedures. A few of them are as follows:

1. A system to estimate the Linac performance over a long period.
2. An AI-based application to estimate the passing rate of IMRT QA procedures and for automatic problem identification with the support of imaging systems.
3. An approach to estimate MLC positional errors and to estimate the QA data abnormalities.
4. A tool to measure the quality control value to detect outliers automatically.
5. Algorithm to estimate the deviation of a final plan from its original goal to find the requirement for re-planning.

It is important to mention that all of the above developments are under research level and not yet implemented for routine clinical applications.

6.6.2 APPLICATIONS OF ML MODELS FOR QUALITY ASSURANCE IN RADIOTHERAPY

A few examples to explain how AI techniques are applied to perform QA in RT are as follows:

1. ATP validation: ATP validation is a complicated task that involves support from clinicians, upgradation from computer professionals, findings of the users, and validation of the results in all the steps of RT workflow. Its main objective is to measure errors and find the suitability of the plan. The error may be caused by a communication gap between the oncologist and the medical physicist, and diversion from the standard practice of the institution due to the participation of the patient in a clinical trial, incorporation of oncologist's literature knowledge to make a decision, medical history of the patient, patient's opinion about the associated risk, etc. However, most of these errors can be easily managed by various approaches such as rule-based methods, Random Forest approach, Bayesian network (BN), etc. Even though rule-based methods perform well, they also have limitations like lack of capacity to do grey area measurement, efficiency, and adaptability. The Random Forest approach can be used to analyze the contours on an image, to classify the region of interest, and use that information in the algorithm to detect the errors in the contours automatically. As it is a probabilistic approach, all the regions are not shown explicitly. BN model can transparently handle the probabilistic events and is considered the best option. Also, AI-based BN

models can mimic the reasoning process of a human to find the suitability of the plan.

2. Knowledge-based planning (KBP): Inverse treatment planning needs a large number of objective functions to indicate dosimetric objectives and each function is specified by relevant parameters. Generally, the TPS algorithm optimizes those functions to perform a process. If the quantity of variables is high, users can not analyze the images and find those functional parameters to achieve the clinical objectives of a treatment plan. Fortunately, KBP can make such a planning process easy by giving a preliminary knowledge of original plans as a reference to compare the current plan. These algorithms were developed to reduce plan complexity and develop novel planning techniques. KBP algorithms have already been implemented in Varian Rapidplan. Many approaches to plan generation and evaluation were demonstrated based on the knowledge collected from internal data and criteria of an institution. If the knowledge base of as many as possible experienced institutions is incorporated into the algorithm, the quality of the plan will be improved. Further, automatic KBP is encouraged to upgrade the planning process automatically in response to physiological changes that occurred during treatment. As mentioned earlier, various ML algorithms have been developed for personalized treatment as well. Therefore, it is recommended to take efforts to enhance the efficiency and confidence of the knowledge-based automatic planning process in the future.

3. To perform dosimetry-related quality assurance: ML-based algorithms can enhance the dosimetric procedures on two aspects. The first aspect is to develop models based on ML to estimate long term procedures like IMRT QA. Accordingly, various models such as regression algorithms, CNN-based models, etc. were developed recently. Regression algorithms can reduce the time required for plan measurement when the plan has more chance to be failed through multi-institutional validation. However, CNN based models don't need extra domain knowledge. The second aspect is to develop ML-based models by using the data collected from routine QA measurements and machine performance. The presently available software in TPS is also collecting data regarding machine failure and its performance rate to prepare a chart of machine repair and maintenance. It will enable the model to predict the issues associated with machine performance and induce the user to take preventive measures without wasting time. Regarding proton therapy, there are very few ML-based techniques to validate its dosimetric procedures which create an opportunity for future development.

6.6.3 QUALITY ASSURANCE OF ML ALGORITHMS IN RADIOTHERAPY

QA of ML algorithms is an unsolved and interesting issue. When the data sources are increased and new ML algorithms are developed, the process of evaluating those models have also been grown correspondingly. To evaluate a model few basic principles should be followed that include the requirement of checking and validating the algorithms. Generally, three data sets are used during the model learning phase, testing phase, and validation phase which are from different sources/institutions. If there are no outside data sets or matching data sets, the user must perform all the processes using homogeneous data. But, it increases the risk of an unprecedented effect on its outcome since many variables may not be denoted explicitly. Under the extreme situation, "leave-one data-out" tactics can be adopted where the model is built by leaving one data and its performance is checked with the remaining data points. This process is carried out multiple times by leaving a different data point every time.

Another problem that should be solved is the incorporation of incomplete data sets into the algorithm. It may lead to knowledge scarcity in the particular area or issue of concern which may be solved by validating the algorithm using completely different data sets. Still, there might be issues associated with missing data that is due to the inability of the algorithm to collect all the data. For example, an ML algorithm is designed to give guidance to a patient with pneumonia. But, the algorithm left out one important variable that is the patient's asthma history. If the patient has both pneumonia and asthma, the algorithm will underestimate the risk and provide guidance accordingly. But, the asthma patient is very much aware of his respiratory problem. If the patient is directed to take a test to confirm asthma and its result is included in the algorithm, it can predict the outcome perfectly. Unfortunately, this kind of the variable is very difficult to program and include so that they provide poor advice.

Problem framing is another indicator of low-quality ML algorithms. An interesting example is the "finger of death" explained with the H&N IMRT case where the algorithm failed to include the objective of reducing the dose to the normal tissues. Then, we may get a model with excellent performance but failed to include the objective of the problem. However, this kind of issue can be easily solved by using validation data sets that are different from training data sets.

Also, some of the algorithms do not have transparent approaches like black boxes that create problems while inspecting its quality. For example, CNN models have been demonstrated for many applications but it is difficult to inspect. However, regression models and BN models are preferred sometimes even though their execution is not better than CNN. The decision tree approach can be adapted to enhance the transparency where cases are branched into each node based on their feature. But, this is also not clear to know the sense of a specific feature and the decision basis of the feature.

6.6.4 CHALLENGES ASSOCIATED WITH AI FOR QUALITY ASSURANCE IN RT

A few of the challenges associated with ML for QA in RT are as follows:

1. Data quality:
   a. Data availability is extremely high in medicine and its complexity is also very high. Hence, it challenges the AI-based model development and its decision-making process.
   b. Most of the AI algorithms use numeric data sets. But, the data is not numeric in most of the cases and requires mapping and matric computation for feature selection.

   c. Clinical data sets are sparse that increases the noise level and uncertainty.

   d. Incomplete data containing missing values is also challenging the algorithms as reduces its prediction capacity.

   e. The performance of every algorithm is different and highly depends on the data characteristics. Hence, local data sets should be used to compare all the algorithms before implementing them for clinical use.

   f. Non-standardized and inconsistent terminology usage also causes noise and spoils the reliability of QA algorithms.

2. Model adaptability:

   a. The adaptability and learning frequency of an algorithm plays a major role to make the model practical and flexible for modifications and upgrades.

   b. To evaluate the upgradation, provisions need to be incorporated into the algorithm so that users can arrange data suitable for clinical modifications.

   c. Raw data should be analyzed before its use in any model because clinical data are variable and have specific profiles. Therefore, the model should have adaptability, data standardization, and reproducibility to consider those changes.

3. Modeling limitations:

   a. Lack of complete evaluation to analyze the dependency of a model on the characteristics of data sets in addition to its challenges associated with data usage and stricture.

   b. If the signals are low, more data is needed for feature learning which triggers the requirement for high computing power and in turn reduces the model adaptability. To avoid the same, an "out of box" approach can be followed where the parameters in the model are pre-learned as per the independent data sets, and later the trained values are fine-tuned as per the desired data sets.

   c. The most important challenge is in handling small high-quality data size and its associated complexity. This challenge can be overcome by sharing clinical study results among institutions to increase the sample size.

6.6.5 FUTURE DIRECTIONS TO IMPROVE AI-BASED QUALITY ASSURANCE IN RT

1. Create tools for third-party QA and integrate them to enhance the resource utility and standard of present QA procedures, viz., automatic plan generation, plan testing, and plan evaluation.

2. Integrate ML-based QA procedures into machine-based applications to make suitable QA for adaptive planning.

3. Facilitate objectives for precision medicine in combination with genomics, radiomics, and proteomics to perform more advanced RT plan assessment.

4. Take more efforts to standardize and implement guidelines to effectively use data format, content, structure, and its related terminologies as per TG 263.
5. Instantiate principles and guidelines among institutions having a similar effect on QA procedures to enhance the portability of an algorithm.
6. Ontology knowledge can be used to construct a probability table using the available data and use it clinically.
7. Knowledge formalized in the ontology can be used to direct probability table construction from available clinical data representing instances of how that knowledge was applied clinically to reduce communication errors and to simplify data extraction approaches across institutions.
8. Connect data features into real-world cases through ML to grow its ontology base.
9. Ascertain the independence between the design and validation of ML-based QA tools.
10. Find points to integrate ML tools and human capacity in the decision-making process.

6.7 AI IN RADIATION BIOLOGY

Due to the advancements in computational techniques, many methods have been developed for data analysis at a large scale in the area of molecular screening, proteomics, genomics, etc. In most of these methods, a supervised learning method was used earlier which was further upgraded by using ML and DL techniques. Recently, they have been further enhanced with neural network-based algorithms by utilizing the advantage of AI. Originally, they have been introduced to support decision making in many areas like the detection of benign and malignant tumors. With the enormous efforts of researchers, AI-based algorithms that are capable of detecting various types of cancer from clinical and non-clinical data sets.

Also, AI has the potential of developing algorithms in the area of Radiation biology to simulate the physiology of radiation sickness, and radiation-induced biological effects at molecular, cellular, tissue, and organ level. Since the human system is complex, it is necessary to understand the variation in the biological effects of ionizing radiation among individuals to protect them. If there are many variable and complex factors that influence the outcome, the associated complexity in radiation biology can be understandable by using computational methods. However, these methods should be suitable to predict and process more number of biological events to study life complexity and achieve the desired solution (Indraganti et al., 2019).

6.8 AI IN RADIATION PROTECTION/SAFETY

AI-based systems have been implemented to ensure the protective and effective use of radiation in industry, medicine, and research. The government of Singapore has introduced an AI-based system to help their radiation protection agency to give explanation and suggestions to the public on radiation protection point of view. Originally, it was developed by the combined efforts of scientific officers from radiation protection agencies who are familiar with the associated rules and regulations and computational experts. Even though the scientific officers are playing a major role to maintain the system, it was developed in such a way that even a clerical staff can answer the regular questions and provide suggestions on their regulatory aspects and services.

The system consists of two working teams: an operational team and a development team. The operational team has two subdivisions: one sector is to implement radiation safety standards and legislation by the way of inspection and licensing, and the second sector is to give services to promote radiation protection. The main function of the development team is to confirm the safe handling of radiation devices in the public, perform radiation surveys, conduct awareness programs for safe handling and usage of radiation, and to train the radiation workers (Tan et al., 1989).

6.8.1 Motivations to Develop AI-Based Systems for Radiation Protection

The basic considerations to develop AI-based systems for radiation protection are as follows:

1. Scarcity of experts: Generally, some limited scientific officers are working in radiation protection agencies like Atomic Energy Regulatory Board (AERB), Mumbai with formal education or experience. Additional manpower development in this area is a time consuming and expensive event. Therefore, AI-based systems can be used to manage all the activities with the limited experts and to relieve them from heavy workload by automating some of their routine functions. In this way, the system can use manpower effectively and productively. Also, the same system can be utilized as a teaching tool to strengthen radiation safety professionals to handle various cases practically.
2. Type of the task: To give a small instruction, the scientific officer either depends on the huge volumes of regulations associated with the legislation or their knowledge, experience, and expertise. Identifying and using the correct legislation is not easy always mainly for rare cases. Further, the right rule should be applied at the right time and direction that necessitates an expert's knowledge as well.

6.8.2 Problems Associated with AI-Based Systems for Radiation Protection

A few of the problems related to AI-based systems regarding radiation protection are as follows:

1. Complexity in the decision-making process: Finding a relevant license for a specific radioactive source and directing the exact legal requirement is a

simple process. But, it became a challenging task when a large range of radioactive sources are used for various applications.

2. Unawareness of radiation physics: Lack of knowledge of the end-user about the basics of radiation physics further complicate the automation of the decision making process. In most cases, the end-user may not aware of the difference between a radioactive source and X-ray equipment so that they cannot categorize and understand the characteristics of their source. Hence, a simple one-to-one interaction that deals with sensitive information may not sufficient to complete the task successfully. Under these circumstances, AI-based systems can efficiently handle the installation procedure by providing sufficient information to the end-user without wasting an expert's time.

3. To satisfy all the safety requirements, source details and their applications should be provided. Regulatory authorities need to provide relevant rules and regulations, laboratory dimension, beam delivery and storage criteria, shielding, and manpower requirements based on the activity/quantity of radioactive substance and procedures involved. Also, the requirement for preventive measures to handle radiation hazards and contamination of radioactive substances should be considered while planning a laboratory. Therefore, the system should be capable of determining the type of laboratory-based on the source classification. Even though all the rules and regulations are included in the system, it should be used under the supervision of the expert as it requires more knowledge and experience in decision-making processes. This is termed knowledge engineering.

6.8.3 Benefits and Future Directions

AI-based systems have many benefits at the scientific officer level to train newly appointed scientific officers who have lack practical experience, at the clerical staff level to train them on basic aspects of radiation physics parameters and at the end-user level. If the end-users are scientific officers, the system acts as an assistant and provides immediate response and guidance without any questions. Otherwise, the system behaves as a colleague and provides more guidance to handle tough cases.

Despite this, the present system should be improved to solve the complexity involved in machine- man interface and with different categories of users. Further, its potential may be extended towards non-ionizing radiation applications in the future.

6.9   RADIOMICS IN RADIOTHERAPY

Recently, radiation oncology identified a novel field for quantitative image analysis (QIA) namely Radiomics where the involvement of medical physicists is meager at present but has bright potential in the future. Radiomics have an important role in precision medicine by estimating the treatment outcome and side effect of RT on individual patients. It consists of two major steps: (1) extraction of dynamic and static features from images suitable for a further treatment plan, and (2) integration of those imaging features into a model to estimate the treatment outcome. It helps the radiation oncologists to make a decision on each treatment and to monitor the prognosis of cancer.

If an institution is interested to handle radiomic models, it is essential to form a multidisciplinary team that consists of medical physicists, radiation oncologists, biologists, and computer scientists. To integrate QIA with a particular RT data to make it an individualized radio-oncomics signature, basic knowledge on AI approaches, big data analysis, medical imaging modalities, and molecular and clinical basis of tumor suitable for radiomic analysis should be required. This section discusses the objectives of radiomics, various models used for, impact, and challenges of radiomics in RT (Jan et al., 2018).

6.9.1 RADIOMICS OBJECTIVES AND WORKFLOW

Radiomics was originally implemented in radiology to enhance the efficiency of detection from large CT data sets. Due to advancements in computer applications along with data mining, many features that include physical, biological, and clinical data are extracted from images to predict the treatment outcome. The earlier imaging features are qualitative data that became quantitative with the potential of AI.

Such radiomic concepts were expanded into Radiogenomics with the incorporation of molecular data into imaging features that can characterize cancers, detect genetic changes, and predict the response to the treatment. Also, they have been recently translated into radiation oncology by combining general dose-volume parameters, biomarkers, and radiomic concepts that are termed radio-oncomics.

Radio-oncomics integrate both diagnostic and therapeutic data that includes image data, image-guided data, volumetric dose distribution, and data required to verify the treatment. To establish radiomics in radiation oncology effectively and to evaluate the results, all the members in the multidisciplinary working team should be expertized in their field and have a fundamental knowledge of their related disciplines as well. Typically, the radiomics workflow consists of five steps as shown in Figure 6.2.

6.9.2 INFLUENCE OF RADIOMICS IN RT

1. Radiomics on predicting treatment outcome, individual risk assessment, and treatment response: Researchers developed many radiomics based models to predict patient's survival even though this endpoint is complex. It depends on the properties of the tumor in addition to gender, age, and performance index of patients. Therefore, radiomics models should be capable of comparing those parameters to prove their efficiency. To do so, radiomics features need to be integrated with clinical parameters as given below.
   a. To quantify the radiomic signature of tumors, tumor-specific survival can be considered as an appropriate endpoint. To quantify the patient's risk of tumor recurrence, prognostic endpoints such as local and systematic survival which is free from progression may be considered. Then, these two quantities may be translated into an appropriate therapeutic modality.

```
┌─────────────────────────┐
│   Radiomics Workflow    │
└─────────────────────────┘
            │
            ▼
┌─────────────────────────┐      ┌──────────────────────────────────────────┐
│                         │      │  Acquires data from diagnostic images for  │
│    Image acquisition    │ ──▶  │  treatment planning, delivery, monitoring, │
│                         │      │              and follow-up                 │
└─────────────────────────┘      └──────────────────────────────────────────┘
            │
            ▼
┌─────────────────────────┐      ┌──────────────────────────────────────────┐
│      Segmentation       │ ──▶  │  Contour OAR, and target and then          │
│                         │      │            3D-rendering                    │
└─────────────────────────┘      └──────────────────────────────────────────┘
            │
            ▼
┌─────────────────────────┐      ┌──────────────────────────────────────────┐
│                         │      │  Extract features based on shape, texture, │
│   Features extraction   │ ──▶  │     wavelets, and intensity histogram      │
│                         │      └──────────────────────────────────────────┘
└─────────────────────────┘
            │
            ▼
┌─────────────────────────┐      ┌──────────────────────────────────────────┐
│    Data aggregation     │ ──▶  │ Integrate diagnostic data, physical data,  │
│       and mining        │      │      biological data, and clinical data    │
└─────────────────────────┘      └──────────────────────────────────────────┘
            │
            ▼
┌─────────────────────────┐      ┌──────────────────────────────────────────┐
│                         │      │ Study the combination of radiomic features,│
│        Analysis         │ ──▶  │  physical and biological data with         │
│                         │      │            clinical data.                  │
└─────────────────────────┘      └──────────────────────────────────────────┘
```

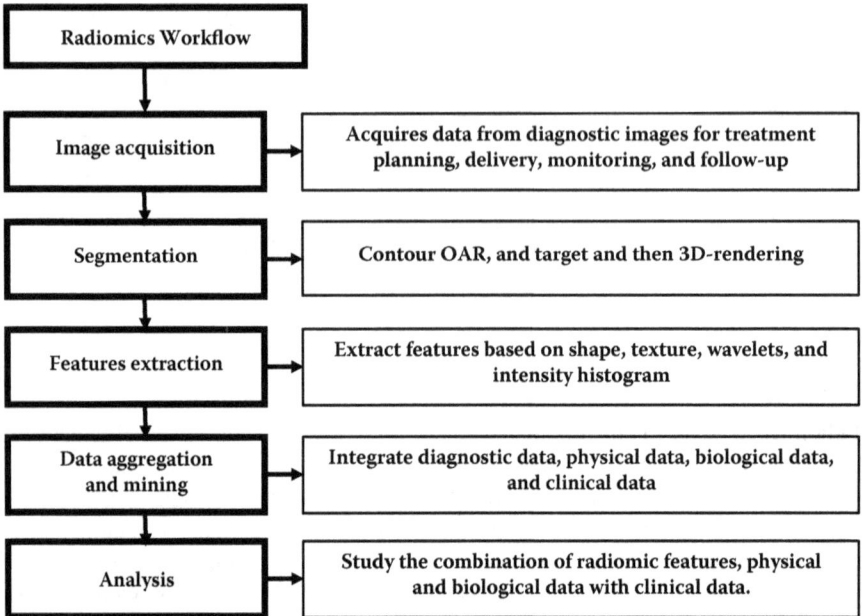

FIGURE 6.2   Activities in radiomics workflow.

   b. Generally, identifying a correct endpoint for RT response assessment is a challenging task. Few analyses were performed by choosing prognostic factors like pathological variation of the tumor as an endpoint but it is not valid for all kinds of tumors. Therefore, radiomics classifiers like delta radiomics have been used to quantify the RT response. Also, radiogenomics have been used for the same by assessing the radiation-induced variation in its oncogene expression.

   c. Earlier, radiomics studies were carried out using the CT data to predict the survival and progression followed by RT. Recently, researchers confirmed that the radiogenomics approach may be suitable to predict the mutational status of few genes like EGFR, KRAS, etc., accurately by combining radiogenomics data with clinical data.

   d. Many researchers analyzed the impact of radiomics in PET imaging to predict the survival rate, pathological variation caused by the treatment, and tumor progression.

   e. The potential of MRI for disease diagnosis, treatment planning, follow-up, and functional imaging has been demonstrated clinically. These potentials of MRI may be enhanced by the incorporation of radiomics data with MRI data to make it an alternative to the invasive biopsy procedure.

2. Radiomics to enhance RT efficiency

   a. As discussed earlier, the definition for target volume to plan any treatment can be advanced and improved using quantitative imaging data. Now a day, CT, MRI, and PET imaging data are used to define target volumes. If radiomics data are integrated with these conventional imaging data, even sub-volumes that need more dose than the nearby region can also be identified for dose painting.

    b. The quantitative feature capacity of imaging modalities enables the potential of semi or completely automatic segmentation, and disease identification which may decrease interpersonal discrepancy.

    c. For segmentation, many unsupervised and supervised models have been developed but they need to be trained to achieve high consistency.

3. Radiomics for patient-specific treatment: Adaptive RT makes the RT procedure specific for each patient as it depends on the intrinsic properties of the tumor and hence implements personalized treatment.

4. Radio-oncomics to predict TCP and NTCP: Radiomics can predict tumor response in addition to normal tissue toxicities due to irradiation. Also, it has the potential to quantify the properties of individual tissues. Many researchers analyzed the potential of radiomics to predict normal tissue complications like pneumonitis, xerostomia, sticky saliva, and sensorineural hearing loss in H&N cancer patients.

5. Radiomics to improve diagnosis: Treatment follow-up and patient care may also be improved by radiomics tools such as CT-based radiomics, and MRI-based classifier.

6.9.3 CHALLENGES FOR MEDICAL PHYSICISTS

The applications of big data analysis approaches in radiation oncology contain image, clinical, physical, and biological data sets that create various novel tasks in research and routine medical practice. It challenges the medical physics professionals as a multidisciplinary radiation oncology team member in the following aspects.

1. Treatment planning: The expected signs of progress in RT planning by the introduction of radiomics are:

    a. Multimodality images are used to diagnose the disease and to plan the treatment by modeling a 3D patient and the same is further supported with quantitative images in this radiomics era.

    b. Radiomics supported IMRT can generate heterogeneous dose distribution to a biologically inhomogeneous tumor by representing a Biological Target Volume (BTV).

    c. Radiomics can be applied to describe the BTV precisely by mapping the genetic information of normal and cancerous tissues on imaging data sets.

    d. The severity of radiation may be predicted by integrating radiomics into volumetric dose distribution.

    e. When we integrate radiomics with TPS, the routine duty of medical physicists in QA of imaging will be extended to consider radiomics tools as well. Since the radiomics tools are under the developmental stage, it will be a challenging task. However, medical physicists should verify whether the treatment planning parameters satisfy the necessary standards to ensure patient safety.

f. Organ motion, variation in patient positioning, and changes in BTV during the treatment may cause uncertainties while correlating the volumetric dose matrix with imaging data sets. Therefore, medical physicists should aware of such limitations and pitfalls.

g. Standardization and evaluation of radiomics parameters would be a tedious task in multi-institutional trials.

2. RT delivery: Generally, Image-Guided Radiotherapy (IGRT) features extracted from their series of images are used to estimate the time-dependent effect of radiation during treatment. In this aspect,

a. Delta-radiomics approach can be applied to measure the response of the tumor to irradiation.

b. CBCT-radiomics can be used to predict the survival of patients.

c. Radiomics tools integrated with IGRT-image data sets can help the clinical decision-making process based on treatment response.

3. Dose distribution: Type of radiation, DVH, 3D (spatial) and 4D (temporal) dose distributions, real dose delivered, and the accumulated dose is the important physical parameters used to predict the outcome of the treatment and response of normal and cancerous tissues to radiation. Combination of these parameters and radiomics signatures can improve such predictions but its dosimetric uncertainties should be analyzed cautiously.

6.9.4   FUTURE DIRECTIONS

A few of the future directions in the area of radiomics are as follows:

1. In this big data digital era, many powerful models have been evolved to analyze a large amount of information which may create opportunities in the future to help for decision making on therapy design and acceptance, enhance the outcome prediction, and to enable patient satisfaction.

2. Accumulation of diagnostic and therapeutic digital big data sets along with genomic data may trigger research in the area of basic and clinical science applied to radiation oncology.

3. Medical physicists should understand the AI-based technological advancements then only they can play an essential part in the radiation oncology expert team.

4. Upgradation of the present curricula by including applications of radiomics in radiation oncology.

5. Medical physics and radiation oncology associations should initiate activities to train the professionals in the area of AI technology.

6.10 AI CONSIDERATIONS FOR RT CURRICULUM DEVELOPMENT

AI techniques are gradually introduced into routine RT clinical practice worldwide. Recently, Varian introduced ETHOS_solution which is an AI-based treatment delivery system to improve the efficiency of adaptive radiotherapy. Further, ML-based TPS, namely research, has been approved for auto organ segmentation and treatment planning. These advancements in AI and its transformation highlight the need for upgradation in the RT curriculum to explain the importance of AI. Particularly, RT professors should interact with budding medical physicists and radiation oncologists regarding the benefits, errors, and pitfalls of AI in the RT profession. Moreover, research on AI technologies should also be reflected in the curriculum to encourage AI-based developments in the future.

Since more research articles have been published in this area, the available data can be utilized to change and make use of the AI models to educate the students. It may allow them to spend more time enhancing the models and patient care. Based on the applications and developments of AI in RT, the following essential elements have been suggested to include in the RT curriculum (Crispen et al., 2020).

1. Basic concepts and potential applications of AI in RT: RT professionals should be trained well to handle AI systems, understand its language, and to manage technological upgradations efficiently and safely. Experts suggested that the curriculum should be designed to target literacy instead of proficiency and to focus on the basics of AI, ML, and DL and their applications in RT. It is also suggested to include courses related to computer science and informatics. Then, the teacher should be trained well to understand the basics and knowledge to extend the same on RT. It is recommended to prefer trained medical physicists to teach those courses even though they can be handled by AI experts. So that they can discuss the basics with simple examples related to their RT practice and share the related ethics, confidentiality, and patient's rights.

2. AI ethics and constitutional requirements: The second essential elements that need to be included in the curriculum of RT are AI ethics and constitutional requirements. Students should aware of the ethical issues and associated risks while using ML and DL algorithms. Even though AI systems duplicate neural networks of a human brain, they think and perform differently. Therefore, more importance should be given to legal and ethical aspects especially during decision-making processes.

3. AI-based quality and safe practices in RT: In addition to the routine quality assurance procedures that are carried out in all the steps of routine RT workflow to ensure accurate and safe dose delivery, QA procedures related to AI technologies should also be performed. As it modifies the routine day-to-day activities, teaching plays a major role to learn and follow the standards related to quality and safe practices, understanding the impact of AI algorithms, limitation of AI-based QA procedures, and reassessing the automation in RT workflow.

4. Influence of AI on multiple disciplines: AI curriculum should also include contents to understand how the AI in RT influences other professionals who are associated with patient care that includes nurses, psychosocial, and nutritional support staff.
5. Research and development: Research to develop new AI methods and their evaluation will be a potential area in the future. If AI may not give a solution to all the RT challenges, it is not advisable to fully rely on AI methods. Presently, AI methods have well-identified problems related to decision making, RT automation, QA models, data analysis, outcome prediction, etc., that triggers novel research in this field.

REFERENCES

Alan M. K., Samuel M. H. L., and Mark H. P. (2019), 'Quality Assurance Tasks and Tools: The Many Roles of Machine Learning', *Medical Physics*, 47(5), e168–e177 [published online ahead of print].

Chunhao W., Xiaofeng Z., Julian C. H., and Dandan Z. (2019), 'Artificial Intelligence in Radiotherapy Treatment Planning: Present and Future', *Technology in Cancer Research & Treatment*, 18, 1–11.

Crispen C., Grad C. A. P., Christopher E., et al. (2020), 'The Impact of Artificial Intelligence and Machine Learning in Radiation Therapy: Considerations for Future Curriculum Enhancement', *Journal of Medical Imaging and Radiation Sciences*, 51(2), 214–220.

Georgios K., Luis A. V., Travis Z. G. P., et al. (2011), 'Toward IMRT 2D Dose Modeling Using Artificial Neural Networks: A Feasibility Study', *Medical Physics*, 38(10), 5807–5817.

Indraganti P. K., Namita I., and Anoushka K. (2019), 'Possible Role of Artificial Intelligence in Radioprotection', *Frontiers in Drug, Chemistry and Clinical Research*, 2, 1–2, DOI: 10.15761/FDCCR.1000133.

Jan C. P., Michael B., Benedikt W., et al. (2018), 'Radiomics in Radio Oncology – Challenging the Medical Physicist', *Physica Medica*, 48, 27–36.

Ramin J., Zahra S., Mahmoud R. A., et al. (2017), 'Artificial Neural Network-Based Gynecological Image-Guided Adaptive Brachytherapy Planning Correction of Intra-fractional Organs at Risk Dose Variation', *Journal of Contemporary Brachytherapy*, 9(6), 508–518.

Reid F. T., Gilmer V., Clifton D. F., et al. (2018), 'Artificial Intelligence in Radiation Oncology: A Specialty-Wide Disruptive Transformation?', *Radiotherapy and Oncology*, 129, 421–426.

Tan C. L., Pang C. M., Chant Y. C., and Starkey C. (1989), 'Applications of Artificial Intelligence in Radiation Protection', *International Journal of Computer Applications in Technology*, 2(3), 166–170.

Vasant K., Jason W. C., Gilmer V., et al. (2018), 'The Application of Artificial Intelligence in the IMRT Planning Process for Head and Neck Cancer', *Oral Oncology*, 87, 111–116.

7 Artificial Intelligence in Systems Biology

Opportunities in Agriculture, Biomedicine, and Healthcare

S. Dhivya[1], S. Hari Priya[2], and R. Sathishkumar[1,2]
[1]Department of Biotechnology, Bharathiar University, Coimbatore, India
[2]DRDO-BU Center for Life Sciences, Bharathiar University campus, Coimbatore, India

CONTENTS

DOI: 10.1201/9781003175865-7

OBJECTIVES

- To introduce artificial intelligence in systems biology
- To explain artificial Intelligence methodologies, tools in systems biology, including machine learning tools used in genome analysis, and variant calling
- To list artificial intelligence applications in systems biology – agriculture, drug discovery, biomedicine, oncology, identifying variants/mutations from genetic data, and workflow analysis for genome analysis
- To use case studies to know the importance of artificial intelligence in Systems Biology towards pharmacogenomics, cancer cure, and COVID-19 pandemic
- To highlight artificial intelligence's future challenges in systems biology, including gene prediction, protein-protein interaction, and neural networks

7.1   INTRODUCTION TO ARTIFICIAL INTELLIGENCE (AI)

The artificial intelligence (AI) concept began in the mid-1950s to understand intelligence, its origin, and creation, in natural and artificial environments. It is a multidisciplinary field that extends out and is stimulated by a great diversity of other fields in perpetual motion. AI generally involves ideas, approaches, and systems as a part of the computer program that exhibits characteristics similar to intelligent behavior. Some degree of intelligence is observed in animals often the same scope of intelligence was observed by human action. For example, the creation of aircraft that is capable of mimic and express human intelligence, thought, consciousness, and emotions. During the mid-1980s, AI received a major boost when applied to create artificial neural networks (ANNs) and currently it bridges the gap between advanced fields like systems biology and synthetic biology. Advances in diverse fields created the environment to apply artificial intelligence to accomplish complicated tasks logically and easily. US National Research Council of the National Academies affirmed numerous sub-disciplines of biology (Figure 7.1) and the integration of AI with diverse sub-disciplines of science to gain knowledge on biological systems (Shukla Shubhendu and Vijay, 2013).

Recent application of AI technology in cybernetics deals with two complementary issues, (1) AI in systems biology have helped to formulate theories, methods, algorithms, and helps to generate big data and its implications for a given task; (2) furthermore, biological systems are so complex it needs inter- and transdisciplinary expertise to understand the principles. Thus, the interdisciplinary collaboration will yield the solution for the unresolved questions (Urban et al., 2013). "Systems biology is a universal approach to decipher the intricacy of *biological systems* while synthetic biology or artificial biology is a blend of engineering and biological sciences with an idea to generate novel biological models" (Bera, 2019).

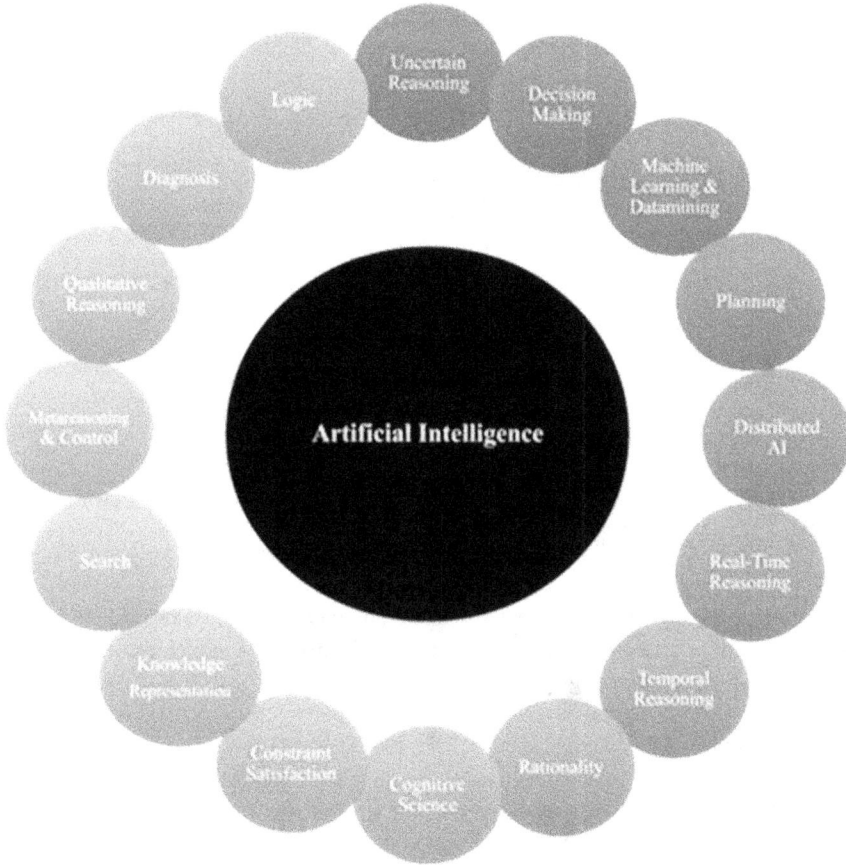

FIGURE 7.1 Sub-disciplines of artificial intelligence (adapted from Shukla, Shubhendu, and Vijay, 2013; with copyright permission from IJSER publisher).

Systems biology can solve the most complex problems in medicine, drug discovery, and biomedical engineering. The basic problem lies in the convolution of biotic systems that have emerged over billions of years. AI technology application in systems biology includes text-mining, qualitative physics, statistical interpretations, machine learning, and deep learning algorithms, etc. Hence, AI technology in systems biology is helping to do quality research leading to solutions that are unresolved until now. The key characteristics of AI are shown in Figure 7.2. For example, AI technology has been widely used to resolve complex problems in diverse areas such as drug discovery and coral reef systems biology. AI also makes a significant contribution to capturing, distributing, developing, and usage of these resourceful data for human welfare.

AI includes machine learning, deep learning, knowledge management, and multiagent systems. AI provides a scientific platform by incorporating and boosting the skills of humans and computers via interaction between the human-machine processor, computational ingenuity analysis, and array recognition. It also provides theoretical

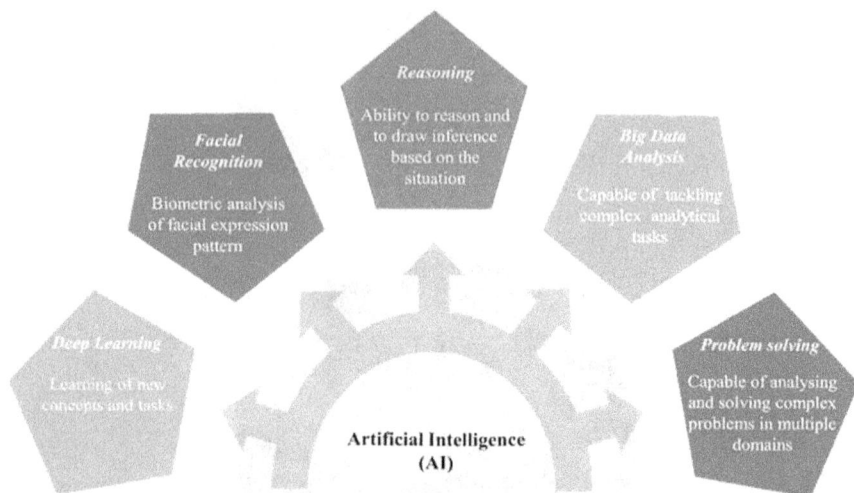

FIGURE 7.2 Characteristics of AI.

and practical knowledge via computer theories and data mining. AI plays a significant role in the pharmaceutical industries for the discovery of novel drugs. Lack of knowledge in AI methodologies and tools are the major problems that exist in systems biology. It has a potential impact on current research and future development in systems biology. The tools and methods developed by AI researchers should help in understanding systems biology as traditional statistical approaches have limitations.

Systems biology in life science has resulted in the construction of a "complete" computational model to capture knowledge about important systematic properties, 3D structures, and functions of each biological unit. It operates on a basic understanding of the system via simulations. To bridge the technological gap between man and machine, computational models play a vital role in better perception of biological systems, collection of integrative data, developing new methods, and tools for systems biology.

7.2 AI METHODOLOGIES AND ALGORITHM FOR SYSTEMS BIOLOGY

Microarray technology is useful in analyzing the expression of multiple genes that leads to various diseases. Using computational methods, it is possible to detect de novo mutations that are generated via sequencing technology. Mutations in the exonic region have been identified through reading processing, aligning, mapping, and variant calling.

Algorithm for read processing such as Next Generation Sequencing (NGS) Data QC toolkit, Cutdapt, and FastX have been used to trim out the low-grade adapters in sequencing. To identify the sequence similarity, the processed reads were compared with the reference genome, followed by multiple sequence alignment using NovoAlign, BWA, STAR, TWAP, TOPHAT, and RNA sequencing. GATKs (Genome Analysis Tool Kits) are widely utilized for intel alignment base quality recalibration, variant calling, and also to find precise mutants from sequencing, mapping, genomic libraries, and sample enrichment. Numerous germline and somatic mutant calling algorithms were developed for detecting low-frequency mutants from the complex system through an error correction technique. Genomic mutants fall under four major groups like insertion, deletion (del), structural variants like duplication, translocation, copy number variants, and SNVs (Single Nucleotide Variants). SNV is ≤10 bp and it is to check non-reference nucleotides from the pile of sequence that covers each position. The tools used for germline variant calling involves GAP and MAG integrated by GATK, whereas CRISP and Thunder are used for the analysis of variant calling and pooled samples data.

7.2.1 Machine Learning (ML)

Machine learning (ML) in artificial intelligence enables the machine to make decisions by themselves without explicit programming. Figure 7.3 portrays the major relationship between diverse computational learning technologies. Machine learning includes the implementation of genetic algorithms (GAs). Genetic algorithms are defined as a perfect algorithm which includes Darwinian evolutionary theory (survival of the fittest) and the easiest form of genetic process. Depending upon the biological operators such as mutation, crossover, and selection, GAs are widely used to produce good solutions to biological problems. The mutational

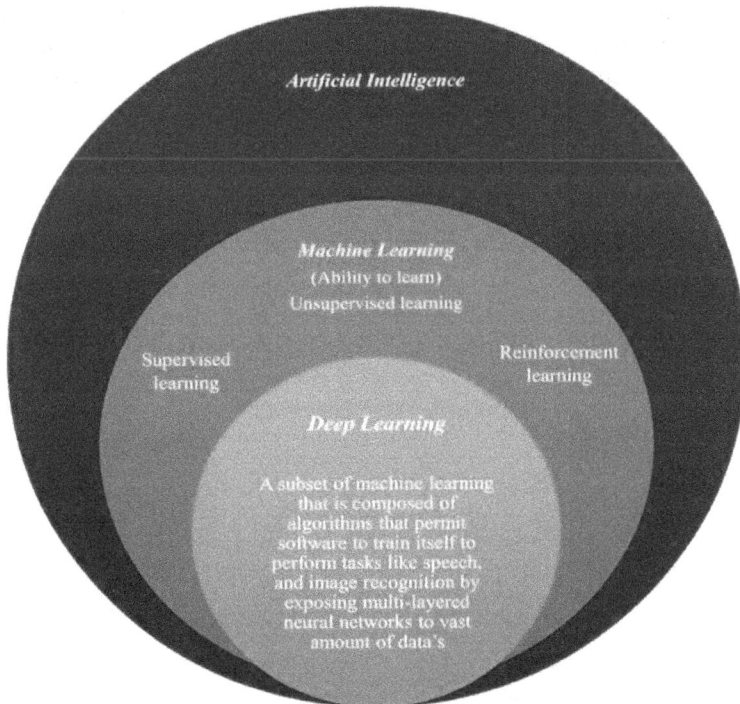

FIGURE 7.3 Relationship between ML, DL, and AI (adapted from Moore and Raghavachari, 2019; copyright permission from Frontiers publishers).

operator instigates a change in the final solution of the problem so that the diversity in the population could be maintained, while a crossover operator mimics biological recombination (Bhasin and Bhatia, 2011).

7.2.2 ML Algorithm Applied in Systems Biology

Cell Profiler: Usually, biological images are analyzed by a single parameter from a group of images. Cell Profiler is a software developed by Anne Carpenter and her colleagues at MIT and Harvard for the quantitative analysis of cell numbers using a fluorescent microscope. Presently, by applying deep learning techniques, a cell profiler can be utilized in an array of biological fields.

Deep Variant: Data mining of whole-genome sequence (WGS) is possible only using Deep learning (DL) algorithm. With the application of a deep learning algorithm, a systems tool called "Deep Variant" was developed by Verily life science and Google to predict common genetic variations in a more accurate and precise manner, contrary to the traditional tools.

Atomwise: "Atomwise" is a biotech firm in San Francisco that has developed an algorithm with atomic accuracy to convert molecules into three-dimensional shapes of amino acids (Webb, 2018). Mahmud et al. (2018) showed a list of deep learning (DL) techniques that are applied in systems biology (Figure 7.4). In biomedicine, the genetic data has been deciphered to confirm the presence of biomarkers but to know the stage of the disease is still a challenging task. Using DNN, the genomic and proteomic data were analyzed to detect the novel biological markers. In cheminformatics, deep learning is used in identifying the target

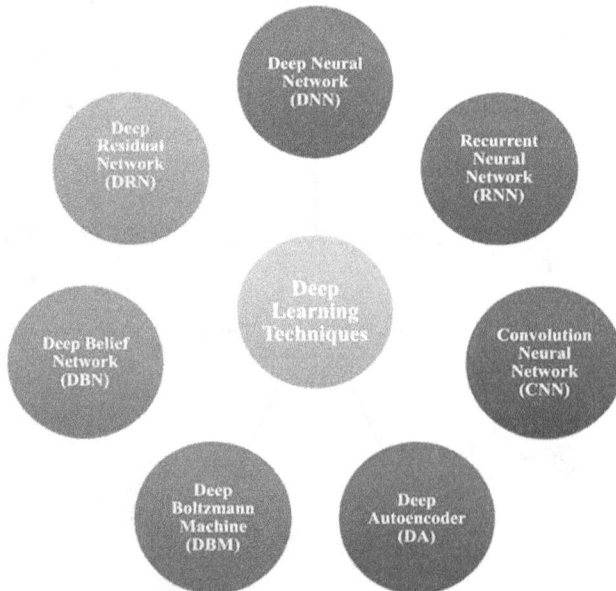

FIGURE 7.4 Deep learning techniques utilized in systems biology.

drug (Mamoshina et al., 2016). In single cells, DNA methylation stages were envisaged using a computational tool called "Deep CpG" that was recently established by CNN. A Deep CpG tool is used for predicting the motifs appropriate for DNA methylation. Deep CpG is predominantly used in studying epigenetic markers (Angermueller et al., 2017).

Tensor Flow: It was first established by Google researchers using a deep learning (DL) algorithm. Currently, Tensor Flow is involved in accelerating neural network strategy. Tensor Flow is employed in various fields for time management and graphical predictions. Recent advancements in Tensor Flow entrenched towards a supporting tool called "Tensor Board" that is used for the visualization of complex models (Rampasek and Goldenberg, 2016).

7.2.3 COMPUTATIONAL NEURAL NETWORKS

Neural networks are the second major bottom-up approach in attaining artificial intelligence, while deep learning comprises an array of neural network that transmits the data from one neuron to the other via hidden layers (Figure 7.5). These hidden layers help to resolve complex problems by naturally mimicking the human brain (Figure 7.6). Artificial Neural Networks (ANNs) require machine learning algorithms to significantly analyze the input data. Artificial neurons comprise various inputs and a single output. Simultaneously, one neuron activates the other

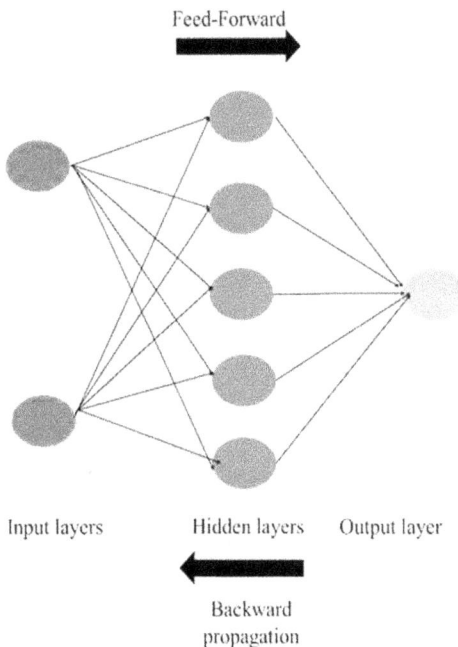

FIGURE 7.5 Artificial neural networks (ANNs).

(a)

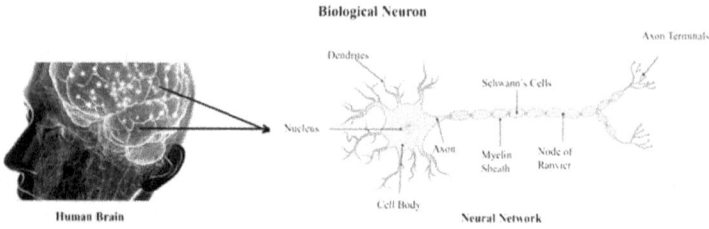

(b)

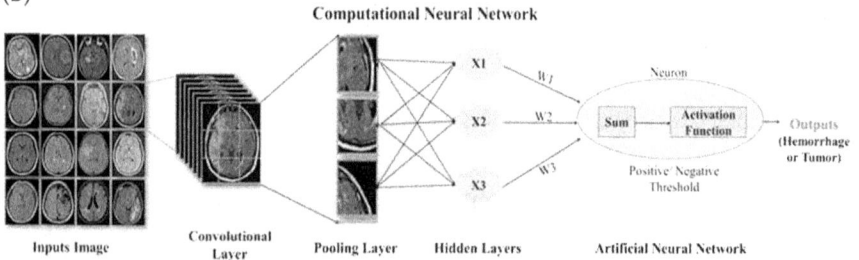

FIGURE 7.6   Schematic representation of biological neuron vs. computational neural network. (a) in the biological system, once the neuronal activation function/signal reaches a certain threshold, it is transmitted to the other neurons via the axon. (b) In a computational neural network, a deep learning algorithm is used to learn the features of the human brain and reflect a hierarchy of structures as output. Here, X1, X2, and X3 are the input signals to the neuron. to adjust the final outputs, the neurons are complemented with a bias node and input signals. Here, W1, W2, and W3 are the weights that are in connection to the signals. the input and product of weight provide the strength of the signal. Typically, a neuron receives several inputs and it uses a mathematical function to attain a single output (modified from Zhu et al., 2019; with copyright permission from Frontiers publishers).

neuron using precise activation functions like (1) sigmoid function, (2) step function, (3) linear function, (4) ramp function, and (5) hyperbolic tangent function.

ANN comprises (1) an input layer that receives the input signals or values; (2) hidden layers, which are a group of neurons separating the input and output layer; and an (3) output layer, which has one neuron and its output value range between 0 and 1 (Shanmuganathan, 2016). A hidden layer in ANN screens the pooled data interconnects with each layer and provides an accurate output. Nowadays, DL techniques are vastly used in biomedicine, cellular imaging, and analysis of whole genome by the mining of huge data sets and creating a computational model. Hence, deep learning in biological big data analysis provides a better knowledge of the high-dimension data set, detecting regulatory mutants, and also analyzing the rate of mutation via DNA sequencing of the whole cell or tissue samples.

7.2.4 Pros and Cons of Artificial Neural Network (ANN)

Figure 7.7 shows the pros and cons of an artificial neural network.

Artificial Neural Network

Pros

- A neural network can perform tasks that a linear program cannot.
- Artificial neural network is self-organized while learning. A normal program is fixed for its task and will not do anything other than what is intended.
- Neural network works in parallel like a human brain.
- Artificial neural network is fault tolerance.
- Can build extremely powerful models by adding multiple layers.
- Artificial neural network is the fastest application than the human brain.

Cons

- The neural network needs training to operate.
- The architecture of neural network is different from the architecture of a microprocessors, therefore need to be emulated.
- Requires high processing time for large neural networks.

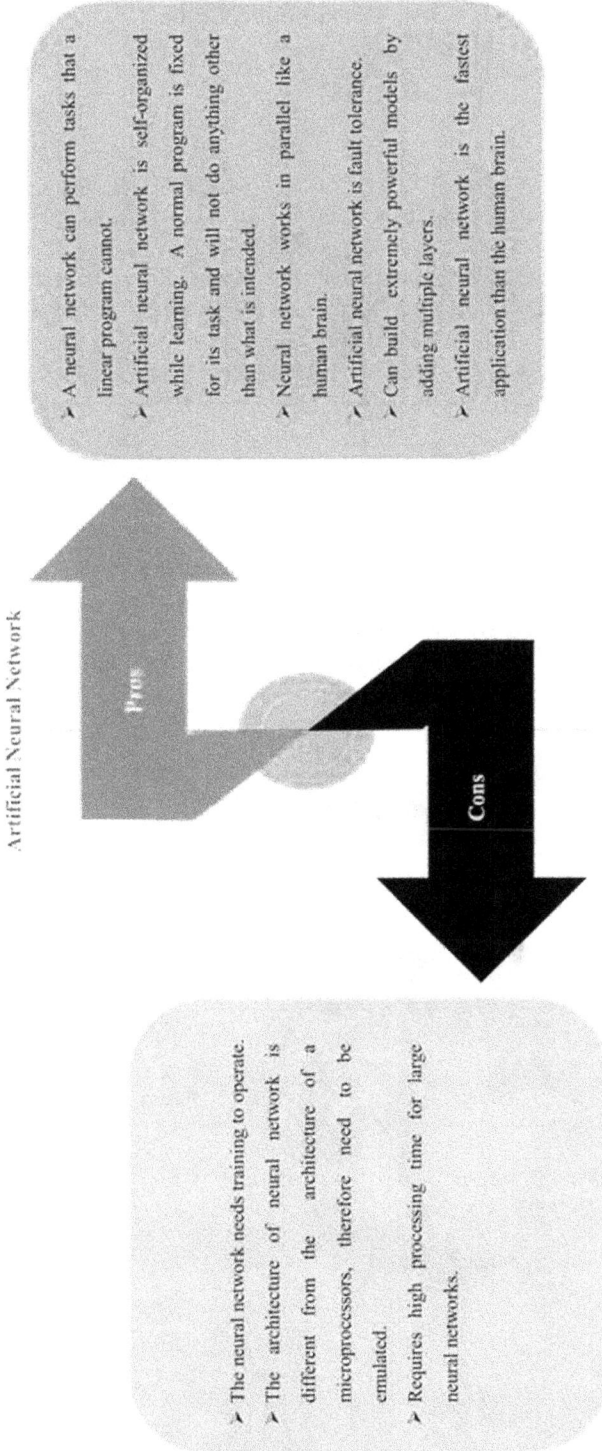

FIGURE 7.7 Pros and cons of artificial neural networks (ANNs).

7.3 APPLICATIONS OF ARTIFICIAL INTELLIGENCE (AI) IN AGRICULTURE, BIOMEDICINE, AND HEALTHCARE

7.3.1 AI IN AGRICULTURE

AI technology is precisely used in agriculture to detect diseases, pests, and proper nutritional supply to the plants in the field. In agriculture, the use of AI falls under three main categories. (1) Agricultural robots are developed to harvest the crops at higher volume and a faster rate than humans; For instance: Initiation of Blue-River Technology has led to the development of "See and Spray Robot" which control weeds in the cotton field. (2) Crop and soil health is monitored using deep learning algorithms and software-based technologies. The development of "Harvest CR00 Robots" has benefited the strawberry growers to gather and box the fruits with less labor cost. In recent times, PEAT a Berlin-based agricultural firm has established an application named "Plantix" which detects diseases, pests, and certain soil defects. Figure 7.8 illustrates the mechanism of disease detection in plants; (3) AI-based machine learning robots were established to forecast the crop yield and weather changes. "aWhere" is a Colorado-based firm that is involved in analyzing crop sustainability, climatic conditions and to detect diseases and pests in the farm using machine learning algorithms (Figure 7.9). Apart from this, AI technology is also employed to analyze altered stress levels in plants. To provide valuable results, the AI machine learning approach under stress is illustrated in Figure 7.10 (Gambhire and Shaikh Mohammad, 2020).

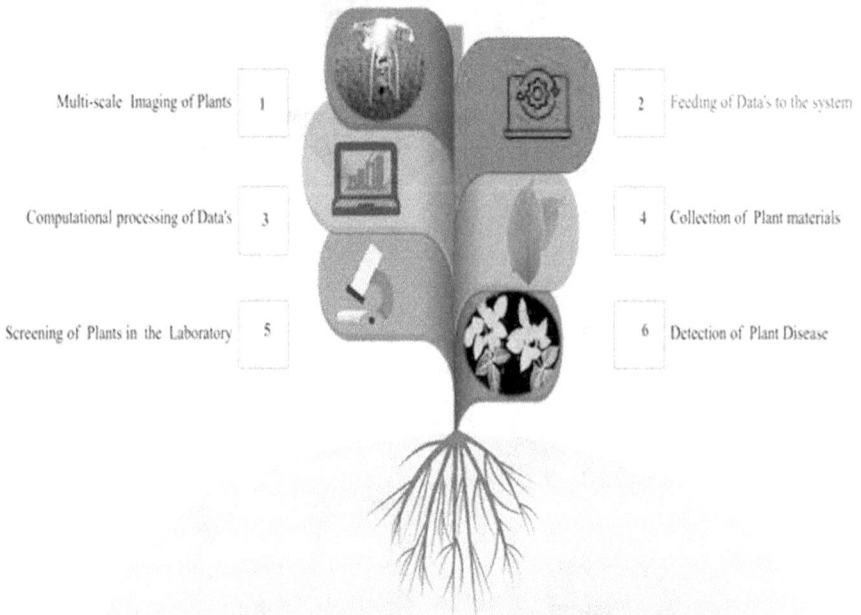

Multi-scale Imaging of Plants 1	2 Feeding of Data's to the system
Computational processing of Data's 3	4 Collection of Plant materials
Screening of Plants in the Laboratory 5	6 Detection of Plant Disease

FIGURE 7.8 Disease detection in crops using AI technology.

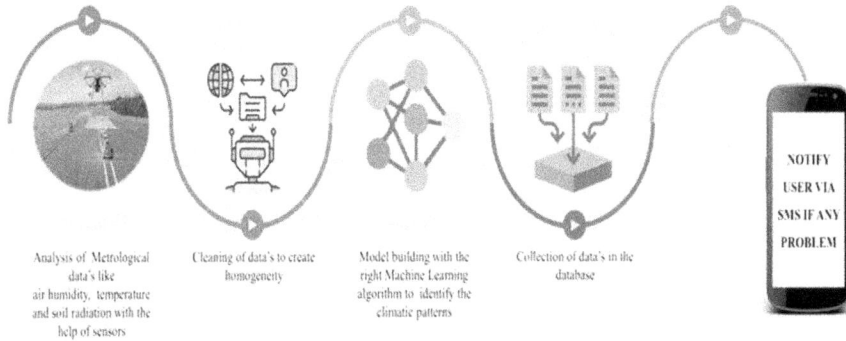

FIGURE 7.9 Sensing of meteorological data using machine learning algorithms.

7.3.2 AI IN BIOMEDICINE

Recent advancement in biomedicine and medical informatics has laid the foundation for the evolution of complex biomedical systems. Implementation of machine learning (ML) algorithms in biomedicine help in disease diagnosis, biomedical data processing, analyzing the function of living organisms, and biomedical research. In disease diagnosis integration of machine learning algorithms, Point-of-Care Testing (POCT), and biochips can easily spot cardiac ailments at a very early stage (Rong et al., 2020). AI can also be used to analyze the survival rate of cancer patients. In biomedical imaging, AI technology can be implemented with electroencephalography (EEG) for an exact prediction of the epileptic seizure (Usman and Fong, 2017). Apart from this, AI technology is adapted to process huge complex clinical data, by incorporating logical reasoning and providing valuable conclusion within a short period.

7.3.3 AI IN DNA EXPRESSION PROFILING

Microarray technology is extensively used for studying the expression pattern of multiple genes concurrently. Series of experimental conditions enabled us to gather a huge amount of gene expression data at a varied time point. At present, it is a tough challenge for the researchers to scientifically interpret the gene expression data, owing to their robustness and huge data sets. By using computational tools, it is possible to convert the DNA expression profiles into theoretical data. Like clustering algorithms that display metabolic regulation of certain genes, concept learning is also vital for analyzing the sequential expression pattern of genes. The use of AI technology in gene expression profiling displays the progressive stages of the microarray data and it also defines the actual behavior of the model. It also provides a license for the users to identify the variants that naturally exist in the model via statistical analysis (Dubitzky and Azuaje, 2004).

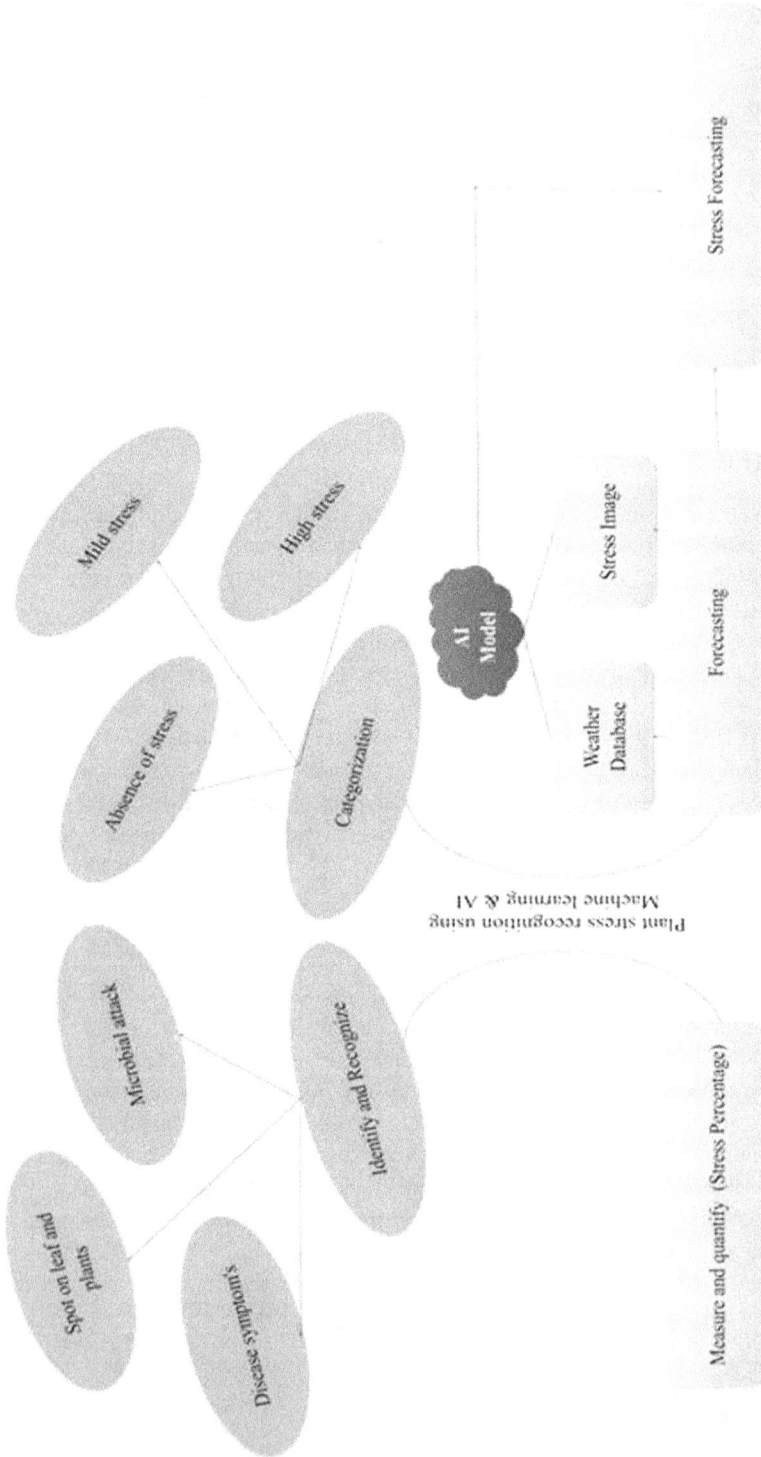

FIGURE 7.10 Recognition of plant stress using machine learning and artificial intelligence (copyright permission from Research Gate publisher).

7.3.4 AI FOR IDENTIFYING EXONIC REGIONS

In the era of genomics, the development of high-throughput techniques like Next-Generation Sequencing (NGS) has fastened the sequencing of a whole genome in a short period. At present, AI with machine learning has been implemented to recognize the exonic regions in a genome. Henceforth, the application of machine learning algorithms in gene prediction tools would be more complex than traditional homology-based predictions. Presently "MethBank" database is used for whole-genome sequencing that affords configurable and interactive data analysis. It is a user-friendly database that works well on diverse computer platforms like Java, Linux, and MySql (Zou et al., 2015).

7.3.5 AI IN IDENTIFYING VARIANTS/MUTATIONS FROM GENETIC DATA

Genetic variants and various human diseases were detected using high-throughput genome sequencing technology like Whole-Exome Sequencing (WES). In humans, missense variants cause genetic disorders like cancer, Mendelian diseases, and other unidentified ailments. Experimental validation of these genetic diseases is quite complex, which is laborious and needs huge resources, while this problem can be solved using computational approaches like analysis of sequence similarity, phylogenetic relationship, and 3D protein structural homology. Apart from this, some of the common methods used for predicting genetic diseases are shown in Figure 7.11.

VarCards is a database that holds all the potential information associated with exonic mutants and the classification of human genetic variants with consequences of allele frequencies. It is well studied by Receiver Operating Characteristic (ROC) curves that include diverse factors like precision, sensitivity, and Area under the Curve (AUC). The cutoff values are utilized to detect the deleterious missense mutants that were observed from the ANNOVAR and the dbNSFB database. CNN (Convolutional Neural Network) is a machine learning technique that is commonly used to detect genetic mutants. Campagne and Torracina software use the CNN method to analyze genomic data and identify indel's (Nagarajan et al., 2019).

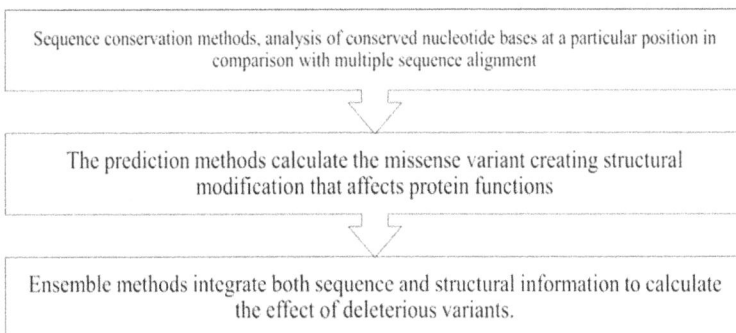

FIGURE 7.11 Steps involved in predicting genetic disorders via computational methods.

Genomic data were categorized into three groups as training data (60%), model testing data (30%), and model validation data (10%). The deep variant method is used for detecting SNPs while the mutation in a gene is identified using deep sequence software.

7.3.6 AI Workflow Method for Genomic Analysis

Ensemble project updates comparative genomics resources every year and generates alignments and protein homology predictions. eHive, an AI tool to maintain comparative genomics, is built on blackboard systems, network distribution, graphs, and block branch diagrams. MySQL database functions as a core processing unit while Perl script inquiries the system and performs the job. It works on three main steps (1) pairwise whole-genome alignments, (2) multiple whole-genome alignments, and (3) creation of gene trees. Here, the pairwise alignment pipeline is explained. It consists of the following steps for comparing human and pika genomes. The first step involves the alignment of raw data; unit Chunk and to collect information on each genome using Group DNA. The other two programs Create Pair Aligner Jobs and Create Filter Duplicate Jobs using BlastZ, Filter Duplicates, and Target Filter Duplicates run for the input DNA query. The BlastZ analysis runs the entire BLAST program (Altschul et al., 1990). The variations in the chunk sequences are removed via Query Filter Duplicate and Target Filter Duplicate analysis. The efficient query regions were identified using the updated Max Alignment Length module in a MySQL database. Furthermore, the raw data was connected and netted using the pairwise sequence alignment method. In the axtChain program, the input data are formatted using Dump Large Nib for Chains module. The Create Alignment Chain Job generates one Alignment Chain job for each genomic region. The netting is also executed using the above-mentioned chain alignment strategy. Latter, the sanity test analysis with the input query sequence was performed using Pairwise Health Check analysis. The third and final step includes the alignment of human and pika genomes (Severin et al., 2020).

7.3.7 AI in Structure Prediction

The prediction of protein structure and folds are vital for recognizing the natural role of the cell. Experimental analysis of the structure and folding pattern of numerous protein sequences that are deposited in the public databases is a tedious process. So to overcome this problem, the implementation of the machine learning technique would rapidly analyze the protein sequences and predict their function (Soding, 2017). The use of AI technology in the prediction of genome modification, protein-protein binding sites, and protein-protein networks is precisely about 70–80%. To identify a novel drug target, the application of ML in data mining is quite favorable in retrieving the data from secondary databases and journals (Suthaharan, 2014).

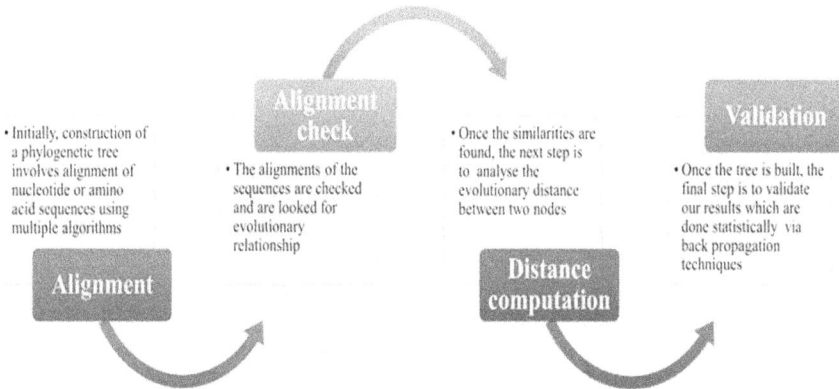

FIGURE 7.12   Steps involved in the construction of an evolutionary tree.

7.3.8   AI IN PHYLOGENY

A phylogeny is a branching tree model that confines the evolutionary origin of any biological entity. Clade and clade length signifies the evolutionary time taken for a precise evolution. Multiple steps implicated in the construction of an evolutionary tree are shown in Figure 7.12. The distance between each sequence is calculated using the Distance Matrix method. It works by building a correlation matrix in two comparable modes, i.e., Unweighted Pair Group Method with Arithmetic Mean (UPGMA) and Neighbor Joining (NJ) method. A recent development in computational biology has provided the base for automated analysis and tree building using AI algorithms. AI algorithms for a standard tree construction are k-nearest neighbor, Bayes theorem, decision trees, and neural network.

7.3.9   AI IN HEALTHCARE

AI technology along with the machine learning approach is widely used in healthcare centers to satisfy the patients, predict the correct diseases, and to improve the patient's health via personalized drugs. AI in healthcare can be used to predict the functions of various organs such a urinary bladder volume, and stroke. It is also being used to accelerate drug discovery methods and supply in a cost-effective manner (Rong et al., 2020). Apart from this, AI plays a vital role in the expert system (ES) that mimics the decision-making ability of a human expert (Patra et al., 2010). ES aims in solving complicated biological problems with the usage of IF-THEN rules rather than using the traditional coding method. The architecture of the expert system is shown in Figure 7.13. ES is widely used in diverse areas of medicine like MYCIN, CADUCEUS, eye, hypertension, pregnancy, leukemia, and several other human diseases to provide the solution for human health. Earlier, the MYCIN system was used for the diagnosis of blood-clotting disease, while CADUCEUS was developed to diagnose thousands of diseases (Oluwafemi et al., 2014).

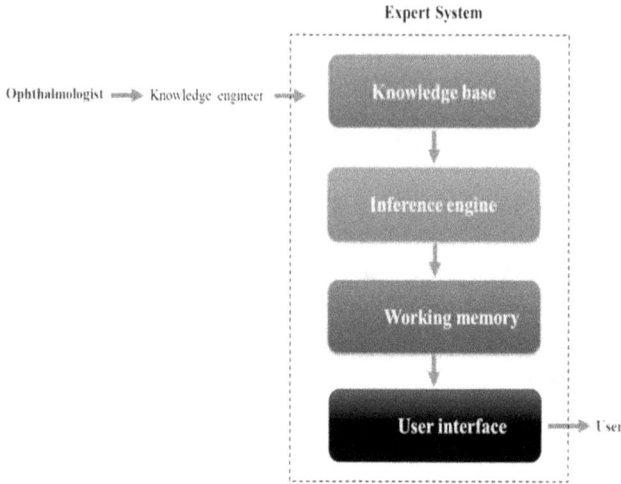

FIGURE 7.13 Architecture of the expert system.

7.4 CASE STUDIES ON AI IN SYSTEMS BIOLOGY

7.4.1 AI TECHNOLOGIES IN SYSTEMS BIOLOGY TOWARDS PHARMACOGENOMICS

In pharmacogenomics, AI technology plays a vital role in converting the accumulated raw data into a readable format. At present, pharmaceutical and nutraceutical industries have started using systems biology and machine learning algorithms to determine the molecular mechanism of the drug thereby reducing the time and cost of the experiment. The development of a novel drug is generally based on clinical studies, electronic medical imaging, medical records, and DNA expression profiling. In hospitals, a huge volume of clinical reports can be analyzed via machine learning algorithms. A case study involves the implementation of AI in systems biology towards pharmacogenomics. For instance, the application of computational tools and machine learning techniques in pharmacogenomics helps in the discovery of a precise drug for cancer treatment with the help of patient details, drug resistance, NGS data, and gene expression profiling. Accurate and efficient drug molecules are being developed by a virtual screening approach. Machine-learning methods and AI technology have been functionalized in diverse stages of virtual screening. There are two stages of virtual screening: (1) ligand-structure based virtual screening and(2) ligand-receptor based binding. Potential AI algorithm generates ligand-structure based virtual screening methods, which are based on non-parametric scoring functions. To identify the exact ligand site, various non-predetermined AI-based scoring functions are utilized (RF-score, ID score, and NN score). Intending to improve the performance of scoring functions in AI technology uses four algorithms: (1) SVM, (2) Bayesian, (3) RF, and (4) DNN methods. Nagarajan et al. (2019) detected the mutants and identified a precise drug target using a computational approach (Figure 7.14).

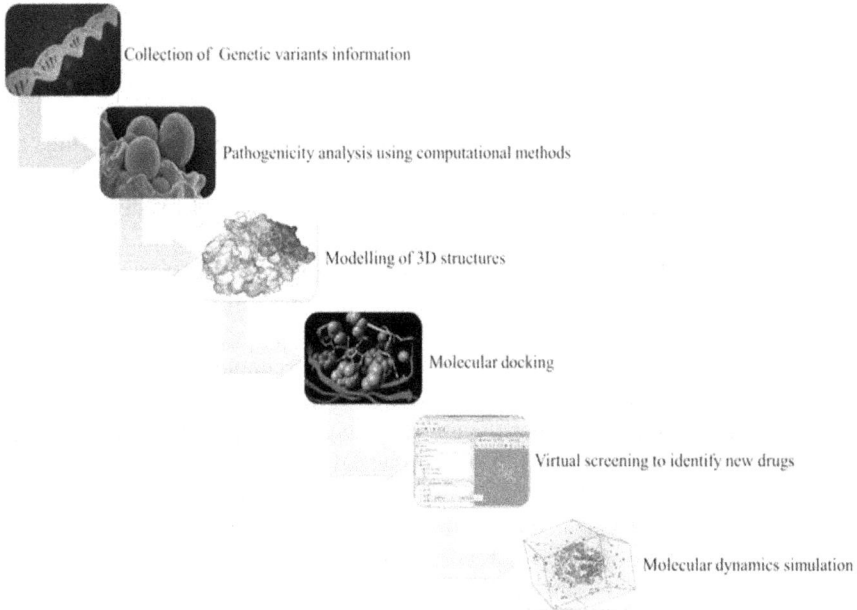

FIGURE 7.14   Steps involved in analyzing the variants and finding a suitable drug for the disease via systems biology approach (modified from Nagarajan et al., 2019; with copyright permission from Hindawi publisher).

7.4.2   AI IN SYSTEMS BIOLOGY FOR CANCER CURE

The incorporation of AI technology in cancer imaging would produce abundant scientific records, which would help the oncologist to speed up the treatment process for life-threatening cancer diseases (Kantarjian and Yu, 2015). In cancer imaging, AI is used to discriminate against normal cells and metastatic cancer cells. AI in medicine brings a societal revolution in healthcare centers by analyzing the key regulatory genes involved in lung, breast, and thyroid cancer. The *Predictive Modeling for Pre-Clinical Screening* mainly focuses on developing novel drugs to treat cancer patients at the pilot-scale. AI technology is also implemented for the discovery of cancer cells and lymph node metastasis in women breast cancers. With the aid of suitable computational models, AI in oncology uses Ordinary Least Square methodology for medical imaging. In silico machine learning approach offers a better vision into the omics concept, next-generation sequencing, molecular dynamics simulation, imaging, and clinical data. Conversely, there are certain limits in designing a machine learning approach for cancer, (1) to access, share, label, and integrate multi-modal data's of diverse types of cancer; (2) to develop AI models for cancer research that can be scaled up using next-generation processors; and (3) to assess complexity and consistency in the AI models. Among various types of cancer, the occurrence of lung cancer is quite predominant in many countries and its mortality rate varies from one nation to the other. The identification of a desired lung cancer type is either by mutations of epidermal growth factor receptor and anaplastic lymphoma receptor tyrosine kinase rearrangements or via sequential mutations of T790 is a serious process in the diagnostic treatment of critical cancer patients with gefitinib, erlotinib, nivolumab, and atezolizumab (Coccia, 2020).

Convolutional Neural Network (CNN) technology is utilized for differentiating the type of cancer like breast, bladder, and lung via complex visual recognition. It also helps the oncologist to detect the type of cancer and provide suitable treatment for the sufferers. During laboratory screening, the performance levels of cancer cells were detected using computational modeling. Depending upon the lung pattern of CT scan (Computerized tomography), CNN's technology can be applied. ImageNet developed by the GoogleNet architecture that would increase the robustness of the biological systems thereby decoding and improving their dissimilar functions. Coudray et al. (2018) observed that DL algorithms can be utilized for automated examination of tumor slides with the help of The Cancer Genome Atlas (TCGA) database. Henceforth, novel AI technology can help pathologists to detect precise gene mutation or cancer subtypes quickly.

7.4.3 Applications of AI for COVID-19 Pandemic

Preventive medicine requires the provision of novel technologies like artificial intelligence (AI), machine learning (ML) approach, Big Data, and the Internet of Things (IoT) to combat today's emerging deadly diseases (Haleem et al., 2020). COVID-19 (Coronavirus) is one such pandemic disease that has a threat to the world. The medical industry is now looking for new technologies that can be used to monitor and control the spread of the COVID-19 pandemic. AI is one such technology that can be implemented to detect the spread of coronavirus, mortality rate, diagnosis, monitoring and it is also useful in controlling the infection (Hu et al., 2020). AI technology can boost the design strategy, medications, and testified data outcomes of the COVID-19 patient. A detailed procedure for AI and non-AI based diagnosis of COVID-19 symptoms is shown in Figure 7.15.

7.5 FUTURE CHALLENGES IN ARTIFICIAL INTELLIGENCE

Artificial intelligence uses computing machines that accomplish the tasks intelligently and expressively. It succeeds in driving robots, filtering mails, medical diagnosing, predicting the weather, and playing a game, etc. (Crevier, 2002). Practitioners and researchers of AI have claimed that machines are working as humans as they can think, feel the response, and have emotions. It accepts data, makes some process, stores, manipulates, and returns the information. Nowadays, it is a great competitor to the human brain (Thomson, 1999). Machines are the simulation of humans where they can talk, walk, and some operations. Artificial Intelligence of any device, computer, robot, or machine that cannot substitute the human and it is preprogrammed (Crevier, 2002). AI has a great challenge in understanding the human brain and mimics it. AI researchers face a lot of

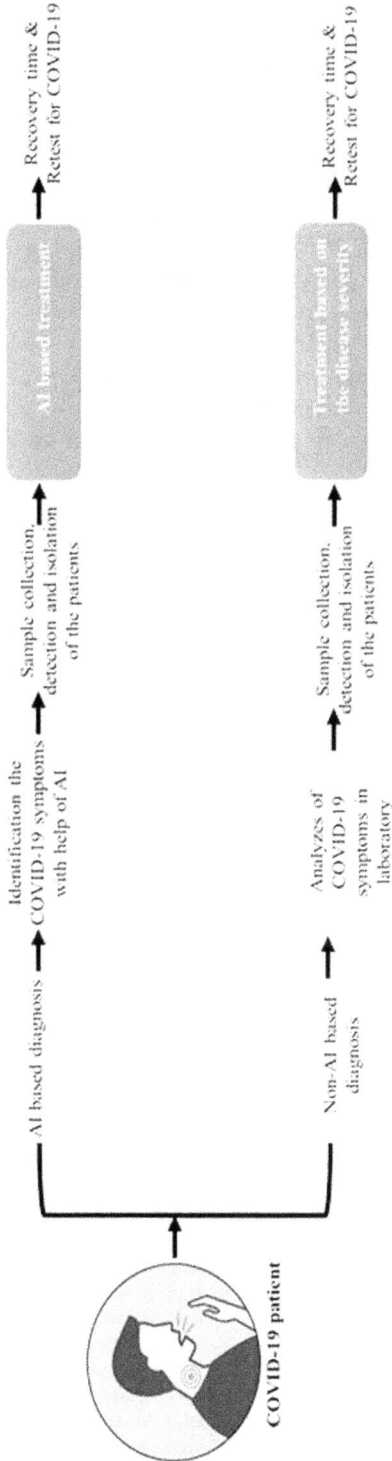

FIGURE 7.15 AI and non-AI-based detection of COVID-19.

encounters in mimicking the human brain and turning it into devices (Tatchell and Bennett, 2009). Artificial Intelligence research is implemented in an expert system, robotics, cybercrime, agriculture, and biomedicine. The expert system is a program that mimics the human in a specific area. MYCIN, an example of an expert system, diagnoses the blood infection. The first expert system was designed in 1970 (Dennet, 2008). Robotics is another application of AI, which is extensively used in science and technology in the manufacture, application, and design (Hunt and Shelley 2009). "Artificially Intelligent Robots can mimic humans in real-life (Perez et al., 2018). A perfect robot has certain abilities like self-evolve, self-diagnose, filtering mails, medical self-repair, sensing, perception, and reasoning, etc." Artificial intelligence has a great challenge due to its direct impact on society. A lot of great outcomes are currently hidden in the future. It is growing with the understanding of the human mind and works in two dimensions (1) it understands the human brain working process and (2) it mimics the human mind artificially.

ACKNOWLEDGMENTS

Our lab is funded by Bharathiar University, UGC-SAP, and DST-FIST. Dr Dhivya. S thanks University Grant Commission Women's Post-Doctoral Fellowship (PDFWM-2015-17-TAM-34021) and Hari Priya. S acknowledges DST-INSPIRE, New Delhi (IF180901) for the fellowship support. We would also like to acknowledge the copyright permissions given by the respective publishers to reproduce the part/modified/full images.

REFERENCES

Altschul, S.F., Gish, W., Miller, W., Myers, E.W., & Lipman, D.J., 1990. Basic local alignment search tool. Journal of Molecular Biology, 215, 403–410.

Angermueller, C., Lee, H. J., Reik, W., & Stegle, O., 2017. DeepCpG: Accurate prediction of single-cell DNA methylation states using deep learning. Genome Biology, 18(1), 67.

Bera, R. K. , 2019. Synthetic Biology, Artificial Intelligence, and Quantum Computing, Synthetic Biology-New Interdisciplinary Science, IntechOpen, pp. 1–28.

Bhasin, H., & Bhatia, S., 2011. Application of genetic algorithms in machine learning. International Journal of Computer Science and Information Technologies, 2(5), 2412–2415.

Coccia, M., 2020. Artificial intelligence technology in oncology: A new technological paradigm. JEL Codes: O32, O33. Technology in Society, 60, 101198.

Coudray, N., Ocampo, P.S., Sakellaropoulos, T., Narula, N., Snuderl, M., Fenyö, D., Moreira, A.L., Razavian, N., & Tsirigos, A., 2018. Classification and mutation prediction from non-small cell lung cancer histopathology images using deep learning. Nature Medicine, 24(10), 1559–1567.

Dennet, D., 2008. Brainchildren: Essays on Designing Minds, MIT Press.

Dubitzky, W., & Azuaje, F., 2004. Artificial Intelligence Methods and Tools for Systems Biology. Computational Biology, vol. 5, Springer Netherlands. eBook ISBN 978-1-4020-2865-6. 10.1007/978-1-4020-5811-0.1568-2684

Gambhire, Akshaya, & Shaikh Mohammad, Bilal N., April 2020. Use of Artificial Intelligence in Agriculture. Proceedings of the 3rd International Conference on

Advances in Science & Technology (ICAST) 2020. Available at SSRN: https://ssrn.com/abstract=3571733 or http://dx.doi.org/10.2139/ssrn.3571733

Haleem, A., Javaid, M., & Vaishya, R., 2020. Effects of COVID 19 pandemic in daily life. Current Medicine Research and Practice.

Hu, Z., Ge, Q., Jin, L., & Xiong, M., 2020. Artificial intelligence forecasting of covid-19 in China. Frontiers in Artificial Intelligence, 3, 41. arXiv preprint arXiv:2002.07112

Hunt, R., & Shelley, J., 2009. Computers and Commonsense, Prentice Hall of India Private Limited: New Delhi.

Kantarjian, H., & Yu, P., 2015. Artificial intelligence, big data, and cancer. JAMA Oncology, 1(5), 573–574. DOI:10.1001/JAMAOncol.2015.1203

Mahmud, M., Kaiser, M.S., Hussain, A., & Vassanelli, S., 2018. Applications of deep learning and reinforcement learning to biological data. IEEE Transactions on Neural Networks and Learning Systems, 29(6), 2063–2079.

Mamoshina, P., Vieira, A., Putin, E., & Zhavoronkov, A., 2016. Applications of deep learning in biomedicine. Molecular Pharmaceutics, 13(5), 1445–1454.

McKevitt, P., & Crevier, D. 2002. AI: The Tumultuous History of the Search for Artificial Intelligence, Basic Books, London and New York, 1993. Pp. xiv+ 386. ISBN 0-465-02997-3. The British Journal for the History of Science, 30(1), 101–121.

Moore, J.H., & Raghavachari, N., 2019. Artificial intelligence based approaches to identify molecular determinants of exceptional health and life span-An interdisciplinary workshop at the National Institute on Aging. Frontiers in Artificial Intelligence, 2, 12.

Nagarajan, N., Yapp, E.K.Y., Le, N.Q.K., Kamaraj, B., Al-Subaie, A.M., & Yeh, H.Y., 2019. Application of computational biology and artificial intelligence technologies in cancer precision drug discovery. BioMed Research International, 12, 8427042. DOI: 10.1155/2019/8427042.

Oluwafemi, J.A., Ayoola, I.O., & Bankole, F., 2014, August. An expert system for diagnosis of blood disorder. Intertnational Journal of Computer Applications, 100(3), 36–40.

Patra, P.S.K., Sahu, D.P., & Mandal, I., 2010. An expert system for the diagnosis of human diseases. International Journal of Computer Applications, 1(13), 71–73.

Perez, J. A., Deligianni, F., Ravi, D., & Yang, G. Z. 2018. Artificial intelligence and robotics. arXiv preprint arXiv:1803.10813, 147.

Rampasek, L., & Goldenberg, A., 2016. Tensorflow: Biology's gateway to deep learning? Cell Systems, 2(1), 12–14.

Rong, G., Mendez, A., Assi, E.B., Zhao, B., & Sawan, M., 2020. Artificial intelligence in healthcare: Review and prediction case studies. Engineering, 6(3)291–301.

Shanmuganathan, Subana., 2016. Artificial neural network modeling: An introduction. Artificial Neural Network Modeling. Springer: Cham, 1–14.

Shukla Shubhendu, S., & Vijay, J., 2013. Applicability of artificial intelligence in different fields of life. International Journal of Scientific Engineering and Research, 1(1), 28–35.

Soding, J., 2017. Big-data approaches to protein structure prediction. Science, 355(6322), 248–249.

Suthaharan, S., 2014. Big data classification: Problems and challenges in network intrusion prediction with machine learning. ACM SIGMETRICS Performance Evaluation Review, 41(4), 70–73.

Tatchell, J., & Bennett, B., 2009. Usborne "Guide to Understanding the Micro". In Watts Lisa (Ed.), Usborne Electronics.

Thomson,R., (Ed.), 1999. Philosophical Logic and Artificial intelligence, Kluver Academic.

Urban, J., Cisar, P., Pautsina, A., Soukup, J., & Barta, A., 2013. Artificial Intelligence in Biology, Technical Computing Prague, 326.

Usman, S.M., & Fong, S., 2017. Epileptic seizures prediction using machine learning methods. Computational and Mathematical Methods in Medicine, 2017, 1–10.

Webb, S., 2018. Deep learning for biology. Nature, 554(7693), 555–557.

Zhu, G., Jiang, B., Tong, L., Xie, Y., Zaharchuk, G., & Wintermark, M., 2019. Applications of deep learning to neuro-imaging techniques. Frontiers in Neurology, 10, 869.

Zou, D., Sun, S., Li, R., Liu, J., Zhang, J., & Zhang, Z., 2015. MethBank: A database integrating next-generation sequencing single-base-resolution DNA methylation programming data. Nucleic Acids Research, 43(D1), D54–D58.

8 Artificial Intelligence Applications in Genetic Disease/Syndrome Diagnosis

P. Vinayaga Moorthi
Department of Human Genetics and Molecular Biology,
Bharathiar University, Coimbatore, India

CONTENTS

OBJECTIVES

Artificial intelligence (AI) applications in this genetic disease and syndrome chapter aims to address the following:

- To trace out the emergence of AI
- To understand the algorithms used for machine or deep learning
- To find out the application of AI involved in disease diagnosis
- To find out the application of AI involved in diagnosis psychiatric disorder
- To list out the AI devices/software approved by Food and Drug administration (FDA)

8.1 INTRODUCTION

Inculcating cerebration in a machine is called artificial intelligence (AI). It uses a set of algorithms to perform better in achieving its goal as a good predictor/evaluator in its assignment. This is due to machine learning (ML) and uses different neural networks for delivering its services (Huang et al., 2015; Hopfield, 1982). With the evolution of advanced AI systems with incredible software, AI now becomes inevitable in electrical and electronic engineering fields (Nguyen et al., 2018; Yang et al., 2018; Chiang and Zhang, 2016; Guo et al., 2016; Alshahrani and Kapetanios, 2016; Kim, 2010; Schaal, 1999). In medicine, AI implementation was started for the early error-free diagnosis and treatment (Yu et al., 2018; Mamoshina et al., 2016; Peng et al., 2010; Thian et al., 2019). So this chapter addresses the involvement of AI in various disease/syndrome diagnoses with different software systems and databases.

8.2 MILESTONES

In history, non-human objects that are performing like human beings were used by people. The Greek god Hephaestus has had mechanical servants (Gera, 2003). It was assumed that robots (mechanical) had been used for protecting the leftovers of Buddha, as pointed out by Lokapannatti (Strong, 2007). A humanoid automata was used by al-Jazari as a waitress in the 12th century (Carbonell et al., 2015), while human automata were created in Japan during the 18–19th century (Carbonell et al., 2015). Alan Turing (1950) recognized computers as a device that could be created with the power of thinking like a human being, and he created a Turing test named after him to find out the capability of computers to mimic human intelligence (Searle, 1982; Russell and Norvig, 2003). In 1956, the term artificial intelligence (AI) was created and the era of AI was unveiled at the end of the Second World War (Russell and Norvig, 2010).

8.3 ALGORITHMS

The development of the oldest algorithms, Hebbian learning, dated back to 1949 (Hebb, 1949) and was originated as the outcome of inspiration from the neuronal architecture of the brain. It leads to the formation of a single layer artificial neural network, the perception (Rosenblatt, 1958), and now subsequently, multilayers are used. In AI, computers can think and take decisions according to the situation. It was due to Machine Learning (ML) and Deep Learning (DL) (Huang et al., 2015). ML is an algorithm that has the potential to be trained and revolutionize through experiences. It induces the systems to decide with advanced algorithms based on the already fed information. The two types of learning algorithms are Supervised and Unsupervised.

Supervised learning algorithms are performing their activity/analysis on unknown/unlabeled data based on the experience it has on previously known/labeled data hence they are used for sorting out data as 1, -1, or 0 or for regression. Logistic regression is an AI algorithm (Schmidhuber, 2015; Hosmer et al., 2013; Ng, 2000; Pregibon, 1981; Russell and Bohannon, 2015). Similarly, K-nearest Neighbor (KNN) algorithm helps solve problems of classification and regression. It identifies data based on its close relationship. With similar applications to the KNN, the Support Vector Machine (SVM) algorithm helps in predicting the line (Hyperplane) of the data that separate the data into two (towardsdatascience.com, 2020). Similarly, the deep learning algorithms have Artificial Neural Network (ANN) and Convolutional Neural Network (ConvNet/CNN) essential for AI. Sigmoid neuron (Nielsen, 2015), the man-made neuron used now, are the components and arranged as interconnected input, hidden and output layer to form ANN (Von Neumann and Kurzweil, 2012; Hebb, 2002; Olazaran, 1996; Minsky and Papert, 1998; McCulloch and Pitts, 1943). Training of ANN is an essential process and is met with gradient descent algorithms to map the data through processing as a batch of training and testing (Nielsen, 2015). This trained ANN is following forward pass, the information processing mechanism, and hence become an inevitable tool for regression analysis. Similarly, the CNN arrangement is similar to that of the architecture of the brain neuron (Nielsen, 2015). In CNN, the number of neurons in the layers from the input to hidden is decreasing, and due to which it performs well with complex data such as problems in recognition of speech and images.

8.4 ARTIFICIAL INTELLIGENCE IN THE DIAGNOSIS OF GENETIC DISEASES

8.4.1 CANCER

In cancer, distinguishing tumor severity based data was obtained using preprocessed (trained) ANN (Jhajharia et al., 2016). Based on its interpretation ability certain elastic nets constituted with a lasso and ridge regression have been used for pointing out the biomarkers in cancer (Garnett et al., 2012; Barretina et al., 2012; Shen et al., 2011) and one such member is elastic-net-based prognosis prediction (ENCAPP) algorithm (Das et al., 2015). Similarly, data of transcriptome was well utilized by ANN-based Cox-nnet for prognosis (Ching et al., 2018).

A DL impregnated national lung cancer screening trial (NLST) data set revealed its 94.4% accuracy in Computerized Tomography (CT) image analysis and was better than radiologists (Ardila et al., 2019). A DL algorithm successfully used the image of the tissue slides of non-small cell lung cancer and precisely distinguished Adenocarcinoma from squamous cell carcinoma which helped analyze the existence of mutation (Coudray et al., 2018). Involvement of AI in the generation of data for the prognosis of ovarian cancer patients evidenced by the work of Enshaei et al. (2015). A regression model (DL-Cox proportional hazard (DL-CPH)) can collect all essential biomarker information from the CT images of one type of epithelial ovarian cancer (high-grade serous ovarian cancer) and able find out its recurrence in patients (Wang et al., 2019).

In breast cancer, Decision Tree (DT) rules (Weighted fuzzy DT (wFDT)) have been implemented for survival analysis (Khan et al., 2008; Chi et al., 2007). Breast cancer predicting DNN (multimodel DNN- MDNNMD) was suggested by Sun et al. (2018). Similarly, LYmph Node Assistant (LYNA) (DL algorithm), diminished the errors in the identification of breast cancer from biopsy samples (Sentinel lymph node) (Liu et al., 2018). Similarly, ANN was employed in prostate cancer diagnosis has diminished the errors that occurred in the positive cases (false positive) with 90% sensitivity (Stephan et al., 2002). In prostate cancer, XmasNet programmed by Liu et al. (2017) outperformed other models in lesion classification with 84% accuracy. DCNN bound DL has learned better differentiation criteria in distinguishing prostate cancer patients from its benign condition cases (Wang et al., 2017). In breast cancer, the DeepSEA transcription factor binding classifier unravels the close interaction of risk locus (SNP: rs4784227) and FOXA1 (Cowper-Sal·lari et al., 2012).

CNN outperformed experts in distinguishing skin cancer (LeCun et al., 2015). ML-based quantitative texture analysis (QTA) has higher visibility and reveals the distinguishing marks between subclinical pheochromocytoma and lipid-poor adenoma (LPA) besides adrenal incidentaloma (Yi et al., 2018). Similarly, the J48 classifier outperformed experts in adrenal lesion diagnosis with Magnetic Resonance Imaging (MRI) (unenhanced) (Romeo et al., 2018). In thyroid cancer, deep CNN (DCNN) has used images of ultrasounds for precise identification (Li et al., 2019). CNN-computer-aided detection (CNN-CAD) was adopted for endoscopic resection screening in patients as well as the depth of the invasion using images of endoscopy (Mori et al., 2019). Similarly, DeepSEA, a DL algorithm using the data of the chromatin profile is supporting the visualization of the observable effect of intron specific variations. In diseases like α-thalassemia, the DeepSEA transcription factor binding classifier identified the change in the nucleotide base (C→T) facilitates the interaction with GATA1 (De Gobbi et al., 2006).

8.4.2 Diabetes

AI can be applied to diagnose and investigate diabetes (Islam et al., 2020; Williams et al., 2020; Oka et al., 2019; Chikh et al., 2012). In diabetes diagnosis, Islam et al. (2020) proposed a DANN and ultra-wideband (UWB) method for measuring the glucose present in the blood without collecting it and its accuracy was also around 88%. An AI-coupled automated nutritional intervention was also used by Oka et al. (2019) in diabetic patients (Type 2 Diabetes) for glucose management/control. Similarly, Williams et al. (2020) DL algorithm was explored for estimating the nerve damage (neuropathy) due to diabetes by using the advanced microscopic (corneal confocal) images. Chikh et al. (2012) used, MAIRS2, a modified artificial immune recognition system (AIRS)2 for accurately classifying diabetes for detection with 89.10% compared to its AIRS2 with 82.69%.

8.5 ARTIFICIAL INTELLIGENCE IN THE DIAGNOSIS OF SYNDROMES

In Down syndrome (DS), the SVM algorithm using triangular kernel function accurately distinguished the left and right loop with 95% and 96.7%, respectively (Wojtowicz and Wajs, 2012). Similarly, a Bayesian neural network (BNN) was suggested for the identification of Turner syndrome (TS) after childbirth (Filho, 2013). An ANN, the multilayer (three layers) perceptron (MLP) has used data of infants with and without the developmental disorder (DD) and identified DD with 93.2% accuracy and was comparatively higher than LR with 92.7% accuracy (Soleimani et al., 2013). The ANN, particularly multilayer, also was involved in the screening of chromosomes (non-invasive method) and found the abnormalities with 85.1% accuracy while it was 42.9% for TS prediction (Nicolaides, 2004). An ANN with metaphase stage chromosome classification was created by Wang et al. (2009). In a study by Catic et al. (2018) ANN was used for the classification of syndromes such as Patau, Down, Klinefelter, Turner, and Edward syndrome based on the data of patients' maternal serum, ultrasound, and their demography. The sensitivity of their neural networks such as feedforward and feedback in these syndrome diagnoses was 92% and 99%, respectively.

In syndrome diagnosis, facial features play a key role in diagnosis (Basel-Vanagaite et al., 2016; Rai et al., 2015; Ferry et al., 2014; Hart and Hart, 2009). In facial recognition, DeepFace (DCNN) involvement is on par with humans (Taigman et al., 2014). With DCNN, approaches and methods have been proposed to use the facial features for the classification using the criteria (age and gender) (Levi and Hassner, 2015) as well as expressions like a smile (Liu et al., 2015). A Deep-Gestalt framework (Liehr et al., 2017) that uses the application of Face2Gene delivers the diversity of disease phenotypes and capable of identifying syndromes of genetic origin. Since their outcomes from the facial images are clear, they are supporting the clinical setting (Hadj-Rabia et al., 2017; Basel-Vanagaite et al., 2016).

8.6 ARTIFICIAL INTELLIGENCE IN THE DIAGNOSIS OF PSYCHIATRIC DISORDERS

Psychiatric research is one important area in health science. It is now enabled with advanced systems for collecting and analysis of data from patients. One such well-advanced technology is AI (Esteva et al., 2019; Zhang et al., 2018; Dwyer et al., 2018; Sarma et al., 2018; Stead, 2018; Xia et al., 2017; Gao et al., 2017).

8.6.1 DEPRESSION

As proposed, the visual and vocal expressions were used as a preliminary tool by AI systems for measuring the Beck Depression Inventory-II Score (BDI-II) which is an essential parameter for understanding the depression severity (Jan et al., 2018). Separation of the patient with normal and depression was possible with 67% accuracy in linear discriminant analysis using EEG data (Field and Diego, 2008) while 70% and 83.3% distinguishing ability was marked with SVM and logistic regression (LR) using EEG data respectively (Bisch et al., 2016; Iosifescu et al., 2009). The integrated mental-disorder genome score (iMEGES) constructed with Tensorflow, the ML base, and DNN was used to generate a score with preference to disorders (psychiatric) (Khan et al., 2018).

8.6.2 ALZHEIMER'S DISEASE

Depth-supervised adaptive 3 Dimensional CNN (3D CNN) has the potential to evaluate the MRI image of Alzheimer's Disease (AD) patients by using a sequential parameter obtained from features of AD (Hosseini-Asl et al., 2018). Koyamada et al. (2015) have constructed a decoder, the subject-transfer decoder, based on deep neural network (DNN) and it outperformed SVM in decoding. AI is now supervising and evaluating the EEG data, i.e., graph using its various models (Hosseinifard et al., 2013; Hannesdóttir et al., 2010; Avram et al., 2010; Thibodeau et al., 2006). Similarly, Haenssle et al. (2018) proved better diagnostic intelligence in CNN than dermatologists. In brain image (MRI) analysis, the application of DL algorithms made significant improvements in image visualization (virtually) and diminished the usage dose of gadolinium since it has an impact on the brain and renal system (Gong et al., 2018; Guo et al., 2018).

8.6.3 AUTISM SPECTRUM DISORDER

DL algorithms are smart enough to perceive the brain functional/activation pattern to diagnose the autism spectrum disorder (ASD) in patients (Heinsfeld et al., 2018). In ASD as well as in spinal muscular atrophy (Xiong et al., 2015), the ML algorithm, Human Splicing Code, has been actively involved in the precise classification of a genetic variant (missense variant) that causes the disease even in the intron.

8.6.4 ANXIETY

A DT algorithm applied Preschool Age Psychiatric Assessment (PAPA) and predicted at 96% the future occurrence of generalized and separation anxiety disorders (SAD) school children (Carpenter et al., 2016). Similarly, another DL algorithm measured the neural damage from the appearance of the retina (fundus photograph) and helps to foresee the condition of optic nerve damage (glaucoma) (Medeiros et al., 2019).

8.6.5 PARKINSON'S DISEASE

In Parkinson's disease patients, cloud-coupled ML mobile applications have been used for assessing the movement of muscles (motor function) and gravity of symptoms (Pan et al., 2015; Stamate et al., 2017). An ML integrated Cloud – unified Parkinson disease rating scale (UPDRS) application (Stamate et al., 32) used in mobile was used for collecting the information about patients involuntary hand movements, walking manner, etc. which are playing a key role in understanding the condition of the patient that gives the outcome the medication and decisions on future treatment (Fisher et al., 2016; Hammerla et al., 2015). Algorithms (ML and DL) (Hammerla et al., 2015) have accurately (84–90%) discriminated the Parkinson disease manifestations such as dyskinesia and bradykinesia (Eskofier et al., 2016; Memedi et al., 2015). In addition to the application of AI algorithms for the diagnosis of different diseases, there are method/approaches (Deconvolution) were also proposed by the researchers (Zhang et al., 2019; Kindermans et al., 2017; Springenberg et al., 2014) to get precise information on the different neural networks (Zhang et al., 2019; Springenberg et al., 2014), how they are the processing/ analyzing the image information (Kindermans et al., 2017) and which part of the layers from which output normally are given.

8.7 ARTIFICIAL INTELLIGENCE IN OTHER DISEASE DIAGNOSIS

8.7.1 INFECTIOUS DISEASE

According to Agrebi and Larbi (2020), ML (High-definition care platform (HDCP)) is used by hospitals (University of Lowa) for curbing the occurrence of infection in the surgical site (74%). SVM and High-Resolution Melt (HRM) were used for the precise identification of bacteria (Fraley et al., 2016). SVM-based Digital In-line Holographic Microscopy (DIHM) information on red blood cells (RBC) was useful for the identification of cells (RBC) infected with malaria (Go et al., 2018). The seasonal autoregressive moving average (SARIMA) and neural network autoregression (NNAR) are used in South Africa for the occurrence of tuberculosis (Walsh et al., 2017). A chest radiograph was also used as a tool by deep learning neural networks for tuberculosis characteristics identification (Lakhani and Sundaram, 2019).

8.7.2 LUNG AND BRAIN DISEASE

The CNN-enabled smoker's thoracic CT helps in identifying their mortality rate as well as acute respiratory distress (ARD) (González et al., 2018). The disease that affects the air sac/interstitium of the lung called infiltrative lung disease was also diagnosed with CNN (Walsh et al., 2016). CNN was given exercises to distinguish the disease of the lung affecting the interstitium called fibrotic lung disease from reports of the CT scans (Walsh et al., 2018). Algorithms designed by Prevedello et al. (2017) and Chen et al. (2016) with AI used CT information for the identification of cerebral hemorrhage and cerebral edema, respectively. Similarly, CT used by SVM estimated the possibility of occurrence of a cerebral hemorrhage in ischemic stroke patients in post thrombolytic therapy (Bentley et al., 2014).

8.8 FOOD AND DRUG ADMINISTRATION APPROVAL AND GUIDELINES

For the implementation and maintenance of AI in the medical field, no regulatory standards were framed and implemented (Yaeger et al., 2019) while FDA published a discussion paper related to AI-related regulatory framework (US Food and Drug

Administration, 2019). Yaeger et al. (2019) listed out the FDA approved AI-enhanced/enriched software/platforms for clinical diagnosis/decision and are given below: In 2018, FDA has given clearance to AI enriched software, Viz Large Vessel Occlusion (LVO) that verifies the angiogram of CT of one type of ischemic stroke (Embolic stroke) (Yaeger et al., 2019). AI-based malignant tissue identifying ProFound AI.

8.9 CONCLUSION

The learning/training knowledge, upgrading ability through algorithms, information-based analysis using unique codes are the reason behind the AI dispersal and existence in a variety of fields. The information in the form of images or data that are inculcated inside the AI algorithms made AI precise in prediction on a prior experience basis compared to the experts of different fields. With the initial implementation in different sectors, (AI) needs to be validated and surveillance should be done for a longer time for understanding its real nature in different fields where AI is applied. Extending the boundaries of AI applications, data security and other protection measures need to be considered. To date, its application, perhaps, is found applicable for a considerable number of diseases while its application in other genetic, developmental, and rare diseases may help the people in the society to get an early diagnosis and live a healthy life.

REFERENCES

Agrebi, S., Larbi, A., 2020. Use of artificial intelligence in infectious diseases. Chapter-18. Artificial Intelligence in Precision Health, 415–438. 10.1016/B978-0-12-817133-2.00018-5

Alshahrani, S., Kapetanios, E., 2016. Are deep learning approaches suitable for natural language processing? In: Métais, E., Meziane, F., Saraee, M., Sugumaran, V., Vadera, S., (Eds). Natural Language Processing and Information Systems. Cham: Springer. 343–349 pp.

Ardila, D., Kiraly, A.P., Bharadwaj, S., Choi, B., Reicher, J.J., Peng, L., Tse, D., Etemadi, M., Ye, W., Corrado, G., Naidich, D.P., Shetty, S., 2019. End-to-end lung cancer screening with three-dimensional deep learning on low-dose chest computed tomography. Nature Medicine 25, 954–961. 10.1038/s41591-019-0447-x.

Avram, J., Baltes, F.R., Miclea, M., Miu, A.C., 2010. Frontal EEG activation asymmetry reflects cognitive biases in anxiety: evidence from an emotional face Stroop task. Applied Psychophysiology and Biofeedback 35(4), 285–292.

Barretina, J., Caponigro, G., Stransky, N., et al., 2012. The Cancer Cell Line Encyclopedia enables predictive modelling of anticancer drug sensitivity. Nature 483, 603.

Basel-Vanagaite, L., Wolf, L., Orin, M., Larizza, L., Gervasini, C., Krantz, I., Deardoff, M., 2016. Recognition of the Cornelia de Lange syndrome phenotype with facial dysmorphology novel analysis. Clinical Genetics 89(5), 557–563.

Bentley, P., Ganesalingam, J., Carlton, J.A., et al., 2014. Prediction of stroke thrombolysis outcome using CT brain machine learning. Neuroimage: Clinical 4, 635–640

Bisch, J., Kreifelts, B., Bretscher, J., Wildgruber, D., Fallgatter, A., Ethofer, T., 2016. Emotion perception in adult attention-deficit hyperactivity disorder. Journal of Neural Transmission 123(8), 961–970.

Carbonell, J., Sánchez-Esguevillas, A., Carro, B., 2015. Assessing emerging issues. The external and internal approach. Futures 73, 12–21.

Carpenter, K.L.H., Sprechmann, P., Calderbank, R., Sapiro, G., Egger, H.L., 2016. Quantifying risk for anxiety disorders in preschool children: a machine learning approach. PLoS ONE 11(11), e0165524.

Catic, A., Gurbeta, L., Kurtovic-Kozaric, A., Mehmedbasic, S., Badnjevic, A., 2018. Application of Neural Networks for classification of Patau, Edwards, Down, Turner and Klinefelter Syndrome based on first trimester maternal serum screening data, ultrasonographic findings and patient demographics. BMC Medical Genomics 11, 19.

Chen, Y., Dhar, R., Heitsch, L., et al., 2016. Automated quantification of cerebral edema following hemispheric infarction: application of a machine-learning algorithm to evaluate CSF shifts on serial head CTs. Neuroimage: Clinical 12, 673–680.

Chi, C.L., Street,W.N., Wolberg, W.H., 2007. Application of artificial neural network-based survival analysis on two breast cancer data sets. AMIA Annual Symposium Proceedings, American Medical Informatics Association, 130 pp.

Chiang, M., Zhang, T., 2016. Fog and IoT: an overview of research opportunities. IEEE Internet Things Journal 3(6), 854–864.

Chikh, M.A., Saidi, M., Settouti, N., 2012. Diagnosis of diabetes diseases using an Artificial Immune Recognition System2 (AIRS2) with fuzzy K-nearest neighbor. Journal of Medical Systems 36, 2721–2729.

Ching, T., Zhu, X., Garmire, L.X., 2018. Cox-nnet: an artificial neural network method for prognosis prediction of high-throughput omics data. PLoS Computational Biology 14, e1006076.

Coudray, N., Ocampo, P.S., Sakellaropoulos, T., et al., 2018. Classification and mutation prediction from non-small cell lung cancer histopathology images using deep learning. Nature Medicine 24(10), 1559–1567. http://www.ncbi.nlm.nih.gov/pubmed/30224757

Cowper-Sal·lari, R., et al. 2012. Breast cancer risk-associated SNPs modulate the affinity of chromatin for FOXA1 and alter gene expression. Nature Genetics 44, 1191–1198.

Das, J., Gayvert, K.M., Bunea, F., et al. 2015. ENCAPP: elastic-net-based prognosis prediction and biomarker discovery for human cancers. BMC Genomics 16, 263.

De Gobbi, M., et al. 2006. A regulatory SNP causes a human genetic disease by creating a new transcriptional promoter. Science 312, 1215–1217.

Dwyer, D.B., Falkai, P., Koutsouleris, N., 2018. Machine learning approaches for clinical psychology and psychiatry. Annual Review of Clinical Psychology 14, 91–118.

Enshaei, A., Robson, C.N., Edmondson, R.J., 2015. Artificial intelligence systems as prognostic and predictive tools in ovarian cancer, Annals of Surgical Oncology 22, 3970–3975.

Eskofier, B.M., Lee, S.I., Daneault, J.F., Golabchi, F.N., Ferreira-Carvalho, G., Vergara-Diaz, G., Sapienza, S., Costante, G., Klucken, J., Kautz, T., et al., 2016. Recent machine learning advancements in sensor-based mobility analysis: deep learning for Parkinson's disease assessment. Proceedings of the Annual International Conference of the IEEE Engineering in Medicine and Biology Society, 655–658 pp.

Esteva, A., Robicquet, A., Ramsundar, B., Kuleshov, V., DePristo, M., Chou, K., et al., 2019. A guide to deep learning in healthcare. Nature Medicine 25, 24–29.

Ferry, Q., Steinberg, J., Webber, C., FitzPatrick, D.R., Ponting, C.P., Zisserman, A., Nellåker, C., 2014. Diagnostically relevant facial gestalt information from ordinary photos. Elife 3, e02020.

Field, T., Diego, M., 2008. Maternal depression effects on infant frontal EEG asymmetry. International Journal of Neuroscience 118(8), 1081–1108.

Filho, H.P.L., 2013. Applicability of data mining technique using Bayesians network in diagnosis of genetic diseases. International Journal of Advanced Computer Science and Applications 4(1), 1–4.

Fisher, J.M., Hammerla, N.Y., Ploetz, T., Andras, P., Rochester, L., Walker, R.W., 2016. Unsupervised home monitoring of Parkinson's disease motor symptoms using body-worn accelerometers. Parkinson and Related Disorder 33, 44–50.

Fraley, S. I., Athamanolap, P., Masek, B. J., Hardick, J., Carroll, K. C., Hsieh, Y-H., Rothman, R. E., Gaydos, C. A., Wang, T-H., Yang, S., 2016. Nested machine learning facilitates increased sequence content for large-scale automated high resolution melt genotyping. Scientific Reports 6, 19218.

Gao, H., Yin, Z., Cao, Z., Zhang, L., 2017. Developing an agent-based drug model to investigate the synergistic effects of drug combinations. Molecules 22 (12), 209.

Garnett, M.J., Edelman, E., Heidorn, S., et al., 2012. Systematic identification of genomic markers of drug sensitivity in cancer cells. Nature 483, 570.

Gera, D.L., 2003. Ancient Greek Ideas on Speech, Language, and Civilization. Oxford University Press.

Go, T., Kim, J.H., Byeon, H., Lee, S.J., 2018. Machine learning-based in-line holographic sensing of unstained malaria-infected red blood cells. Journal of Biophotonics 11 (9), e201800101.

Gong, E., Pauly, J.M., Wintermark, M., et al., 2018. Deep learning enables reduced gadolinium dose for contrast-enhanced brain MRI. Journal of Magnetic Resonance Imaging 48(2), 330–340.

González, G., Ash, S.Y., Vegas-Sánchez-Ferrero, G., Onieva Onieva, J., Rahaghi, F.N., Ross, J.C., Díaz, A., San José Estépar, R., Washko, G.R., 2018. COPDGene and ECLIPSE Investigators, Disease staging and prognosis in smokers using deep learning in chest computed tomography. American Journal of Respiratory and Critical Care 197, 193–203. 10.1164/rccm.201705-0860OC.

Guo, B.J., Yang, Z.L., Zhang, L.J., 2018. Gadolinium deposition in brain: current scientific evidence and future perspectives. Frontiers in Molecular Neuroscience 11, 335. http://www.ncbi.nlm.nih.gov/pubmed/30294259.

Guo, Y., Liu, Y., Oerlemans, A., Lao, S., Wu, S., Lew, M.S. Deep learning for visual understanding: a review. Neurocomputing 2016;187:27–48.

Hadj-Rabia, S., Schneider, H., Navarro, E., Klein, O., Kirby, N., Huttner, K., Wolf, L., Orin, M., Wohlfart, S., Bodemer, C., et al., 2017. Automatic recognition of the XLHED phenotype from facial images. American Journal of Medical Genetics Part A 173(9), 2408–2414.

Haenssle, H.A., Fink, C., Schneiderbauer, R., Toberer, F., Buhl, T., Blum, A., Kalloo, A., Hassen, A.B.H., Thomas, L., Enk, A., Uhlmann, L., 2018. Reader study level, I.I.G. level, Man against machine: diagnostic performance of a deep learning convolutional neural network for dermoscopic melanoma recognition in comparison to 58 dermatologists. Annals of Oncology 29, 1836–1842.

Hammerla, N.Y., Fisher, J.M., Andras, P., Rochester, L., Walker, R., Plötz, T., 2015. PD disease state assessment in naturalistic environments using deep learning. Proceedings of the Twenty-Ninth AAAI Conference on Artificial Intelligence, 1742–1475 pp.

Hannesdóttir, D.K., Doxie, J., Bell, M.A., Ollendick, T.H., Wolfe, C.D., 2010. A longitudinal study of emotion regulation and anxiety in middle childhood: associations with frontal EEG asymmetry in early childhood. Developmental Psychobiology 52(2), 197–204.

Hart, T., Hart, P., 2009. Genetic studies of craniofacial anomalies: clinical implications and applications. Orthodontics and Craniofacial Research 12(3), 212–220.

Hebb, D.O., 1949. The Organization of Behavior. Hoboken: John Wiley and Sons.

Hebb, D.O., 2002. The Organization of Behavior: A Neuropsychological Theory. Mahwah, NJ: L. Erlbaum Associates. 335 pp.

Heinsfeld, A.S., Franco, A.R., Craddock, R.C., Buchweitz, A., Meneguzzi, F., 2018. Identification of autism spectrum disorder using deep learning and the ABIDE data set. Neuroimage: Clinical 17, 16–23.

Hopfield, J.J., 1982. Neural networks and physical systems with emergent collective computational abilities. Proceedings of the National Academy of Sciences USA 79(8), 2554–2558.

Hosmer Jr, D.W., Lemeshow, S., Sturdivant, R.X., 2013. Applied Logistic Regression. 3rd ed. Toronto: John Wiley and Sons, Inc.

Hosseini-Asl, E., Ghazal, M., Mahmoud, A., Aslantas, A., Shalaby, A.M., Casanova, M.F., et al., 2018. Alzheimer's disease diagnostics by a 3D deeply supervised adaptable convolutional network. Frontiers in Bioscience 23, 584–596.

Hosseinifard, B., Moradi, M.H., Rostami, R., 2013. Classifying depression patients and normal subjects using machine learning techniques and nonlinear features from EEG signal. Computer Methods and Programs in Biomedicine 109(3), 339–345.

https://towardsdatascience.com/support-vector-machine-introduction-to-machine-learning-algorithms-934a444fca47, 2.12.2020

Huang, G., Huang, G.B., Song, S., You, K., 2015. Trends in extreme learning machines: a review. Neural Networks 61, 32–48.

Iosifescu, D.V., Greenwald, S., Devlin, P., Mischoulon, D., Denninger, J.W., Alpert, J.E., et al., 2009. Frontal EEG predictors of treatment outcome in major depressive disorder. European Neuropsychopharmacology 19(11), 772–777.

Islam, M., Ali, M.S., Shoumy, N.J., Khatun, S., Karim, M.S.A., Bari, B.S., 2020. Non-invasive blood glucose concentration level estimation accuracy using ultra-wide band and artificial intelligence. SN Applied Sciences 2, 278. 10.1007/s42452-01 9-1884-3

Jan, A., Meng, H.Y., Gaus, Y.F.B.A., Zhang, F., 2018. Artificial intelligent system for automatic depression level analysis through visual and vocal expressions. IEEE Transaction on Cognitive and Developmental System 10(3), 668–680.

Jhajharia, S., Varshney, H.K., Verma, S., Kumar, R., 2016. A neural network based breast cancer prognosis model with PCA processed features, B.U. Department of Computer Engineering, Jaipur, India 304022. 2016 International Conference on Advances in Computing, Communications, and Informatics (ICACCI), IEEE, Jaipur, India, 1896–1901 pp.

Khan, A., Liu, Q., Wang, K., 2018. iMEGES: integrated mental-disorder GEnome score by deep neural network for prioritizing the susceptibility genes for mental disorders in personal genomes. BMC Bioinformatics 19, 501.

Khan, S.H.U., Choi, J.P., et al., 2008. wFDT weighted fuzzy decision trees for prognosis of breast cancer survivability. Proceedings of the 7th Australasian Data Mining Conference, Australian Computer Society, 141–152 pp.

Kim, T.H., 2010. Emerging approach of natural language processing in opinion mining: a review. In: Tomar, G.S., Grosky, W.I., Kim, T.H., Mohammed, S., Saha, S.K., (Eds). Ubiquitous Computing and Multimedia Applications. Berlin: Springer. 121–128 pp.

Kindermans, P.J., Schütt, K.T., Alber, M., Müller, K.R., Erhan, D., Kim, B., et al., 2017. Learning how to explain neural networks: PatternNet and PatternAttribution. https://arxiv.org/pdf/1705.05598.pdf.

Koyamada, S., Shikauchi, Y., Nakae, K., Koyama, M., Ishii, S., 2015. Deep learning of fMRI big data: a novel approach to subject-transfer decoding. https://arxiv.org/pdf/1502.00093.pdf.

Lakhani, P., Sundaram, B., 2019. Deep learning at chest radiography: automated classification of pulmonary tuberculosis by using convolutional neural networks. Radiology 284(2), 574–582. 10.1148/radiol.2017162326

LeCun, Y., Bengio, Y., Hinton, G., 2015. Deep learning. Nature 521, 436–444.

Levi, G., Hassner, T., 2015. Age and gender classification using convolutional neural networks. Proceedings of the IEEE Conference on Computer Vision and Pattern Recognition Workshops, 34–42 pp.

Li, X., Zhang, S., Zhang, Q., Wei, X., Pan, Y., Zhao, J., Xin, X., Qin, C., Wang, X., Li, J., Yang, F., Zhao, Y., Yang, M., Wang, Q., Zheng, Z., et al., 2019. Diagnosis of thyroid cancer using deep convolutional neural network models applied to sonographic images: a retrospective, multicohort, diagnostic study. The Lancet Oncology 20, 193–201.

Liehr, T., Acquarola, N., Pyle, K., St-Pierre, S., Rinholm, M., Bar, O., Wilhelm, K., Schreyer, I., 2017. Next generation phenotyping in Emanuel and Pallister Killian syndrome using computer-aided facial dysmorphology analysis of 2D photos. Clinical Genetics 93(2), 378–381.

Liu, S., Zheng, H., Feng, Y., Li, W., 2017. Prostate cancer diagnosis using deep learning with 3D multi parametric MRI. Proceedings SPIE 10134, Medical Imaging 2017: Computer-Aided Diagnosis, 1013428. 10.1117/12.2277121

Liu, Y., Kohlberger, T., Norouzi, M., Dahl, G.E., Smith, J.L., Mohtashamian, A., Olson, N., Peng, L.H., Hipp, J.D., Stumpe, M.C., 2018. Artificial intelligence-based breast cancer nodal metastasis detection. Archives of Pathology and Laboratory Medicine 143(7), 859–868. 10.5858/arpa.2018-0147-OA

Liu, Z., Luo, P., Wang, X., Tang, X., 2015. Deep learning face attributes in the wild. Proceedings of the IEEE International Conference on Computer Vision, 3730–3738 pp.

Mamoshina, P., Vieira, A., Putin, E., Zhavoronkov, A., 2016. Applications of deep learning in biomedicine. Molecular Pharmaceutics 13(5), 1445–1454.

McCulloch, W.S., Pitts, W., 1943. A logical calculus of the ideas immanent in nervous activity. Bulletin of Mathematical Biophysics 5(4), 115–133.

Medeiros, F.A., Jammal, A.A., Thompson, A.C., 2019. From machine to machine: an OCT trained deep learning algorithm for objective quantification of glaucomatous damage in fundus photographs. Ophthalmology 4, 513–521.

Memedi, M., Sadikov, A., Groznik, V., Žabkar, J., Možina, M., Bergquist, F., Johansson, A., Haubenberger, D., Nyholm, D., 2015. Automatic spiral analysis for objective assessment of motor symptoms in Parkinson's disease. Sensors (Basel) 15(9), 23727–23744.

Minsky, M., Papert, S., 1998. Perceptrons: An Introduction to Computational Geometry. Expanded ed. Cambridge, MA: MIT Press.

Mori, Y., Berzin, T.M., Kudo, S.E., 2019. Artificial intelligence for early gastric cancer: early promise and the path ahead. Gastrointestinal Endoscopy 89, 816–817.

Ng, A., 2000. Linear Regression, CS229 Lecture Notes: Part G. 1–30. https://see.stanford.edu/materials/aimlcs229/cs229-notes1.pdf.

Nguyen, H., Kieu, L.M., Wen, T., Cai, C., 2018. Deep learning methods in transportation domain: a review. IET Intelligent Transport System 12(9), 998–1004.

Nicolaides, K., 2004. The 11–13+6 Weeks Scan. London: Fetal Medicine Foundation.

Nielsen, M., 2015. Neural Networks and Deep Learning. Determination Press. 224 pp.

Oka, R., Nomura, A., Yasugi, A., Kometani, M., 2019. Study protocol for the effects of artificial intelligence (ai)-supported automated nutritional intervention on glycemic control in patients with type 2 diabetes mellitus. Diabetes Therapy 10, 1151–1161.

Olazaran, M., 1996. A sociological study of the official history of the perceptrons controversy. Social Studies of Science 26(3), 611–659.

Pan, D., Dhall, R., Lieberman, A., Petitti, D.B., 2015. A mobile cloud-based Parkinson's disease assessment system for home-based monitoring. JMIR mHealth uHealth 3(1), e29.

Peng, Y., Zhang, Y., Wang, L., 2010. Artificial intelligence in biomedical engineering and informatics: an introduction and review. Artificial Intelligence in Medicine 48(2–3), 71–73.

Pregibon, D., 1981. Logistic regression diagnostics. Annals of Statistics 9(4), 705–724.

Prevedello, L.M., Erdal, B.S., Ryu, J.L., et al., 2017. Automated critical test findings identification and online notification system using artificial intelligence in imaging. Radiology 285, 23–931.

Rai, M.C.E., Werghi, N., Al Muhairi, H., Alsafar, H., 2015. Using facial images for the diagnosis of genetic syndromes: a survey. 2015 International Conference on Communications, Signal Processing, and their Applications (ICCSPA), 1–6 pp.

Romeo, V., Maurea, S., Cuocolo, R., Petretta, M., Mainenti, P.P., Verde, F., Coppola, M., Dell'Aversana, S., Brunetti, A., 2018. Characterization of adrenal lesions on unenhanced MRI using texture analysis: a machine-learning approach. Journal of Magnetic Resonance Imaging 48, 198–204.

Rosenblatt, F., 1958. The perceptron: a probabilistic model for information storage and organization in the brain. Psychological Review 65(6), 386–408.

Russell, S., Bohannon, J., 2015. Artificial intelligence. Fears of an AI pioneer. Science 349, 252.

Russell, S., Norvig, P., 2003. Artificial Intelligence: A Modern Approach. USA: Prentice Hall, 946 pp.

Russell, S.J., Norvig, P., 2010. Artificial Intelligence. A Modern Approach. USA: Prentice Hall.

Sarma, G.P., Hay, N.J., Safron, A., 2018. AI safety and reproducibility: establishing robust foundations for the neuropsychology of human values. In: Gallina B., Skavhaug A., Schoitsch, E., Bitsch F, (Eds). SAFECOMP 2018: Computer safety, reliability, and security, Sep 18–21 2018, Västerås, Sweden. Cham: Springer. 507–512 pp.

Schaal, S., 1999. Is imitation learning the route to humanoid robots? Trends in Cognitive Science 3(6), 233–242.

Schmidhuber, J., 2015. Deep learning in neural networks: an overview. Neural Networks 61, 85–117.

Searle, J.R., 1982. The Chinese room revisited. Behavioral and Brain Sciences, 5(02), 345–348.

Shen, L. Kim, S., Yuan, Q., et al., 2011. Identifying neuroimaging and proteomic biomarkers for MCI and AD via the elastic net. In International Workshop on Multimodal Brain Image Analysis. MBIA 2011. Lecture Notes in Computer Science, vol 7012. Berlin, Heidelberg: Springer, 27–34pp. doi: https://doi.org/10.1007/978-3-642-24446-9_4.

Soleimani, F., Teymouri, R., Biglarian, A., 2013. Predicting developmental disorder in infants using an artificial neural network. Acta Medica Iranica 51, 347.

Springenberg, J.T., Dosovitskiy, A., Brox, T., Riedmiller, M., 2014. Striving for simplicity: the all convolutional net. https://arxiv.org/pdf/1412.6806.pdf.

Stamate, C., Magoulas, G.D., Kueppers, S., Nomikou, E., Daskalopoulos, I., Luchini, M.U., Moussouri, T., Roussos, G., 2017. Deep learning Parkinson's from smartphone data. Proceedings of the IEEE International Conference on Pervasive Computing and Communications, 31–40 pp.

Stead, W.W., 2018. Clinical implications and challenges of artificial intelligence and deep learning. The Journal of American Medical Association 320(11), 1107–1108.

Stephan, C., Jung, K., Cammann, H., Vogel, B., Brux, B., Kristiansen, G., Rudolph, B., Hauptmann, S., Lein, M., Schnorr, D., Sinha, P., Loening, S.A., 2002. An artificial neural network considerably improves the diagnostic power of percent free prostate-specific antigen in prostate cancer diagnosis: results of a 5-year investigation. International Journal of Cancer 99, 66–473.

Strong, J., 2007. Relics of the Buddha. Motilal Banarsidass Publisher.

Sun, D., Wang, M., Li, A., 2018. A multimodal deep neural network for human breast cancer prognosis prediction by integrating multi-dimensional data. IEEE ACM Transactions on Computational Biology, and Bioinformatics 16 (3), 841–850.

Taigman, Y., Yang, M., Ranzato, M., Wolf, L. Deepface: closing the gap to human-level performance in face verification. Proceedings of the IEEE Conference on Computer Vision and Pattern Recognition, 1701–1708 pp.

Thian, Y.L., Li, Y., Jagmohan, P., et al., 2019. Convolutional neural networks for automated fracture detection and localization on wrist radiographs. Radiology: Artificial Intelligence 1(1), e180001. 10.1148/ryai.2019180001

Thibodeau, R., Jorgensen, R.S., Kim, S., 2006. Depression, anxiety, and resting frontal EEG asymmetry: a meta-analytic review. Journal of Abnormal Psychology 115 (4), 715–729.

Turing, A.M., 1950. Computing machinery and intelligence. Mind LIX(236), 433–460.

US Food and Drug Administration, 2019. Proposed Regulatory Framework for Modifications to Artificial Intelligence/Machine Learning (AI/ML)-Based Software as a Medical Device (SaMD)-Discussion Paper and Request for Feedback [Internet][cited May 12 2019]. Available from: https://www.fda.gov/downloads/medicaldevices/deviceregula-tionandguidance/guidancedocuments/ucm514737.Pdf

Von Neumann, J., Kurzweil, R., 2012. The Computer and the Brain. 3rd ed. London, UK: Yale University Press. 136 pp.

Walsh, M.G., de Smalen, A.W., Mor, S.M., 2017. Wetlands, wild Bovidae species richness, and sheep density delineate risk of Rift Valley fever outbreaks in the African continent and Arabian Peninsula. PLoS Neglected Tropical Disease 11 (7), e0005756.

Walsh, S.L.F., Calandriello, L., Silva, M., Sverzellati, N., 2018. Deep learning for classifying fibrotic lung disease on high-resolution computed tomography: a case-cohort study. The Lancet Respiratory Medicine 6, 837–845. 10.1016/S2213-2600(18)30286-8

Walsh, S.L.F., Calandriello, L., Sverzellati, N., Wells, A.U., Hansell, D.M., 2016. UIP Observer Consort, interobserver agreement for the ATS/ERS/JRS/ALAT criteria for a UIP pattern on CT. Thorax 71, 45–51. 10.1136/thoraxjnl-2015-207252

Wang, S., Liu, Z., Rong, Y., Zhou, B., Bai, Y., Wei, W., Wei, W., Wang, M., Guo, Y., Tian, J., 2019. Deep learning provides a new computed tomography-based prognostic bio-marker for recurrence prediction in high-grade serous ovarian cancer. Radiotherepy and Oncology 132, 171–177.

Wang, X., Yang, W., Weinreb, J., Han, J., Li, Q., Kong, X., Yan, Y., Ke, Z., Luo, B., Liu, T., Wang, L., 2017. Searching for prostate cancer by fully automated magnetic resonance imaging classification: deep learning versus non-deep learning, Scientific Report 7, 15415.

Wang, X., Zheng, B., Li, S., Mulvihill, J.J., Wood, M.C., Liu, H., 2009. Automated clas-sification of metaphase chromosomes: optimization of an adaptive computerized scheme. Journal of Biomedical Informatics 42, 22–31.

Williams, B.M., Borroni, D., Liu, R., et al., 2020. An artificial intelligence-based deep learning algorithm for the diagnosis of diabetic neuropathy using corneal confocal microscopy: a development and validation study. Diabetologia 63, 419–430.

Wojtowicz, H., Wajs, W., 2012. Medical decision support system for assessment of der-matoglyphic indices and diagnosis of Down's syndrome. In: Watada, J., Watanabe, T., Phillips-Wren, G., Howlett, R., Jain, L., (Eds). Intelligent Decision Technologies. Smart Innovation, Systems, and Technologies, (16). Berlin, Heidelberg: Springer.

Xia, Y., Yang, C.W., Hu, N., Yang, Z.Z., He, X.Y., Li, T.T., et al., 2017. Exploring the key genes and signaling transduction pathways related to the survival time of glioblastoma multiforme patients by a novel survival analysis model. BMC Genomics 18, 950.

Xiong, H.Y., et al., 2015. RNA splicing. The human splicing code reveals new insights into the genetic determinants of disease. Science 347, 1254806.

Yaeger, K.A., Martini, M., Yaniv, G., Oermann, E.K., Costa, A.B., 2019. United States regulatory approval of medical devices and software applications enhanced by artificial intelligence. Health Policy and Technology 8, 192–197.

Yang, D., Jiang, K., Zhao, D., Yu, C., Cao, Z., Xie, S., et al., 2018. Intelligent and connected vehicles: current status and future perspectives. Science China Technological Sciences 61(10), 1446–1471.

Yi, X., Guan, X., Chen, C., Zhang, Y., Zhang, Z., Li, M., Liu, P., Yu, A., Long, X., Liu, L., Chen, B.T., Zee, C., 2018. Adrenal incidentaloma: machine learning-based quantitative texture analysis of unenhanced CT can effectively differentiate sPHEO from lipidpoor adrenal adenoma. Journal of Cancer 9, 3577–3582.

Yu, K.H., Beam, A.L., Kohane, I.S., 2018. Artificial intelligence in healthcare. Nature Biomedical Engineering 2(10), 719–731.

Zhang, L., Xiao, M., Zhou, J.S., Yu, J., 2018. Lineage-associated underrepresented permutations (LAUPs) of mammalian genomic sequences based on a Jellyfish-based LAUPs analysis application (JBLA). Bioinformatics 34 (21), 624–630.

Zhang, Q., Yang, Y., Ma, H., Wu, Y.N., 2019. Interpreting CNNs via decision trees. Proceedings of 2019 IEEE Conference on Computer Vision and Pattern Recognition, Jun 16–20, 2019, Long Beach. 6261–6270 pp.

9 Artificial Intelligence in Disease Diagnosis via Smartphone Applications

Saradhadevi Muthukrishnan
Assistant Professor, Department of Biochemistry, Bharathiar University, Coimbatore, India

CONTENTS

9.1   INTRODUCTION

AI can create a computer brain for thinking by itself. Thus, the computer gains its own intelligence called AI. Currently, AI enters into medical technology to reduce the burden of the healthcare workers; even suggestions are that AI doctors will replace human doctors in the future. We trust that machines cannot replace the doctor's place. AI can reduce work burden to the healthcare staff. They decide on the patient's health from AI as sometimes a human error will happen. AI includes the most sophisticated algorithms to bring the vast data of healthcare under the single volume that, can be used in the clinical practice. It can correct their errors by specificity and accuracy based on the feedback (Dute et al. 2016).

AI has used in the development of mobile app applications. Mobile health application use extended in chronic diseases diagnosis and health management and includes web-based and smartphone applications (Quinn et al. 2016; Maddison et al. 2015). Using these mobile applications, we can capture the photos, evaluate the diseased patients' signs and symptoms, and store the data as a case history. This information might be providing alerts, suggestions, and medical recommendations according to the severity of the disease (Villarreal et al. 2018). In Singapore, the development of m-Health increased due to the increased usage of smartphones and robust 4G network among the people to diagnose the diseases (Hui Zhang et al. 2017). Globally, the pandemic outbreak is sustaining. In this time, the Indian government introduced the Aarogya setu app to check the nearby coronavirus active cases (Javaid 2020). The mHealth applications are providing health suggestions about the patient, which give an eternal impact on physicians.

Mobile apps with the most sophisticated algorithms help identify deadly diseases like cancer. This sophisticated algorithm is applied to diagnose the early stage of cancer via the signs and symptoms. The early detection of the health status of better treatment options to the cancer patients and to increase the percentage of curing properly (Basch et al. 2016). There are two standard treatments available to cure cancer, like chemotherapy and radiation. But it has a plethora of side effects such as hair loss and loss of appetite. It affects not only the cancer cells but also normal cells. Drott et al. (2016) delineate the use of apps to give information about the side effects of chemotherapy treatment, and the apps give precautionary steps such as nutritious diet that people have to take before undergoing chemotherapy.

Some apps are also used in cardiac rehabilitation and help Coronary Artery Disease patients to know about their health status (Beatty et al. 2013). Kaplan and Haenlein (2010) have delivered the importance of using mobile apps in developing countries to bear remote healthcare and telemedicine. Martinez et al. (2008) has highlighted mobile phones and paper-based microfluidic devices for real-time off-site medical diagnosis. Jin et al. (2009) have developed mobile apps to record the electrocardiograms of the patients. Tan and Masek (2009) have reported about the development of a Doppler device system for fetal ultrasound assessment. Black et al.

(2013) has developed a low-cost pulse oximeter attached to a cell phone, which will help to deal with pneumonia. Chen et al. (2009) have reported the heart sound analyzing app in the mobile phones to determine the heartbeat and variability.

Some of the apps label the problem of patient's medical follow-ups. Bosch Health Buddy System (2009) developed a mobile app that provides sanitary control and reduces the hospitalization process. Bengtsson et al. (2014) and Villarreal et al. (2018) highlighted the mobile app in self-reporting about the patient's hypertension and its treatment process to reduce the disease cruelty. Tahat et al. (2011) reported a mobile application via Bluetooth to monitor the patient's blood pressure. Various telemedicine solutions for blood pressure, hypertension, heart rate, and general healthcare tips developed using mobile applications. Moreover, Ryder et al. (2009) reported a tool to assess the patient's brain strength and memory power. The device also helps to identify the chronically affected mentally ill patients of Parkinson's disease, muscular dystrophy, and multiple sclerosis by means of walking and typing. Thus, the above smartphone-based techniques will help the patients to know about their health status and take care of the clinical report via self-testing from home.

ML technology, which comes under AI is to analyze imaging, genetic disorders and electrophysiological data. ML helps in the identification of genetic disorder diseases by clustering the patient's traits and gives the probability of disease outcomes. There are different types of ML techniques, which include Supervised, Semi-Supervised, Unsupervised, Evolutionary Learning, Reinforcement, and Deep Learning. Using these techniques, we can classify the data sets.

In sophisticated modern hospitals, machines were set for the data collection and examination and to implement of data to share it in the large information systems. ML technologies are likely to be very efficient in analyzing medical data and diagnosing problems. An accurate diagnostic report of a patient is sent to a particular data section of modern hospitals. Then the algorithms can be run using a sophisticated computer as an input of the patient's report. And the results can be obtained automatically by comparing them with the previous patient's record. Doctors interpret the patient's diagnostic report at high speed with more accuracy by taking assistance from the derived classifiers. We can even train non-specialist individuals or students to diagnose the problem with accuracy using these classifiers (Kononenko 2001). ML algorithms more specifically mighty have the capacity to collect large data, from various dissimilar resources and combine all the background information in the study (Rambhajani et al. 2015).

The concern is to increase the usage of mobile apps in healthcare and medicine sector, although the research on its impact is limited. However, many apps focus on hardly any diseases and a plethora of diseases yet to be analyzed. We aim to enable everyone to download an app immediately on their smartphone and to diagnose the abnormalities at any time. So, the focus of this systematic review is to identify and evaluate the commercially available apps for promoting early diagnosis of diseases.

9.2 SMARTPHONE APPLICATIONS AND ML ALGORITHMS IN DISEASE DIAGNOSIS

9.2.1 DIAGNOSIS OF DISEASES BY USING SMARTPHONE APPLICATIONS

Many researchers have undergone research to find different types of smartphone apps to identify and diagnose the various diseases and accepted that apps for working well in the diagnosis process. This application helps to capture and process the significant signs and symptoms of the patients. After capturing the vital signs within the mobile phones, this may help within the storage of patient's data and permit to match that data from the already stored history. This will help in the recommendations and alertness to the patients based on the severity of their diseases (Villarreal et al. 2018; Figure 9.1). During this review, we specialize in the detection of anemia, Parkinson's disease, cancer, disorder, tuberculosis, urinary sepsis, acute Otitis, Covert Hepatic Encephalopathy, child health monitoring media, etc., by using different smartphone applications.

9.2.1.1 Smartphone App for Noninvasive Detection of Anemia

Image-based smartphone app with complete blood count-validation was used in the measurement of hemoglobin (Hgb) level very accurately. Compared to the conventional Hgb measuring devices, these mobile apps are cost-effective, with proved accuracy and specificity. With this smartphone image-based, Hgb estimating instrument, medical care authorities inside the far-off zones may benefit from this innovation to search out the people with iron-deficient gripes. Additionally, this application would likewise provide a proposal to the rational nourishment supplement like folate and iron for the patients (Robert et al. 2018). Using these non-invasive programs can screen, diagnose, and monitor the anemic patients globally.

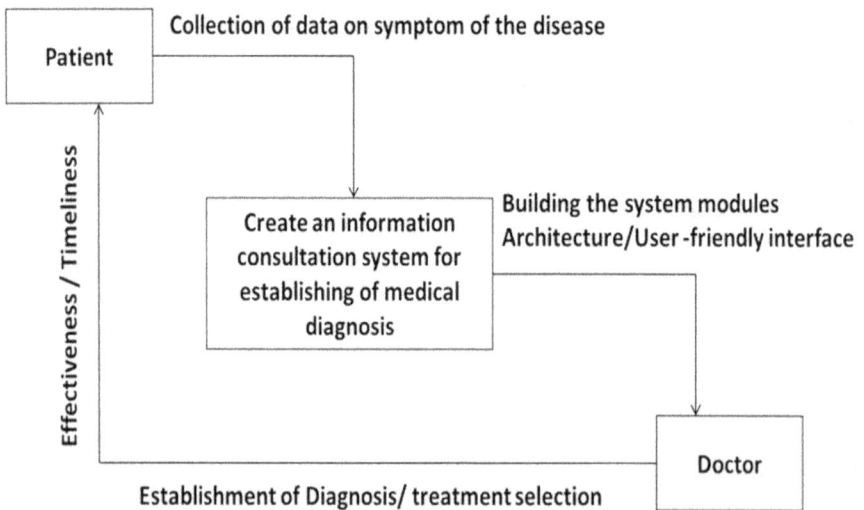

FIGURE 9.1 Mobile Application for Preliminary Diagnosis of Diseases.

9.2.1.2 Mobile Touch Screen Typing in the Detection of Motor Impairment of Parkinson's Disease

A calculation is to distinguish and screen the engine weakness like Parkinson's illness by assessing the composting action of the patients exclusively of the composed content substance on cell phones. It is a more accurate, objective, and modern tool to quantify the Parkinson's-related disorders. It is a home-based, high-compliance, and high-frequency motor test by analyzing the routine typing on touch screens (Arroyo-Gallego et al. 2017). Related to motor impairment, there have been 125 apps; of this, 56 apps are directly related to Parkinson's disease and 69 apps exclusively designed for Parkinson's disease (among this, 23 are data-collecting apps, 29 evaluation apps, 13 apps for treatment, and 4 evaluation and treatment apps). Numerous portable applications are specially planned in determination and sickness of Parkinson's illness (Linares-del Reya et al. 2019).

9.2.1.3 Screening Services for Cancer on Android Smartphones

An intelligent ubiquitous healthcare screening android app was developed for screening cancer disease, consistent with the rules framed by the American Cancer Society, US Preventive Services Task Force and American College of Gastroenterology. In view of the above models, a Decision Tree (DT) investigation portable application was produced for colorectal malignant growth screening. It helps the individual in self-testing, early determination, and with the treatment alternatives (Zubair Khan et al. 2018). An android app of version 4.4.2, for oral cancer detection was developed, which includes JAVA language with videos and data collection interfaces (Gomes et al. 2017). Interactive Information and Communications Technology (ICT) platform (Interaktor) was framed for the patients with breast and prostate cancer who were under the treatment of chemotherapy and radiation. A bile duct cancer is caused by *O. viverrini* infection correlated with cholangio carcinoma (Shin et al. 2010). OvApp is a special mobile application developed with iOS and Android platforms for screening *O. viverrini* affected peoples. This OvApp includes number of special features and three modules, which includes knowledge module (basic knowledge of *O. viverrini*), personal information module (gender, age, body mass index, occupation, educational level, income), and screening module (for *O. viverini* screening; Seneviratne et al. 2018).

9.2.1.4 Detection of Cardiovascular Disease Using Smartphone Mechanocardiography

A "Sim application" and "Care4Heart" were extraordinarily intended for cardiovascular patients to take prudent steps during the sickness seriousness. Especially Care4Heart may be a smartphone-based mindfulness application, which includes a 4-week coronary illness anticipation program. Among the working population of Singapore, and to urge changes in their lifestyle (Hui Zhang et al. 2017). Sim app is particularly designed to know the heart rate. So, these apps are used handy both by the doctors to recognizes the heartbeat of the cardiac patients. By using this technology, the patients themselves will take recordings of their heart rate. These intelligent apps can separate the heartbeat rates from normal sinus rhythm, coronary artery disease, atrial fibrillation, and myocardial infarctions using the multilevel settings. From the app, we can immediately get accurate results. This app with six-axis smartphone built-in inertial sensor works similar to seismocardiography and gyrocardiography for analyzing multiple heart conditions (ZuhairIftikhar et al. 2018). In the global market, several mobile ECGs apps are now available based on different evaluating techniques which include, Zenicor EKG, AliveCore Kardia, Mydiagnostick, Zio Patch, Wearable SEEQ™ mobile cardiac telemetry, and Medtronic implantable loop recorders; Omron M6 blood pressure monitors for AFib detection; and Microlife A200 iPhone photo plethysmographs (Tuominen 2017). Open heart medical procedure patients after re-visitation of their homes from hospitals, a cardiovascular adhere to up and instructions can be done through these smart phone apps (Johnston 2016). Because of this innovation advancement at the worldwide levels, it is feasible for the early identification; determination and anticipation of heart sicknesses by the therapy measures get simpler (Chong et al. 2016).

9.2.1.5 Mobile-Enabled Expert System for Diagnosis of Tuberculosis in Real Time

Tuberculosis is generally identified dependent on the strategy of Enzyme-Linked Immunosorbent Assay (ELISA). The android app was developed to detect tuberculosis based on the same technology using antigen-specific antibody detection. This app has developed ease in our Samsung mobile phones with the minimum target of Software Development Kit (SDK) 21. This android app with open CV features, which includes data pre-processing techniques. After the component extraction and preparation are done, the instance is put away as text and moved to Waikato Environment for Knowledge Analysis (WEKA) to organize the classifier within the disconnected mode. The offline training was conducted with Intel® Core™ i7-4770 CPU at 3.40 GHz processor and 16 GB RAM on a 64 bit Windows system. An Ensemble classifier and Random Forest algorithms built-in mobile platforms were used to give 98.4% accuracy in tuberculosis antigen-specific antibody detection (Antesar et al. 2018).

9.2.1.6 Smartphone-Based Pathogen Detection of Urinary Sepsis

A smartphone-based real-time loop-mediated isothermal amplification (smaRT-LAMP) system has modulated to identify pathogen ID of urinary sepsis patients. It is a standalone device with a custom-built mobile phone app. The analysis done from the app is purely based on quantitative to determine the bacterial pathogens genome copy-number in real time. The smaRT-LAMP system is more accurate in separating the gram-positive bacteria from gram-negative ones. It is cost-effective to fabricate (in addition to the smartphone), and it can detect multiple pathogens samples simultaneously (Barnes et al. 2018). A disposable diagnosing kit and companion Android app are available to diagnose urinary tract infection (UTI) patients even in remote areas. UTI test results accurately identified using 868 MHz Low power wide area network (LoRaWAN) enabled personalized monitor that might disperse to the cloud server. All the test results of UTI were collected robustly at the base station and allow the server inspection. Even the test strips for UTI can sometimes give cent percent correct results based on the color change. Internet of Things (IoT) as a medical solution can be used by the peoples even in the remote areas with weak broadband connections, mobile signals, and landlines. It can apply to any sort of home or regional areas. It can give subscription-free long-range biotelemetry to doctors by offering savings by the regular home visit and the regular clinical visit by the patients (Catherwood et al. 2018).

9.2.1.7 Detecting Acute Otitis Media Using a Mobile App

Acute otitis media is a painful type of ear infection that is caused by bacteria or virus pathogens. The pathogens cause inflammation and infection in the area behind the eardrum called the middle ear. An improved technology called smart "diary app" was developed to find a case study of acute otitis media. Usually, the common infectious diseases cannot detect by the healthcare services and won't attract the attention much like other chronic diseases. But this technology can accurately estimate the disease burden caused by these pathogens. Simultaneously this "diary apps" could also be used in the evaluation of vaccine technologies to detect both the diseases caused and side effects of vaccine used (Annemarijn et al. 2017).

9.2.1.8 Diagnosis of Covert Hepatic Encephalopathy via Encephal App, a Smartphone-Based Stroop Test

Covert hepatic encephalopathy is a neuro cognitive dysfunction in cirrhosis. Because of its difficulty in diagnosis and manifestation are subtle, covert hepatic encephalopathies might be ignoring. Smartphone Encephal App is another version of the Stroop App, to detect covert hepatic encephalopathy. Encephal App has test-retest reliability, good face validity, and external validity for diagnosing covert hepatic encephalopathy in patients with cirrhosis. Encephal App accuracy was correlated and compared with Model end stage liver disease (MELD) score. From the app, it has been assessed that covert hepatic encephalopathy patients stay cognitively impaired despite having a healthy mental condition, which is detected by the app (Jasmohan et al. 2015).

9.2.1.9 Mobile-Based Nutrition and Child Health Monitoring

Evaluating maternity and child healthcare is very important in developing countries like India. Most of the rural people have not conscious of balanced nutrition. And they were unaware of their vital conditions undernutrition and deficiency disease. It is not always possible to track and intervene the nutritional status, daily feeding practices of a mother, and young child. Therefore, we want reliable routine information assortment to spot the gaps within the program method. And to observe behavior trends in the period. Digital knowledge assortment platforms will play a significant role in improving the routine program to make awareness of child nutrition and health monitoring. The people will be half-tracked over time, employing a mobile tool combined with a well-built database. And that was developed with data knowledge, availableness, and visibility, and cut back on resources (Guyon et al. 2016).

9.2.1.9.1 Other Mobile Apps in Healthcare

Mole Mapper is an iPhone-based observational study has developed using the Apple Research Kit framework to spot and measure the moles in our body using the collected images of participants to evaluate the risk of melanoma (Dan et al. 2017). "Sunface app" may be a sun-protective app, a freely available phone app aimed to prevent melanoma. By downloading the app in our mobile phones, an individual can take selfies, photographs were pre-processed to administer the results in step with the Fitzpatrick skin sort, size of the mole, and conjointly offer data regarding totally different levels of UV protection. The app provides visual outcome and provides ability regarding the hindrance of carcinoma. It conjointly provides information and recommendation regarding ABCDE rule for malignant melanoma self-detection. Photoaging mobile phone app (Sunface) and photoaging intervention productivity in output activity changes for UV protection in Brazilian adolescents.

AIGkit app significantly developed for Pompe disease patients, aimed to reduce the disease burden, provide clinical support by continuous tracking of the patients, and give everyday life ambient conditions. The novel "TMT Predict" app has developed to predict the result of Treadmill Test. It is a straightforward, user-friendly app based on six parameters like age, body mass index, sex, dyslipidemia, diabetes, and systemic hypertension. This app could be a useful tool to "rule out" coronary artery disease. The app's prophetic price was high, indicating that it is an honest screening tool to rule out coronary artery diseases.

9.2.2 Machine Learning Technology in the Diagnosis of Various Diseases

Different ML algorithms in the diagnosis of various diseases such as heart disease, diabetes, liver disease, dengue, hepatitis, and acromegaly were discussed in this paper as follows (Figure 9.2; Table 9.1).

9.2.2.1 Heart Disease

Coronary artery disease is a common type of cardiovascular disease that is the leading cause of death for both men and women. Three algorithms like Bayes Net, SVM, and FT have performed to detect coronary artery disease (Otoom et al. 2015). Heart diseases have also diagnosed using the different ML algorithm like Naive Bayes algorithm (Vembandasamy et al. 2015). Data processing studies have additionally used for the above disease evaluation (Chaurasia and Pal 2013). Some of the ML algorithms like Naive Bayes and SVM were applied using WEKA to evaluate the heart diseases in diabetic patients (Parthiban and Srivatsa 2012). SVM and Genetic Algorithm (G.A) are the combinational algorithm-based technique of the wrapper technique approach (Tan et al. 2009). WEKA and Library for Support Vector Machines (LIBSVM) data mining tools has also used here in the analysis (Figure 9.2).

9.2.2.2 Diabetes Disease

Diabetes is a condition that results from evaluating the glucose level in the blood. The ML algorithms such as DT and Naive Bayes have used predicting (Iyer et al. 2015).

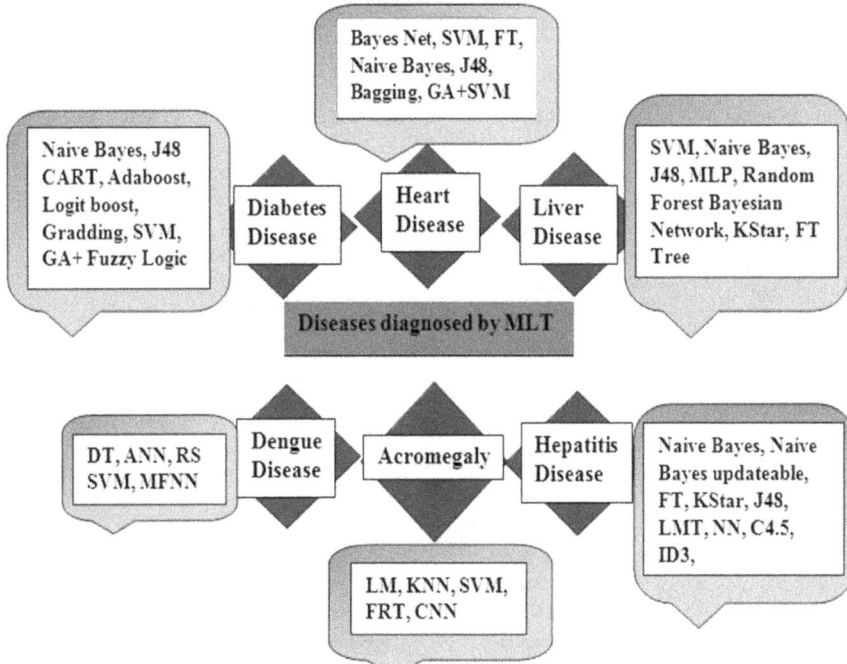

FIGURE 9.2 Diagnosis of Diseases by ML Techniques.

Another algorithm for predicting elevated blood sugar levels is the meta-learning algorithm (Sen and Dash 2014). Grading algorithms along with CART, Adaboost, and Logiboost are the most significant techniques to analyze diabetes (Kumari and Chitra 2013). RBF kernel along with SVM is used in the classification of type-1 or type-2 diabetes. Type-2 diabetes was analyzed using Naive Bayes (Sarwar and Sharma 2012). GA and fuzzy logic models constructed for disease diagnosis (Ephzibah 2011; Figure 9.2).

9.2.2.3 Liver Disease

Liver disease has diagnosed by using the classification algorithms of SVM and Naive Bayes (Vijayarani and Dhayanand 2015). Naives Bayes take less time to predict the disease. Compared to SVM, whereas with more accuracy as against to Naives Bayes (Gulia et al. 2014). Naive Bayes, Kstar, and FT tree analysis are the data mining algorithms used to analyze the liver disease (Rajeswari and Reena. 2010; Figure 9.2).

9.2.2.4 Dengue Disease

Dengue is a severe, contagious disease as compared to other maladies. Malaysia Dengue outbreak detection was done using the peculiar algorithms of Data mining models along with some classification algorithms like Artificial Neural Network (ANN), DT, and Rough Set Theory (RS) (Tarmizi et al. 2013). Arbovirus-Dengue

TABLE 9.1

Specification and Advantage of ML Algorithms

Sl No	Types of ML Algorithms Used	Specification	Advantages	Ref.
1	Bayes Net	Compact and spontaneous graphical illustrations of joint probability distributions. Conduct causal reasoning, risk prediction analysis and regression-based methods.	The causal structure precisely designed for individual-level risk prediction. Can be operated with approximately all statistical software packages.	Otoom et al. (2015)
2	SVM	Used for both classification and regression problems. It converts the primary training data into higher dimension using non-linear mapping.	SVM classifies the unknown sample into different categories and also predicts the risk of heart disease based on the statistical learning theory.	Tan et al. (2009)
3	Functional Trees (FT)	Measures the myocardial strain without the extra sequence acquisition and analyzed rapidly, opening the possibility of use in adult congenital heart disease.	The end-diastolic LV wall segmentations were used as a region of interest for the FT algorithm.	Otoom et al. (2015)
4	Naive Bayes algorithm	Highly scalable with the number of predictors and data points.	Examines both continuous and discrete data.	Vembandasamy et al. (2015)
5	DT	The typical algorithms of decision tree are Iterative Dichotomiser 3 (ID3), C4.5, Classification And	Predicts hyperglycemia.Used for predicting the 9 years risk of developing type-2 diabetes.	Sen and Dash (2014)

(Continued)

TABLE 9.1 (Continued)
Specification and Advantage of ML Algorithms

Sl No	Types of ML Algorithms Used	Specification	Advantages	Ref.
		Regression Tree (CART), and so on.		
6	Radial Basis Function (RBF) kernel along with SVM	Analysz higher-dimensional data. Classification accuracy, sensitivity, and specificity of the SVM and RBF have found to be high.	Used in the classification of type 1 or type 2 diabetes.	Parthiban and Srivatsa (2012)
7	CART	Data obtained from CART used to estimate prediction accuracy, sensitivity and specificity.	Uses a combination of exhaustive searches and computer-intensive testing techniques to unveil patterns and correlations hidden in data.	Kumari and Chitra (2013)
8	Kstar	Provides a uniform procedure to the handling of real-valued attributes, symbolic attributes and missing values.	Great data mining algorithm concerning understandability, transformability and accuracy gives 100%.	Rajeswari and Reena (2010)
9	Artificial Neural Network (ANN)	Three-layered feed forward technique.	ANN itself creates its commands by learning from the data sets this makes pattern recognition and classification of dengue.	Tarmizi et al. (2013)
10	Reed-Solomon (RS)	It uses reducts and core to reject the unnecessary information attributes and help in acquiring essential knowledge out of the information systems.	Used to determine an imprecise concept with the help of a pair of sets related to as lower and upper approximations.	Tarmizi et al. (2013)

(Continued)

TABLE 9.1 (Continued)

Specification and Advantage of ML Algorithms

Sl No	Types of ML Algorithms Used	Specification	Advantages	Ref.
11	C4.5 DT	It is a classifier for analysis of all clinical, hematological, and virological data.	The algorithm can be applied separately in different disease predominance to yield clinically useful positive and negative predictive values.	Fathima and Manimeglai (2012)
12	NN	Sets of algorithms intended to recognize patterns and interpret data through clustering or labeling.	NN can be used to implement nonlinear statistical modeling and give new options to logistic regression.	Karlik (2011)
13	EM	Generate multiple models and then combine them to deliver improved results.	Ensemble methods are meta-algorithms that connect different ML techniques into one predictive model to decrease variance and bias.	Xiangyi Kong et al. (2018)
14	K-Nearest Neighbors (KNN)	Used both for classification as well as regression analysis.	KNN algorithm to obtain the k nearest instances in the training images and computed the mean outcome as the final prediction.	Xiangyi Kong et al. (2018)

disease prediction has done by data mining algorithm (Fathima and Manimeglai 2012). ANN system and MATLAB's® neural network toolbox have used to analyze the Dengue fever (Ibrahim et al. 2005; Figure 9.2).

9.2.2.5 Hepatitis Disease

Hepatitis is a condition of liver infection, which is caused by the hepatitis B virus. The liver condition monitor by software has developed like FT Tree, K Star algorithm, J48, Logistic model tree (LMT), Naive Bayes, Naive Bayes updatable, and NN (Ba-Alwi and Hintaya 2013). The comparative analysis of Naive Bayes (Karlik 2011) and ID3, C4.5, and CART algorithms (Sathyadevi 2011) was altogether used in the diagnosis of hepatitis disease (Figure 9.2).

9.2.2.6 Genetic Disorders (Acromegaly) from Facial Photographs

Recently, AI was used to identify unusual genetic defects or genetic disorders using the facial features of patient images (Hamet and Tremblay 2017; Esteva 2017; Kanakasabapathy et al. 2017). Acromegaly is a rare genetic disorder caused due to secretion of more growth hormones from pituitary glands. This rare genetic disorder was more efficiently detected using AI. The facial characteristics of acromegaly are typically prognathism, widening teeth spacing, nose enlargement, frontal-bone enlargement, brow ridge, zygomatic-arch prominence and forehead protrusion, soft tissue swelling of lips, nose, ears enlargement, and skin thickening. Based on these facial features of acromegaly an automatic and handy face-recognition system has developed. This system will allow the doctors or patients to early detection of acromegaly using the integrated ML technique. The integrated technique of Generalized Linear Models, SVM, K-nearest neighbors, Convolutional Neural Network, and forests of randomized trees to create an Ensemble Method (EM) for the facial detection of acromegaly (Xiangyi Kong et al. 2018; Figure 9.3).

9.3 CONCLUSION

This paper focuses on medical solutions for doctors about patient's health using the web and mobile-based applications. Android smartphones with an intelligent app for the early detection of diseases have discussed in this chapter. Patients who have

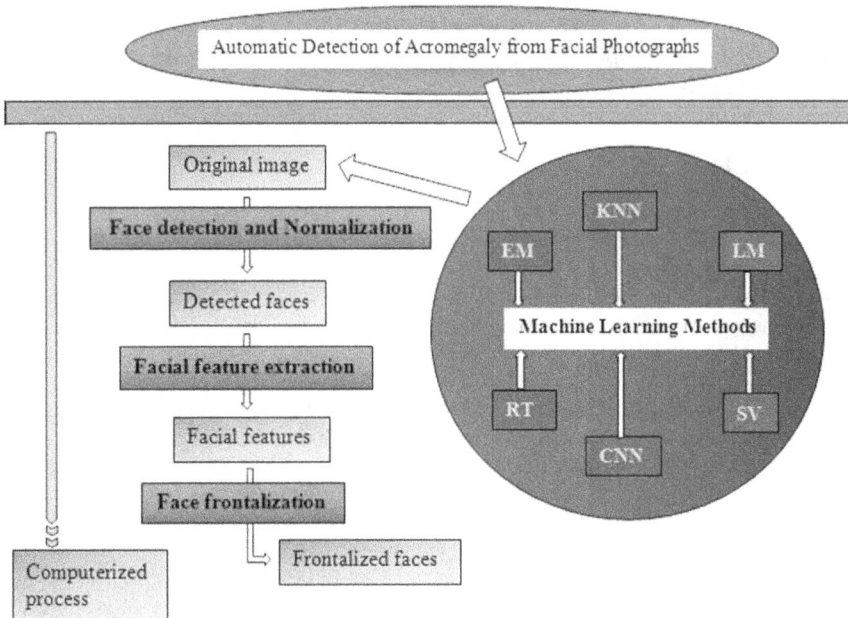

FIGURE 9.3 Machine Learning Techniques in the Automatic Detection of Acromegaly Using Facial Photographs.

engaged with these channels will manage their disease progress by themselves at different stages accompanying their day-to-day activities. Apps can also provide a simple and effective way to screen patients for high-risk groups. The goal of AI has promoted the keep tracking the patient condition after their hospital treatment. This architecture helps to monitor the patient's health continuously through communication between the patients and the doctors. AI has allowed creating an automatic profile generation about the person and education modules for their chronic diseases. The mobile app has the option to capture and record the signs and symptoms of the patients, typically in the diseases of anemia, Parkinson's disease, cancer, carcinogenic liver fluke infection, urinary sepsis, tuberculosis, child health monitoring, acute otitis media, cardiovascular disease, covert hepatic encephalopathy, etc.; an ML algorithm is used in disease diagnosis of heart, diabetes, liver, dengue, hepatitis, and acromegaly. This approach will shift the pathogen screening paradigm worldwide by empowering patients to test themselves from the comfort zone of houses, wherever and whenever they desire.

ACKNOWLEDGMENT

This review work is supported by the Department of Biochemistry, Bharathiar University, Coimbatore.

We declare that we have no financial and personal relationships with other people or organizations that can inappropriately influence our work, there is no professional or other personal interest of any nature or kind in any product, service and/or company that could be construed as influencing the position presented in, or the review of, the manuscript entitled, "Artificial intelligence in Disease Diagnosis Via Smartphone applications."

REFERENCES

Amutha, A.J., Padmajavalli, R., Prabhakar, R., 2018. A novel approach for the prediction of treadmill test in cardiology using data mining algorithms implemented as a mobile application. Indian Heart Journal. 70(4), 511–518.

Annemarijn A.C., Prins-van Ginkel, C., de Hoog, M.L., Uiterwaal, C., Smit, H.A., Bruijning-Verhagen, P.C.J., 2017. Detecting acute otitis media symptom episodes using a mobile app: cohort study. JMIR MhealthUhealth. 5(11), e181.

Antesar A.M., Shabut, M., Taniaa, M.H., Lwina, K.T., Evans, B.A., Yusof, N.A., Abu-Hassane, K.J., 2018. An intelligent mobile-enabled expert system for tuberculosis disease diagnosis in real time. Expert Systems with Applications. 114, 65–77.

Arroyo-Gallego, T.A., Ledesma-Carbayo, M.J., Sanchez-Ferro, A., Butterworth, I., Mendoza, C.S., Matarazzo, M., 2017. Detection of motor impairment in Parkinson's disease via mobile touchscreen typing. IEEE Transactions on Biomedical Engineering. 64(9), 1994–2002.

Ba-Alwi, F.M., Hintaya, H.M., 2013. Comparative study for analysis the prognostic in hepatitis data: data mining approach. International Journal of Scientific & Engineering Research. 4, 680–685.

Barnes, L., Heithoff, D.M., Mahan, S.P., Fox, G.N., Zambrano, A., Hoe, J., Fitzgibbons, J., 2018. Smartphone-based pathogen diagnosis in urinary sepsis patients. EBioMedicine. 36, 73–82.

Basch, E., Deal, A.M., Kris, M.G., Scher, H.I., Hudis, C.A., Sabbatini, P., 2016. Symptom monitoring with patient-reported outcomes during routine cancer treatment: a randomized controlled trial. Journal of Clinical Oncology. 34(6) 557–565.

Beatty, A.L., Fukuoka, Y., Whooley, M.A., 2013. Using mobile technology for cardiac rehabilitation: a review and framework for development and evaluation. Journal of the American Heart Association. 2(6) e000568.

Bengtsson, U., Kasperowski, D., Ring, L., Kjellgren, K., 2014. Developing an interactive mobile phone self-report system for self-management of hypertension. Part 1: Patient and professional perspectives. Blood Pressure. 23, 288–295.

Black, J., Sonenberg, L., Scheepers, R., 2013. Cell phone technology is key to better health in Africa. Available at http://research.microsoft.com/en-us/collaboration/focus/health/smartphone_clinical_diagnosis.aspx.

BOSCH Health Buddy System, 2009. Available at http://www.bosch-telehealth.com. (2009).

Brinker, T.J., Brieske, C.M., Schaefer, C.M. Buslaff, F., Gatzka, F., Petri, M.P., 2017. Photoaging mobile apps in school-based melanoma prevention: pilot study. Journal of Medical Internet Research. 19(9) e319.

Catherwood, P.A., Steele, D., Little, M., Mccomb, S., Mclaughlin, J.A., 2018. Community-based IoT Personalized Wireless Healthcare Solution Trial. IEEE Journal of Translational Engineering in Health and Medicines. 8(6), 2800313. doi: 10.1109/JTEHM.2018.2822302. eCollection 2018.

Chaurasia, V., Pal, S., 2013. Data mining approach to detect heart disease. International Journal of Advanced Computer Science and Information Technology (IJACSIT). 2, 56–66.

Chen, T., Kuan, K., Celi, L., Clifford, G.D., 2009. Intelligent Heart Sound Diagnostics on a Cellphone Using a Hands-Free Kit. Association for the Advancement of Artificial Intelligence (www.aaai.org).

Chong, J.W., Cho, C.H., Esa, N., McManus, D.D., Chon, K.H., 2016. Motion and noise artifact-resilient atrial fbrillation detection algorithm for a smartphone. Biomedical and Health Informatics (BHI), IEEE-EMBS International Conference, 591–594.

Dan, D.E., Webster, E., Suver, C., Doerr, M., Mounts, E., Domenico, L., Petrie, T., 2017. The MoleMapper Study, mobile phone skin imaging and melanoma risk data collected using ResearchKit. Scientific Data. 4(1), 1-8, [170005]. doi: 10.1038/sdata.2017.5

Denise Jantine Dute, D.J., Bemelmans, W.J.E., Breda, J., 2016. Using mobile apps to promote a healthy lifestyle among adolescents and students: a review of the theoretical basis and lessons learned. JMIR MhealthUhealth. 4(2), e39.

Drott, J., Vilhelmsson, M., Kjellgren, K., Bertero, C., 2016. Experiences with a self reported mobile phone-based system among patients with colorectal cancer: a qualitative study. JmirMhealth and Uhealth. 4(2), 182–190.

Dute, D.J., Bemelmans, W.J.E., Breda, J., 2016. Using mobile apps to promote a healthy lifestyle among adolescents and students: a review of the theoretical basis and lessons learned. JMIR MhealthUhealth. 4(2), e39.

Ephzibah, E.P., 2011. Cost effective approach on feature selection using genetic algorithms and fuzzy logic for diabetes diagnosis. International Journal on Soft Computing (IJSC). 2, 1–10.

Esteva, A., 2017. Dermatologist-level classification of skin cancer with deep neural networks. Nature. 542, 115–118.

Fathima, A.S., Manimeglai, D., 2012. Predictive analysis for the arbovirus dengue using SVM classification. International Journal of Engineering and Technology. 2, 521–527.

Gomes, M.S., Bonan, P.R., Ferreira, V.Y., de Lucena Pereira, L., Correia, R.J., da Silva Teixeira, H.B., 2017. Development of a mobile application for oral cancer screening, Technology and Health Care. 25(2), 187–195. doi: 10.3233/THC-161259

Gulia, A., Vohra, R., Rani, P., 2014. Liver patient classification using intelligent techniques. International Journal of Computer Science and Information Technologies. 5, 5110–5115.

Guyon, A., Bock, A., Buback, L., Knittel, B., 2016. Mobile-based nutrition and child health monitoring to inform program development: an experience from Liberia. Global Health: Science and Practice. 4(4), 661–670. doi: 10.9745/GHSP-D-16-00189

Hamet, P., Tremblay, J., 2017. Artificial intelligence in medicine. Metabolism. 69S, 36–40.

Hui Zhang, H., Jiang, Y., Hoang, D., Nguyen, H.D., Poo, D.C.C., Wang, W., 2017. The effect of a smartphone-based coronary heart disease prevention (SBCHDP) programme on awareness and knowledge of CHD, stress, and cardiac-related lifestyle behaviours among the working population in Singapore: a pilot randomised controlled trial. Health and Quality of Life Outcomes. 15, 49.

Ibrahim, F., Taib, M.N., Abas, W.A.B.W., Guan, C.C., Sulaiman, S.A., 2005. Novel dengue fever (DF) and dengue haemorrhagic fever (DHF) analysis using artificial neural network (ANN). Computer Methods and Programs in Biomedicine. 79, 273–281.

Iyer, A., Jeyalatha, S., Sumbaly, R., 2015. Diagnosis of diabetes using classification mining techniques. International Journal of Data Mining & Knowledge Management Process. 5, 1–14.

Jasmohan, J.S., Bajaj, S., Heuman, D.M., Sterling, R.K., Sanyal, A.J., Siddiqui, M., 2015. Validation of EncephalApp, smartphone-based Stroop test, for the diagnosis of covert hepatic encephalopathy. Clinical Gastroenterology and Hepatology. 13 1828–1835.

Javaid, A., May 6, 2020. Aarogya Setu App: What Is It, Its Benefits, How to Download, Privacy Issues and More. Available at: https://www.jagranjosh.com/general-knowledge/aarogya-setu-app-1586848268-1

Jiang, F., Jiang, Y., Zhi, H., Dong, Y., Li, H., Ma, S., 2017. Artificial intelligence in healthcare: past, present and future. Stroke and Vascular Neurology, 2(4) 230–243.

Jin, Z., Sun, Y., Cheng, A.C., 2009. Predicting cardiovascular disease from real-time elec-trocardiographic monitoring: an adaptive machine learning approach on a cell phone. ConfProc IEEE Eng Med Biol Soc2009, 6889–6892.

Johnston, N., 2016. Effects of interactive patient smartphone support app on drug adherence and lifestyle changes in myocardial infarction patients: a randomized study. American Heart Journal, 178, 85–94.

Kaewpitoon, N., Kaewpitoon, S.J., Meererksom, T., Chan-Aran, S., Sangwalee, W., Kujapun, J., 2013. Detection of risk groups for carcinogenic liver fluke infection by Verbal Screening Questionnaire using a mobile application. Asian Pacific Journal of Cancer Prevention, 19, 2013–2019.

Kanakasabapathy, M.K., Sadasivam, M., Singh, A., Preston, C., Thirumalaraju, P., Venkataraman, M., 2017. An automated smartphone-based diagnostic assay for point-of-care semen analysis. Science Translational Medicine. 9(382), eaai7863. doi: 10.112 6/scitranslmed.aai7863

Kaplan, A., Haenlein, M., 2010. Users of the world, unite! The challenges and opportunities of social media. Business Horizons. 53(1) 59–68.

Karlik, B., 2011. Hepatitis disease diagnosis using back propagation and the naive Bayes classifiers. Journal of Science and Technology. 1, 49–62.

Kononenko, I., 2001. Machine learning for medical diagnosis: history, state of the art and perspective. Journal of Artificial Intelligence in Medicine. 1, 89–109.

Kumari, V.A., Chitra, R., 2013. Classification of diabetes disease using support vector ma-chine. International Journal of Engineering Research and Applications. 3, 1797–1801.

Langius-Eklof, A., Craafoord, M.T., Christiansen, M., Fjell, M., Sundberg, K., 2017. Effects of an interactive mHealth innovation for early detection of patient-reported symptom distress with focus on participatory care: protocol for a study based on prospective, randomised, controlled trials in patients with prostate and breast cancer. BMC Cancer. 17, 466.

Linares-del Reya, M., Vela-Desojo, L., Cano-de la Cuerda, R., 2019. Mobile phone applications in Parkinson's disease: asystematic review. Neurología. 134(1), 38–54.

Maddison, R., Pfaeffli, L., Whittaker, R., Stewart, R., Kerr, A., Jiang, Y., 2015. A mobile phone intervention increases physical activity in people with cardiovascular disease: results from the HEART randomised controlled trial. The European Journal of Preventive Cardiology. 22(6) 701–709.

Martinez, A.W., Phillips, S.T., Carillho, E., Thomas, S.W., Sindi, H., Whitesides, G.M., 2008. Simple telemedicine for developing regions: camera phones and paper-based microfluidic devices for real-time, off-site diagnosis. Analytical Chemistry. 80, 3699–3707.

Otoom, A.F., Abdallah, E.F., Kilani, Y., Kefaye, A., Ashour, M., 2015. Effective diagnosis and monitoring of heart disease. International Journal of Software Engineering and Its Applications. 9, 143–156.

Parthiban, G., Srivatsa, S.K., 2012. Applying machine learning methods in diagnosing heart disease for diabetic patients. International Journal of Applied Information Systems. 3, 25–30.

Quinn, C.C., Shardell, M.D., Terrin, M.L., Barr, E.A., Park, D., Shaikh, F., 2016. Mobile diabetes intervention for glycemic control in 45- to 64-year-old persons with type 2 diabetes. Journal of Applied Gerontology. 35(2), 227–243.

Rajeswari, P., Reena, G.S., 2010. Analysis of liver disorder using data mining algorithm. Global Journal of Computer Science and Technology. 10, 48–52.

Rambhajani, M., Deepanker, W., Pathak, N., 2015. A survey on implementation of machine learning techniques for dermatology diseases classification. International Journal of Advances in Engineering &Technology. 8, 194–195.

Ricci, G., Baldanzi, S., Seidita, F., Proietti, C., Carlini, F., Peviani, S., 2018. A mobile app for patients with Pompe disease and its possible clinical applications. Neuromuscular Disorders. 28(6), 471–475.

Robert, R.G., Mannino, G., Myers, D.R., Tyburski, E.A., Caruso, C., 2018. Smartphone app for non- invasive detection of anemia using only patient-sourced photos. Nature Communications. 9, 4924.

Ryder, J., Longstaff, B., Reddy, S., Estrin, D. 2009. Ambulation: a tool for monitoring mobility patterns over time using mobile phones. 2009 International Conference on Computational Science and Engineering (Vol. 4, pp. 927–931). IEEE.

Sarwar, A., Sharma, V., 2012. Intelligent naïve Bayes approach to diagnose diabetes type-2. Special Issue of International Journal of Computer Applications (0975-8887) on Issues and Challenges in Networking, Intelligence and Computing Technologies-ICNICT 2012. 3, 14–16.

Sathyadevi, G., 2011. Application of CART algorithm in hepatitis disease diagnosis. IEEE International Conference on Recent Trends in Information Technology (ICRTIT), MIT, Anna University, Chennai, 1283–1287.

Sen, S.K., Dash, S., 2014. Application of meta learning algorithms for the prediction of diabetes disease. International Journal of Advance Research in Computer Science and Management Studies. 2, 396–401.

Seneviratne, M.G., Hersch, F., Peiris, D.P., 2018. Health Navigator: a mobile application for chronic disease screening and linkage to services at an urban primary health network. Australian Journal of Primary Health. 24(2), 116–122. doi: 10.1071/PY17070

Shin, H. R., Oh, J. K., Masuyer, E., Curado, M. P., Bouvard, V., Fang, Y. Y., Wiangnon, S., Sripa, B., and Hong, S. T. (2010). Epidemiology of cholangiocarcinoma: An update focusing on risk factors. Cancer Science. 101(3), 579–585.

Tahat, A., Sacca, A., Kheetan, Y., 2011. Design of an integrated mobile system to measure blood-pressure. Proceedings of the IEEE 18th Symposium on Communications and Vehicular Technology in the Benelux (SCVT), Ghent, Belgium, 1–6.

Tan, A., Masek, M., 2009. Fetal heart rate and activity monitoring via smart phones. mHealthSummit 2009, Washington, DC. Available at http://research.microsoft.com/en-us/events/mhealth2009/tan-masek-presentation.pdf

Tan, K.C., Teoh, E.J., Yu, Q., Goh, K.C., 2009. A hybrid evolutionary algorithm for attribute selection in data mining. Journal of Expert System with Applications. 36, 8616–8630.

Tarmizi, N.D.A., Jamaluddin, F., Bakar, A., Othman, Z.A., Zainudin, S., Hamdan, A.R., 2013. Malaysia dengue outbreak detection using data mining models. Journal of Next Generation Information Technology. 4, 96–107.

Tuominen, J., 2017. A miniaturized low power biomedical sensor node for clinical research and long term monitoring of cardiovascular signals. IEEE International Symposium on Circuits and Systems (ISCAS), 1–4.

Vembandasamy, K., Sasipriya, R., Deepa, E., 2015. Heart diseases detection using naive Bayes algorithm. International Journal of Innovative Science. Engineering & Technology. 2, 441–444.

Vijayarani, S., Dhayanand, S., 2015. Liver disease prediction using SVM and naïve Bayes algorithms. International Journal of Science Engineering and Technology Research. 4, 816–820.

Villarreal, V., Nielsen, M., Samudio, M., 2018. Sensing and storing the blood pressure measure by patients through a platform and mobile devices. Sensors (Basel). 18(6), E1805. doi: 10.3390/s18061805

Wu, H.C., Chang, C.J., Lin, C.C., Tsai, M.C., Chang, C.C., Tseng, M.H., 2014. Developing screening services for colorectal cancer on Android smartphones. Telemedicine and e-Health. 20(8) 687–695.

Xiangyi Kong, X., Gong, S., Su, L., Howard, N., Kong, Y., 2018. Automatic detection of acromegaly from facial photographs using machine learning methods. EBioMedicine. 27, 94–102.

Zubair Khan, Z., Darr, U., Khan, M.A., Nawras, M., Khalil, B., Aziz, Y.A., 2018. Improving internal medicine residents' colorectal cancer screening knowledge using a smartphone app: pilot study. JMIR Medical Education. 4(1), e10.

ZuhairIftikhar, Z., Lahdenoja, O., Tadi, M.J., Hurnanen, T., Vasankari, T., Kiviniemi, T.O., 2018. Multiclass classifer based cardiovascular condition detection using smartphone mechanocardiography. Scientific Reports. 8, 9344.

10 Artificial Intelligence in Agriculture

M. Sakthi Asvini[1] and T. Amudha[2]
[1]Research Associate, Interdisciplinary Centre for Water Research, Indian Institute of Science (IISc), Bangalore, India
[2]Associate Professor, Department of Computer Applications, Bharathiar University, Coimbatore, India

CONTENTS

10.1 INTRODUCTION TO ARTIFICIAL INTELLIGENCE

We all have a curiosity of knowing, "Can a machine think and work as humans do?"

Artificial Intelligence (AI) is an intelligent system or software developed from how the human brain thinks, learns, works, and decides to solve a particular problem. Such an intelligent system will also exhibit intelligent behavior in learning, remembering, understanding, applying, analyzing and evaluating, thereby assisting its users, e.g., intelligent chatbots, robots used in restaurants to receive and get orders, intelligent sensors used in autonomous cars, etc. It is also said to be learning cognitive abilities through the ways of computational models. AI is widely used in the fields of philosophy, mathematics, science, psychology, business, linguistics, engineering, and so on. The AI system needs some representations that are manipulated by cognitive processes and which in turn translate into actions. Representation describes the knowledge or information from the real world, in which computer can understand and utilize the knowledge to solve complex problems same as how humans do. It is kind of designing agents that can think and act like a human which is called an agent's behavior. Cognitive science is a higher form of human thinking which includes language, perception, memory, emotion, attention and reasoning. It also has the problem space to allow an efficient search to bring out the best solutions. The process of AI is depicted in Figure 10.1. There are numerous applications of AI such as gaming, education, transport, media, retail spaces, communication, workplace, hospitality, sports, entertainment, mobile, healthcare, Aerospace, agriculture, online shopping, real estate, insurance, social networks, cybersecurity, defense, smart homes, events and politics, and government. This chapter deals with the use of AI in the Agriculture sector.

10.2 AGRICULTURE – NEVER DIE BUSINESS UNTIL HUMANS EXIST

Agriculture is one of the important and oldest professions in the world. There are main factors to be considered in growing crops such as, the crop to be cultivated is

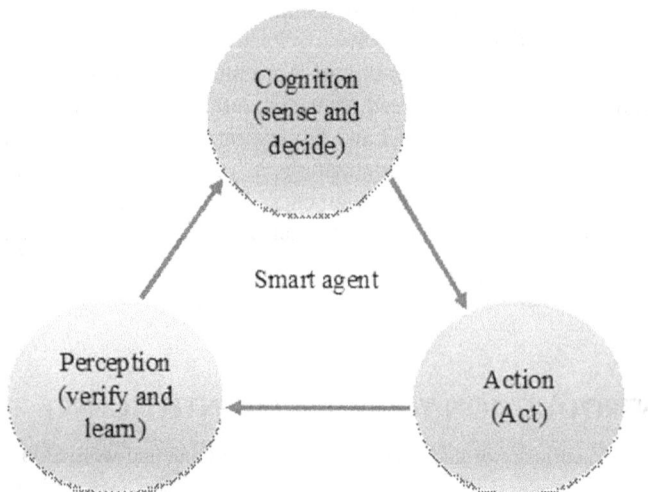

FIGURE 10.1   Representation of the artificial intelligence agent.

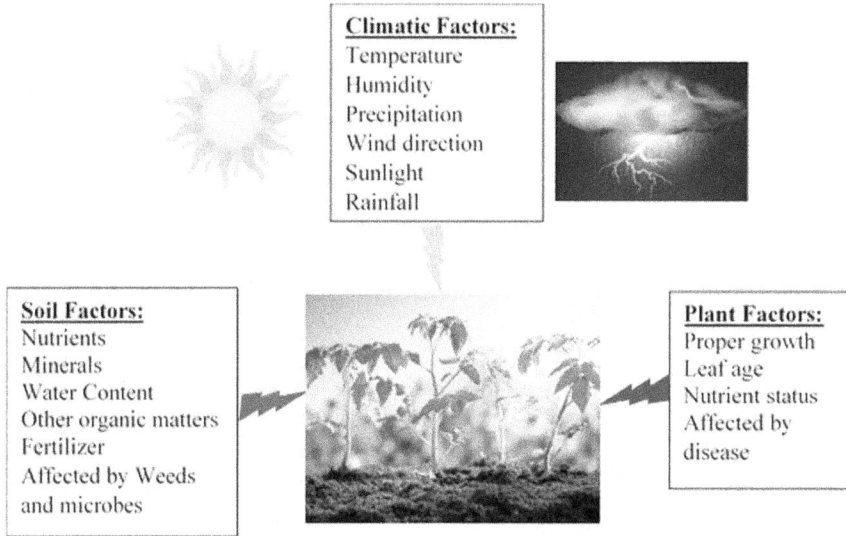

FIGURE 10.2   Important factors to be maintained for proper plant growth.

chosen based on the type of soil, availability of water in the agriculture land, the climatic condition of the place and season which we initiate the cultivation process and seed availability. These factors are very important since certain crops will grow only in a particular type of soil and climate. There are different types of soil such as red soil, black soil, alluvial soil, loamy soil, etc., and each soil has its characteristics. The next factor to be considered is the quality of the soil. A crop needs enough nutrients, water content, sunlight, and good weather conditions for its growth [1]. The soil quality varies based mainly on weather condition. Certain factors need to be considered in agriculture. It is depicted in Figure 10.2.

The climate factors such as temperature, humidity, precipitation, sunlight, wind, and rainfall should be monitored. The soil factors such as the presence of nutrients, minerals, water, and other organic matters should also be monitored. The need for fertilizers in case of soil affected by weeds or other microbes should be checked frequently. The plant factors include proper growth, nutrient status of plants, and leaf age should be monitored to know the health of crops. The technologies play a major role in all these activities in less amount of time.

All the plants have five main phases of its growth: (a) early growth, (b) vegetative, (c) flowering, (d) fruit formation, and (e) ripening, as mentioned in Figure 10.3. At each stage, the plant needs a different level of water and nutrient contents. The root of crops sucks the water and nutrients from the soil at various levels at its different growth stages and also based on weather condition [2]. When the crop grows, the root also grows larger and penetrates deep into the soil. At the initial growth stage, every plant will need less amount of water and nutrients. When the plant grows to its next forthcoming stages, it needs some more water and nutrient content and so on. There are periods for each of its growth stages. If fertilizers or manures are to be supplied to plants for its proper growth, the farmers have to

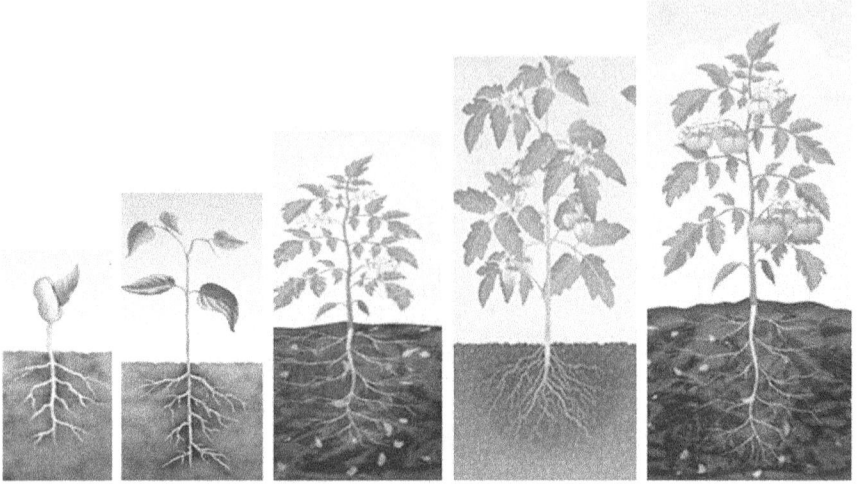

FIGURE 10.3   Growing stages of the crop.

keep watching on agricultural land and take care of plants from the effects of disease caused by insects, rats, bugs, etc., and also should watch on weed and pests grown near the crops. The farmers should take care of crops at each of their growing stages. Recent technologies simplify the work of farmers by monitoring plants at each growth stage, which is discussed below.

The other important parameters to be taken care are price and agricultural products forecasting, pest and weed management, crop productivity, land utilization, fertilizer optimization, soil management, and irrigation management. To monitor all these factors, the utilization of technologies have helped the farmers in many ways to make their work easy and in an efficient manner. Over the years, humanity has found various ways on how to do farming and grow crops with the invention of different technologies. Each of the following is described in detail in the following sections and shown in Figure 10.4.

10.3   NEED FOR AI IN AGRICULTURE

As the human population increases, the land utilization becomes high and there occurs a scarcity of land to do farming. People are in the situation to find creative and efficient ways for better use of land and also to gain more productivity of crops. To help the farmers, the industry has transformed into AI techniques and data science in developing tools to manage all the agriculture practices. The advanced techniques are used for assessing the quality of soil, weather forecasting, identifying disease in the plants, sensing moisture level in the area, etc. Most farmers are still practicing old methods, and they lack in knowledge of using recent technologies. The farmers use trial-and-error method or predict on their own to yield maximum crop productivity which fails at times and farmers meet huge loss and end up losing their life. Several technologies are helping farmers in the form of mobile applications, agriculture robots, drones, smart machines, etc. The combined technologies of artificial intelligence frame all these, Internet of Things, machine learning, data

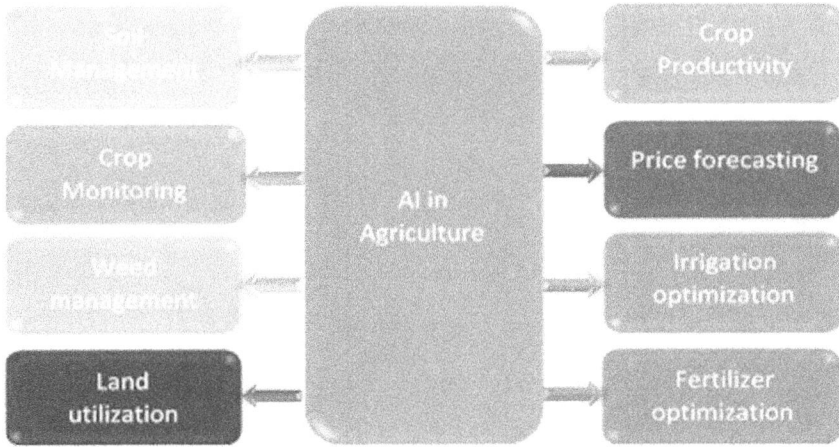

FIGURE 10.4   Factors to be taken care of in the field of agriculture.

science, mobile applications, hardware and software systems, satellite technologies, etc. eAgriculture is a new concept that has a drastic impact on food production and farming. Cloud computing companies focused much on digital agriculture. It uses RFID (Radio Frequency Identification) and OR tags to collect data in less time, which replaces machine technology. Apart from the above-mentioned factors (in Section 10.2), technologies are also used in various sectors. Agricultural data are accessed in the cloud database. Cloud applications help the farmers to create budgets and operational schedules. It also helps to manage the mapping of field-work to the weather condition, monitoring the process of crop growth and to manage the workforce efficiently. There are smart tools to measure operations of machines and software to track costs, production yields, and profit against the benchmark established [3].

Crop infection is predicted and the farmers can also be given awareness about the potential risk of plant disease. The AI system can learn and predict everything from the disease before we conclude from the agricultural data. The AI system has more reliable monitoring and good management of natural resources which helps the farmers in assessing the amount of water, fertilizers, pesticides required for each plant. They can use minimum quantities and yield high crop productivity. It also helps in less impact of natural ecosystems and increased safety of workers. The smarter system with AI technologies can also predict the climatic conditions and helps farmers to navigate shifts according to environmental conditions. Genetic Engineering (GE) is one of the recent technologies that helps in the plant breeding process. Farmers have used traditional breeding techniques by selecting the correct plants for the improvement of crop yield. Germplasm has been improved to develop seeds with different characteristics of other seeds to give the improved crop yield based on specific soil and climate conditions. GE helps the most in this process which provides the plant with high insect and disease resistance, drought and herbicide tolerance. Improved robotic machines, tractors, feeders, and planters help the farmers gain more profit with fewer labors [4]. Thus, with the help of AI

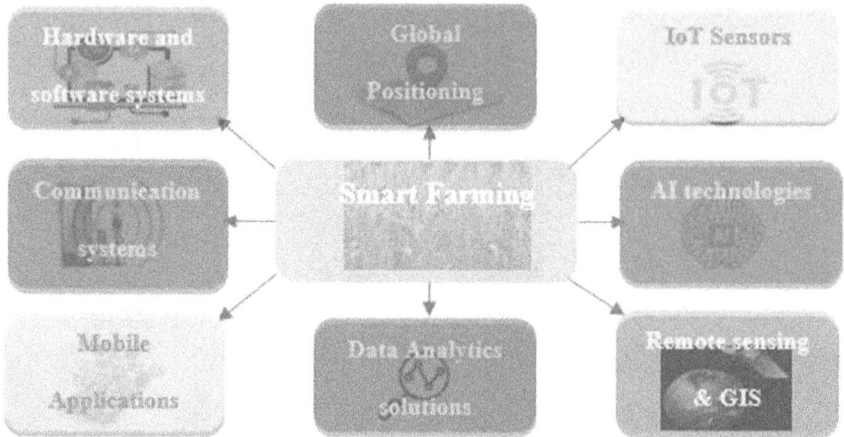

FIGURE 10.5 AI in agriculture.

systems, the field of agriculture adopts a rapid growth in terms of agricultural products and farming techniques.

Figure 10.5 shows the technologies used in smart farming. AI is used as a separate system along with all other technologies to improve sustainable agriculture.

10.4 EMERGING AGRICULTURAL TECHNOLOGIES

There is always a demand for innovative farm technologies and modern farmers show interest in emerging new technologies [5]. There are a few emerging techniques to enhance modern agricultural practices.

10.4.1 SOIL AND WATER SENSORS

Good quality soil and proper, sufficient amounts of water play a major role in the proper growth of crops. This sensor detects moisture, minerals, and nitrogen in the farmland, which helps the farmers to find when to water and fertilize the land rather than depending on a predetermined schedule of watering. As a result, the resources are efficiently used and lowered the cost and also keeps farm eco-friendly by limiting fertilizers and conserving of water.

10.4.2 WEATHER TRACKING

Weather condition is an important factor to be considered in agriculture. The moderate weather condition is always welcoming in the agricultural field. Rainfall plays a major role in crop maintenance. Heavy rainfall may even damage crops at the initial stage. Prediction of rainfall helps the farmers to protect their land. Temperature, humidity, and precipitation sensors help in weather prediction.

10.4.3   SATELLITE IMAGING AGRICULTURE

Remote sensing and GIS technology have many effects on the agricultural field. It is helpful to detect soil quality and crops in real-time. Vegetation maps help the farmers to monitor the crop growth and examine the areas in the field where crops get diseased. It helps them to protect the crop in every step if it has been affected and to ensure the maximum crop yield. It also monitors the soil surface area and identifies the defects in soil quality that occurs due to climate change. Satellite images along with IoT can forecast agricultural yield.

10.4.4   AUTOMATION SYSTEMS

If agricultural equipment like barrels and tractors are automated and equipped with IoT sensors, it makes work easier for farmers and reduces the workload and cost. There are 10 agricultural automation companies that provide new insight for the agricultural field [6]. They develop and manufacture robots, drones, smart tractors, and smart barrels to make a better precision farming.

  i. **Abundant Robotics**
     They invent robots for the hardest problems in agriculture.
 ii. **Agrobot**
     They developed the first robot for harvesting strawberries no matter of where and how they are grown up. By working with farmers and 24 robotic manipulators, Agrobot delivered a robot to pick contactless fruit. It has reduced the labor force engaged in picking the fruit.
iii. **American Robotics**
     This company has developed an autonomous drone, base station and analytics platform through innovations in AI and robotics. This unique drone in a box is named a scout.
 iv. **Bear Flag Robotics**
     They developed an automated tractor which enables the farmers to retrofit the existing tractors to implement control over the tractors by using cutting edge driverless technology.
  v. **Blue River Technologies**
     They built an intelligent solution using robotics and computer vision to spray herbicides only when needed with the exact amount. This is named as See & Spray technology which enables the farmers to prevent and control weeds. Weeds are the wild plants grown unnecessarily in competition to cultivated crops.
 vi. **ecoRobotix**
     They developed an automated weeding robot for the most effective weeding practice of Row crops, meadows and intercropping cultures. It serves as a most ecological and economical intelligent system that requires low energy reduces the negative impact of precision agriculture.

vii. **Rabbit Tractors**

They developed a compact, multipurpose, autonomous, swarm-enabled tractor that gives a new era to farmers who cultivate crops in rows to increase efficiency in agricultural land and to increase the yield by smart cultivation.

viii. **Rowbot**

They developed the first machine that is small with a multi-use platform and self-driving that travels between rows of corn crops, by neglecting the height constraint imposed by the rapidly growing crop.

ix. **Small Robot Company**

They built a small robot that improves crop yield by providing a needed amount of nutrients and supports every individual crop. As a result, it gives an effective method to monitor soil, environment and more production of yield.

x. **Soft Robotics**

They built a soft robot that is called a soft robotic gripper, a software-based control system to manipulate items of varying weight, size, and shape.

10.4.5 RFID TECHNOLOGY

Radio Frequency Identification has digital data about any product in the form of RFID tags or smart labels. The reader can read it using radio waves. It uses electromagnetic fields to find the details of an object attached to it. In Agricultural field, the RFID tags can be attached to the agricultural products to enhance the safety, to predict the health condition of vegetables and traceability. It also helps the processing companies to find useful information like the date of processing, package weight, and batch processing. AI is capable of processing even the uncertain and incomplete data in the real world. Integration of RFID with web-based information and AI can give more accurate information.

10.5 POTENTIAL AGRICULTURAL DOMAINS FOR MODERNIZATION

The plant needs water, minerals, nutrients, sunlight, and space for better growth. AI systems help in agricultural processes' inefficient ways as discussed below.

10.5.1 AI IN CROP MONITORING

Different plants need various amount of water, different types of minerals, nutrients, sunlight, and space for better growth. It also depends on the growing area and its climatic conditions. According to each location of the irrigation land, soil water test and crop water test can be made to calculate the amount needed for the crop to be grown [7–9]. AI systems help the farmers to best select the crops to be grown based on climate and soil conditions where crop yield can be optimized. It is done by using the data collected by drones or any software-based technology. Satellite images can be used as input and GIS software can be used to analyze the crops and soil conditions. With the help of image recognition software, data are collected and smart software is designed using deep learning algorithms and neural network to predict the health of crops and find the disease affected crops. Remote sensing satellite data and IoT sensors help in finding plant nutrient deficiencies also. Leaf sensor finds the water deficit in the plant by monitoring the moisture level in the leaves. The fruit size sensors detect the size of fruits in each of its growing phases and also detects the rate of intact of rounded fruits based on varying diameter size. There are numerous other sensors like temperature sensor, humidity sensor, precipitation sensor, etc., to predict the climate conditions in agricultural land. The data collected from these sensors are stored in the cloud database. These data can be accessed by machine learning models to classify the data and AI predictive techniques can be used to predict the needs of crops and it can also be used to find the future uncertain conditions using ANN from the data obtained from the sensors [10].

AI intelligent systems with IoT sensors best understands the climatological data such as temperature, humidity, solar radiation and wind speed. The analysis of these data will ensure the exact crop water requirement. It also identifies the growth of crops and condition of each crop periodically, where farmers will be aware of any viral or fungal disease that affects the plant, nutrient deficiency, attack of insects, etc. It helps farmers to make arrangements like using of fertilizer or manure to protect the crop. The AI system along with an IoT sensor identify the extreme temperature, stress level of the plant, uncontrolled use of chemicals, and scarcity of water in the soil [11]. The smart application is created to send a message to the farmers in case of any crop deficiency. Figure 10.6 depicts the operations in a smart system.

10.5.2 AI IN SEED GERMINATION

The best crops are obtained from the genetics of the seeds. AI systems are also used to scan the DNA sequence of seeds to make cross-mutations of the seeds. It is one of the methods to get the best crops where the genetics of the seeds are studied and cross mutated. Each seed will have its desirable characteristics. There are intelligent

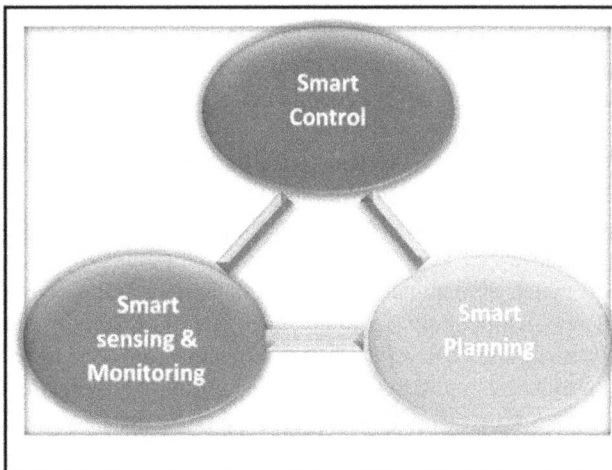

FIGURE 10.6 Smart system.

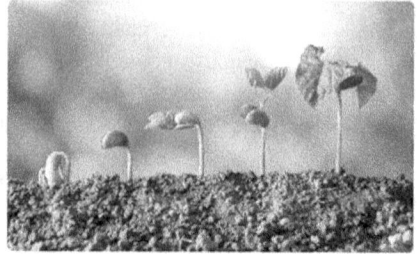

	RY	Ry	rY	ry
RY	RRYY	RRYy	RrYY	RrYy
Ry	RRYy	RRyy	RrYy	Rryy
rY	RrYY	RrYy	rrYY	rrYy
ry	RrYy	Rryy	rrYy	rryy

Round/Yellow: 9

Round/green: 3

wrinkled/Yellow: 3

wrinkled/green: 1
9:3:3:1 phenotypic
ratio

FIGURE 10.7   Phenotype example [13] and seed germination [14].

computer systems to perform this analysis. AI techniques are also used in the seed germination process, where heat and moisture levels are found and enable the crops to grow sooner than the actual expected time. Phenotypes of the seeds are also tested to choose the best seed to use [12]. Figure 10.7 shows the example of phenotype and seen the germination process. Machine learning using k-NN is used to find the different phenotypes found in the seed. Phenotype is the information about seed height and observational characteristics of the seed.

ImageJ application is used to identify hidden data in the image and machine learning application is used to preprocess, classify and visualize the data. AI with the embedded system is used in seed recognition and germination through image processing technique. The low-power sensing system is designed with AI onboard. Convolution neural network is applied and seed germination at different stages image datasets is used to train the system [15]. An ultrasonic sensor helps to develop fissures in seed coat and raises seedling moisture. AI combined with fuzzy logic and genetic algorithms also helps in better seed germination.

10.5.3 AI IN SOIL MANAGEMENT

Farmers aim to maintain the proper health of crops. Healthy soil plays a major role in maintaining the hygiene of plants. Good soil must retain water, releases nutrients, minerals when needed, and it should contain optimum pH and organic matter. It is important in the field of agricultural to best maintain the soil characteristics in which we cultivate the crops. AI systems are used to measure the health of the soil before plantation and during the growth stage. The soil quality can be calculated only based on the soil parameters. AI systems help in predicting the parameters of the soil. It is characterized as stable and dynamic properties. Soil depth, nutrient content, heavy metal contamination, and organic mass are considered stable properties, whereas temperature, humidity, and microbial activity are considered dynamic properties of soil [16]. AI prediction techniques are used to predict the soil fertility using nutrients as input, to predict water infiltration problem in the soil, and to predict the soil resistance to penetration [17]. AI techniques are also used for soil classifications, to estimate organic carbon. An artificial neural network, genetic engineering, and support vector machine are some of AI techniques used in soil classification [18,19]. Soil erosion and degradation is the decline or removal of soil due to poor management. It can also be solved using AI intelligent systems. Soil pollution is another major problem faced in agriculture due to overpopulation and intensive farming. AI combined with IoT and AI-based drones can make use of the computer vision system to monitor the soil on how and when it gets polluted.

To test the quality of the soil, the farmers take a sample of soil from their agricultural land and send it to the soil laboratory to test the soil. It is a time-consuming process and they get results a few days later. For some farmers, it is a difficult process to do. An IBM researcher in Brazil has developed an AI-based paper device which is in the size of a business card called AgroPad. The card contains microfluidics chip embedded into for performing chemical analysis and gives results in less than 10 seconds [20]. As shown in Figure 10.8, the circles in card provide the result. The five-color indicator changes the color based on the amount of pH, nitrogen dioxide, aluminum, magnesium, and chlorine that are present in the sample. Using the dedicated mobile application in the smartphone, which performs machine vision on the strip, it predicts the results by the machine learning algorithm and the farmers can take a snapshot of the card and receive the chemical results.

10.5.4 AI IN CROP PRODUCTIVITY

Crop production is defined as the ratio of agricultural outputs to the agricultural inputs. It is the final yield obtained from growing crops as food and fiber. There are four main classifications of crops, i.e., food crops, cash crops, plantation crops, and horticulture crops. Different crops grow well in different soils and areas. Crop productivity varies from place to place based on the areas they are planted and environmental conditions of each area. The intelligent models are designed to read the impact of changes in climate and weather conditions [22]. Soil erosion also affects the production of crops which also suspected by intelligent systems. It is necessary to save the plants from diseases and weeds to obtain good production.

The proper maintenance of crops, soil, land reforms also leads to increases in crop productivity. We can maintain the above mentioned parameters with the help of IoT sensors, satellite images and AI systems as we have seen earlier. Production may get affected if the climate changes suddenly. Heavy rainfall and flood may damage the food crops and horticulture crops. So, it is at the most necessary to predict climate conditions. The sudden change in climate and weather conditions are unpredictable. An accurate prediction system is required to avoid damages that occur due to climate

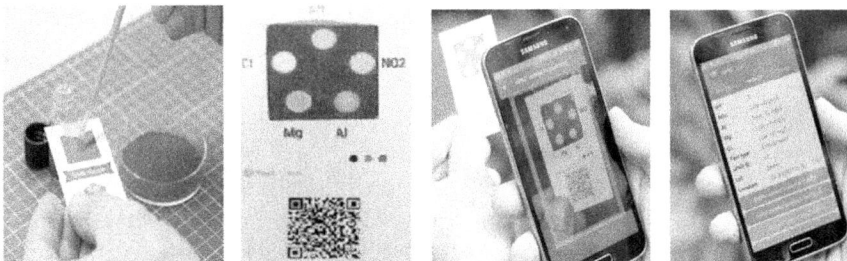

FIGURE 10.8 Agropad [21].

change. There are numerous models and methods to predict the climate; mathematical models, climatic models, weather satellites, IoT sensors, etc., are used as prediction systems. Weather prediction is a big deal as it requires effective analysis and decodes of huge datasets obtained from weather satellites and sensors. It is impossible to control the weather. The meteorologist should use past and present data to predict the future. The accuracy of climate prediction has improved in the modern period, but it cannot be said as 100% accuracy. Some estimated says as the weather prediction is done for 5 days is 90% accurate and for 7 days it is 80% accurate and more than 10 days is only 50% accurate. The AI system tries to give more accurate prediction than other prediction models and systems. AI is capable of accessing a huge amount of data than any other models can do. AI operates simulated mathematical programs, computational methods to work on a huge amount of data. Weather prediction incurs many meteorological parameters including the rotation of the earth to find the best pattern and to make a relevant hypothesis. Trying out many other models, scientist now using AI for better and fast weather prediction. By the use of deep learning mathematical models, the AI system is capable of predicting the future by learning and training the records. Many companies now rely mostly on AI development for accurate weather prediction. IBM developed Deep Thunder, an AI-based system to predict local weather conditions within a 0.2–1.2 miles resolution. Monsanto's climate corporation uses an AI-based solution to provide agricultural weather forecast [23]. These weather prediction measures help the farmers to take protective measures in case of sudden changes to be happened in their land, thus leading to the proper maintenance of crop productivity.

An AI-based sowing app has been developed to predict the correct sowing date. It comprises more than 30 years of meteorological data along with present weather data to predict the perfect sowing date to farmers. A pilot study was carried out in Andhra Pradesh, a state in India. It was carried out by Microsoft in collaboration with International Crops Research Institute for the Semi-Arid Tropics (ICRISAT) and with the Government of Andhra Pradesh. It is proven that farmers who followed the instruction from the sowing app are 30% more productive than farmers who don't follow [24]. The farmers should use weather prediction app, sowing app, etc. to attain maximum crop production from their land. Figure 10.9 represents weather prediction process in agriculture and the role of AI algorithms and techniques used for it.

10.5.5   AI in Price Forecasting of Agricultural Products

All the farmers will have expectations on the price of the crops they cultivated. They used to judge the cost by themselves by their experience on the field and crop they cultivated and another way is to judge with the historic data available in which different price predictions are recorded and used to predict the future price of the crop. It also helps the vegetable and fruits vendors to decide which vegetables to purchase based on the cost. Changes in agricultural food products will be a distress for both producers and consumers. It is one of the challenging problems in the agricultural field [25]. When there is a demand for food crops, the price will be increased. The other factors like climate, location, demand indicators, crop health, and oil prices are also important to predict the price of the product. Time series analysis has been used traditionally to forecast the price. AI forecasting models and

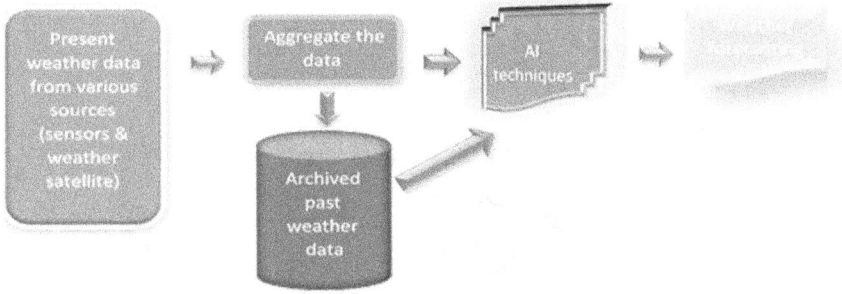

FIGURE 10.9   Role of AI in weather prediction.

feature selection methods are used to predict the price in recent years. Autoregressive Integrated Moving Average (ARIMA), Computational Intelligence models, Artificial Neural Networks (ANN), Support Vector Regression, Multivariate Adaptive Regression Splines (MARS), etc., are used to predict the agricultural products [26]. ANN model has widely been used for cost forecasting of agricultural products for a short-term. The data such as daily wholesale price, weekly wholesale price, the monthly wholesale price of each vegetable or fruits are collected for more than 30 years to run the model. Moreover, agricultural product cost relays on the biological structure of crop production. Indian government runs an official website called the Agricultural Marketing Information Network to provide daily data on market prices and volumes of vegetables and fruits arrived from across 1,514 market places in the country. The retail prices can be obtained from the portal run by the National Horticulture Board which provides retail prices from 30 districts across the country. The forecasting can be done with varying statistical data and with a minimum of 20 years of data is required for the betterment of results [27].

10.5.6   AI IN PEST AND WEED MANAGEMENT

Weed control is the topmost challenging problem for the farmers. Weeds are the unwanted plants that suck up all the water, nutrients, sunlight and space that are intended for the crops. The plants get affected by the disease carriers like rats, mosquitoes, mice, ticks, etc., which destroy the plants. Pesticides are used in agricultural land to control various pests. There are various types of pesticides which are an effective defender of certain pests. Algae, virus, bacteria, and insects are a different pest that affects plant growth. Each has its pesticides to control the damages it occurs to the crops. These pests also create health problems like asthma and allergies to farmers who work in agricultural land. Herbicides are used to kill the unwanted plants grown in between the crops cultivated. Autonomous sprayers can be made with AI techniques so that it drives themselves in the field to hunt the weeds. Robotic weed control is also used in Australia, which helps the farmers to save their time [28].

Figure 10.10 is the smart system used for weed management. The camera is fitted on the tractor which will recognize the weed plants when the sprayers drive over them. The intelligent software in the sprayer will adjust the treatments while

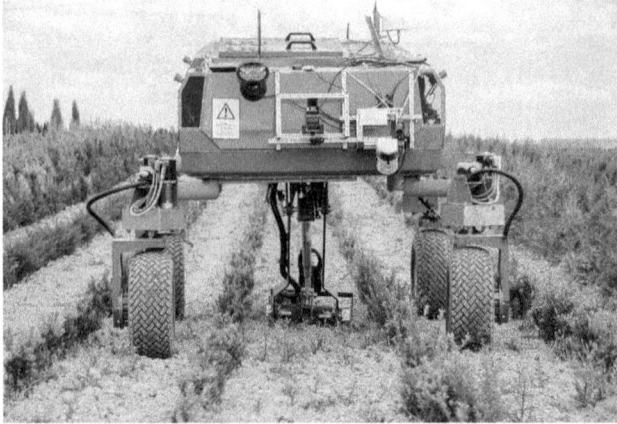

FIGURE 10.10   Weed management with robotics and AI [32].

driving. Through this kind of methods weed plants are identified and herbicides are used to control the weeds on the specific problematic spot. The data captured in the camera are stored in the computer and intelligent system is trained to recognize the place of the weeds available in the field [29]. The other intelligent system for weed management is building an automated robot using Lego MindstormEV3 which will be connected to the computer. The camera will be attached to the robot which consists of motors and servo motors that are used to capture the image of weeds and crops. The robot is designed to accurately distinguish the weed and the crops irrigated. AI system using convolution neural network algorithm is used to process the image captured in the camera. The robot's control will be provided and sprays the herbicides directly to the affected area only [30]. Since the adequate use of herbicide is not much good, intelligent systems help in spraying only to the affected area. The right amount of herbicide is used in the infected area and at the right time. In this way, farmers will benefit from the ill effects of weeds to the crops in irrigation land. A self-organizing neural network is also used to identify the original field crop's discrimination and the weed plant [31]. An artificial neural network is the foundation of AI, a computing device designed to simulate the human brain.

10.5.7   AI in Agricultural Land Utilization

The agricultural cultivating area is decreasing and the world's human population is growing very fast, which leads to an increase in the need for food and increase in land occupancy by the people. The intelligent system has to be developed for the optimum use of land and to gain more crop productivity to solve this critical problem. The land is the biggest asset for farmers. Selection of suitable crops for their agricultural land is a crucial problem for farmers. It is based on significant factors such as the weather condition, rate of production, type of soil, food requirements, yield rate, accessibility of fertilizers, agricultural inputs, spatial factors, and stakeholders. The farmers can only be benefitted if they follow optimal cropping patterns. Crops have to be categorized as seasonal crops and annual crops. For example, onion, corn, wheat, rice, and vegetables, which can be harvested in a maximum of 8 months because seasonal crops and co-conut, mango, coffee, etc. come under annual crops that take years to harvest. The farmer should choose plants that are economic in value. The farmer should check for rooting condition, water content soil erosion, and other land climatic conditions before planting the crops [33,34]. Decision making is a very risky process for farmers.

There are many mathematical models like linear programming, regression models used for optimal land use and cropping. There are many land use models and opti-mization techniques for solving land allocation problems. There are limitations in these methods and advancement in technology is needed to get better results than traditional methods. An intelligent expert system is designed by integrating sensors and AI technology like Multi-Layer Perceptron (MLP) and neural networks. This helps the farmers to check whether the land is suitable for cultivation. Sensor devices sense the climatic conditions and soil quality and that is taken as input for the training systems in MLP system to use land optimally [35]. Optimization algorithms help to use land optimally also by improving proper cropping patterns.

10.5.8 AI IN FERTILIZER OPTIMIZATION

Fertilizers are necessary to prevent nutrient losses to soil, air, and water. Optimum use of fertilizer leads to an increase in crop yield. The majority of farmers depend on the estimation method or trial and error method in the use of fertilizer. If it is not used correctly, the farmers cannot get more yield and leads to increased environmental pollution. Fertilizer usage considers factors such as type of crop planted, area of crops planted, soil type, expected selling price of crops, cost of fertilizers and budget invested for fertilizer products. Based on the response of crops after the usage of fertilizers, the farmers can calculate the profitable combinations of fertilizers [36]. Nitrogen, phos-phorus, potassium, sulfur, calcium, and magnesium are the major fertilizers needed by the crops. Types of fertilizers produced in India are Ammonium Sulfate (AS), Calcium Ammonium Nitrate (CAN), Ammonium Chloride, Urea, Single Super Phosphate (SSP), Triple Super Phosphate (TSP), Urea Ammonium Phosphate, Ammonium Phosphate Sulfate, Diammonium Phosphate (DAP), Mono Ammonium Phosphate (MAP), Nitro Phosphate, and Nitro Phosphate with Potash [37]. Whenever the crop is under stress, the farmers should make use of right fertilizer at the right amount to maintain the yield. The more usage of fertilizer will also result in loss. The stress may be caused due to change in weather condition, poor soil quality, lack of water content, nutrients, lack of weed management, poor maintenance of pesticides, herbicides, fer-tilizers, etc. With the help of computer vision technology, sensors, drone data, and satellite vegetation map helps to find the agricultural land data and weather condition. The infected crops can be taken by snapshot or satellite images of crops can be given as input to the AI model to predict the reason and cause of stress level in the crops. The test results can be given to farmers stating the reason for the stress level in crops and to take necessary steps like feeding with fertilizers to protect the crops. These are framed as many mobile applications taking varying inputs to provide the best combination of fertilizer. Figure 10.11 shows the process involved in fertilization.

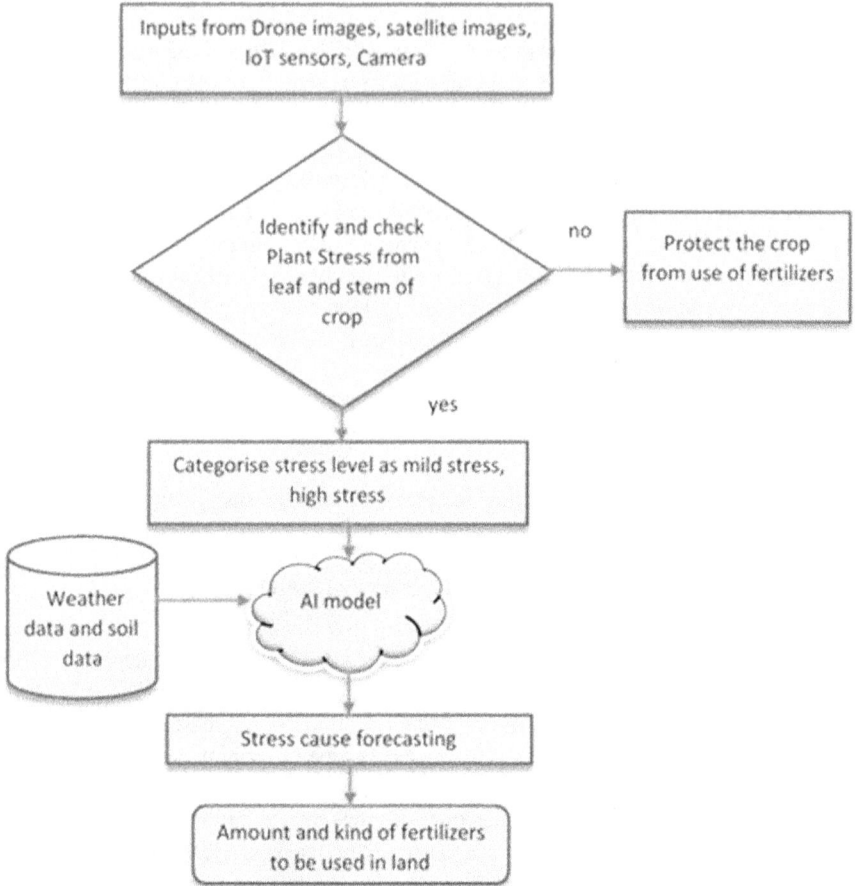

FIGURE 10.11 Fertilizer optimization using AI technique.

10.5.9 AI IN IRRIGATION MANAGEMENT

Water management is most essential in the present world. Water consumption from various sectors is the biggest problem. Irrigation water management system is defined as the regulation of water applied to farms by satisfying the water requirements of crops, also considering the intake characteristics of soil without wasting water, plant, and soil nutrients. It is also important to consider the rainfall events before supplying water to the farm. Irrigation frequency should be based on the stress level of crops to moisture, soil moisture reduction and evaporation, and soil and crops' transpiration rate. The water requirement is mainly based on the evapotranspiration rate and there are many models to find the evapotranspiration rate of a region for given climatic parameters. It is important to supply water to all crops equally by knowing how much water is available to supply [38]. Each crop requires a different level of water requirement. Each crop has a different level of transpiration rate. If a farmer has cultivated different kinds of crops in his land, the moisture content of each kind of plant and soil, water required for each crop has to be calculated to supply water. Crops in different stages of growth require a varying level of water. The farmers use bore well water and the water supplied from the water reservoirs through the canal system to supply to their irrigated lands.

There are different irrigation systems such as

(i) drip irrigation, (ii) sprinkler irrigation, (iii) surface irrigation, (iv) localized irrigation,

(v) center pivot irrigation, (vi) lateral move irrigation, (vii) sub irrigation, and (viii) manual irrigation

All of the above irrigation systems can be made automated by intelligent systems. Many robotics have been designed and empowered to irrigate the land. AI plays a major role in inefficient water use by optimizing the water use in the irrigation system and recreational fields. An automatic irrigation system can be designed by using sensors and deep learning predictive algorithms to predict the weather condition and rainfall which can automatically send required water by calculating soil moisture and climate conditions. Arduino or any other platform can be used to process the sensor data and weather data to predict the water requirement as shown in Figure 10.12.

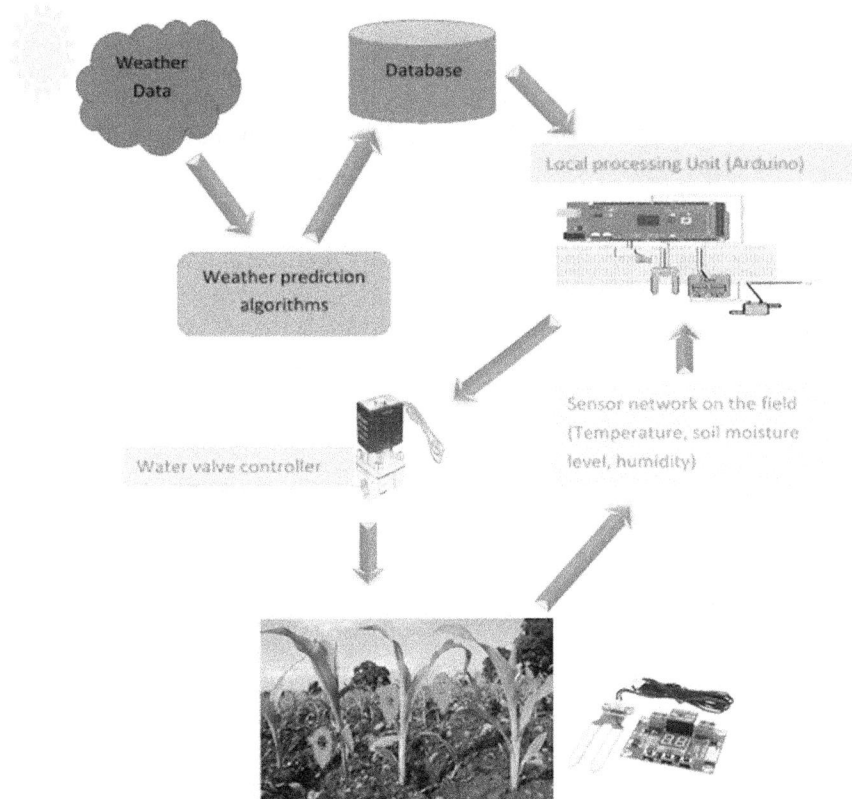

FIGURE 10.12   Irrigation optimization by intelligent systems.

10.6　CAN AI TRANSFORM AGRICULTURAL SCENARIO?

AI is becoming a boon to agriculture scenario. The term *precision agriculture* is known for the applications of AI in agriculture. AI technology helps in identifying plant nutrition level, to monitor diseases in plants, pest, soil moisture, components in soil, to predict weather conditions, etc. The drones with AI-enabled cameras capture the entire agricultural land to find the affected land areas and take preventive measures. IoT sensors and satellite images combined with AI technology and processing algorithms are mainly used to transform the agricultural field. Robots are used in many ways and reduce human resources in the agricultural field. AI has also helped farmers decide what crops can be cultivated, the time and duration of sowing seeds, to predict the yield and cost of crop production and quantity and kind of fertilizer to be used in farmland. Overall, AI helps farmer and guides through the process of sowing, growing, harvesting, and producing. AI technologies do not require constant supervision.

In future, it is expected to be digital farming, which will increase farmers' income to 1,100 million US$ by the end of 2025. AI is expected to take over all the farming farmers who still follow the traditional methods of farming. The researchers have predicted the world population growth will be 10 billion in the year 2050 where 70% more food has to be produced and the world's farmland is becoming unsustainable. Twenty-five percent of farmland is highly degraded, where 44% of farmland is moderately degraded and more than 40% of rural people are living in water scarcity condition. About 80% of deforestation makes degradation. All of these problems are due to poor management of agriculture. The government, industries, and investors should focus on improved and innovative agricultural practices [39].

Agriculture 4.0 – "The future of farming technology" is the next big trend facing the industry focused on precision agriculture. In the future, it aims at focusing on climate change, demographics, food waste, and scarcity of natural resources. The idea behind Agriculture 4.0 is to run agricultural operations with the advancements in technology such as machines, devices, sensors, and information technology. It focusses on cultivating crops with limited and required quantities of fertilizer, pesticides, and water rather than applying to the entire field. Future agriculture will be more advanced with superpower robots, aerial images, and Global Positioning System (GPS) technologies [40,41]. This will lead to optimal land use with more profit to farmers, efficient, and eco-friendly environment. Agriculture 4.0 is expected to solve the food scarcity and climate change problem. It aims to focus on the demand and supply chain using innovative technologies not for the sake of new invention rather than satisfy consumers' needs.

10.7　SUMMARY

Artificial intelligence is playing a vital role in all the agricultural field operations from choosing a crop to cultivating, from the sowing stage to the harvest stage. This chapter describes the tremendous improvement in agriculture with the use of AI technologies combined with the Internet of Things, data analytics, remote sensing, and geographic information system. Many companies innovated agricultural robots for various operations in the farmland. The invention of drones has specific improvement in weed management, crop monitoring, watering, fertilizing, and pesticides. Prediction algorithms have its great advantage in weather prediction, which was very useful information for farmers to plan their cultivation processes. A small climate change has a big impact on crop growth. Hence it is the greatest advantage for farmers to know the climate conditions in their farmland. Many mobile applications help farmers with every information and choose the best method of crop cultivation. The automated system reduces the human resources in the agricultural field. A lot more improvements are expected in the future to improve the lifestyle of farmers with emerging technologies.

REFERENCES

[1] https://www.gardeningknowhow.com/special/children/how-plants-grow.htm
[2] https://www.geeksforgeeks.org/crop-monitoring-smart-farming-using-iot/
[3] https://www.nsiserv.com/blog/how-technology-in-agriculture-is-shaping-the-future-of-the-industry
[4] https://iowaagliteracy.wordpress.com/2018/06/02/5-ways-technology-has-changed-farming/
[5] https://www.ayokasystems.com/news/emerging-agriculture-technologies/
[6] https://www.plugandplaytechcenter.com/resources/10-agriculture-automation-companies-shaping-future-farming/
[7] http://en.cnki.com.cn/Article_en/CJFDTotal-NKDB200701001.htm
[8] Manish K. Nema, Deepak Khare and Surendra K. Chandniha, "Application of Artificial Intelligence to Estimate the Reference Evapotranspiration in Sub-humid Doon Valley", Applications of Water Science, (7): 3903–3910, 2017.
[9] Online document cited at http://www.fao.org/docrep/X0490E/x0490e04.htm#evaporation
[10] https://www.researchgate.net/publication/326988635_IoT_and_AI_methods_for_plant_disease_detection_ in_Myanmar
[11] Zhao Liqiang, Yin Shouyi, Liu Leibo, Zhang Zhen and Wei Shaojun, "A Crop Monitoring System Based on Wireless Sensor Network", Procedia Environmental Sciences, 11: 558–565, 2011.
[12] https://apro-software.com/artificial-intelligence-in-agriculture/
[13] https://www.toppr.com/ask/question/the-ratio-of-phenotype-in-f2-generation-of-a-dihybrid-cross-is/
[14] https://www.news-medical.net/whitepaper/20180828/NMR-and-MRI-Technology-Identifies-Factors-in-Seed-Germination.aspx
[15] Dmitrii Shadrin, Alexander Menshchikov, Dmitry Ermilov and Andrey Somov, "Designing Future Precision Agriculture: Detection of Seeds Germination Using Artificial Intelligence on a Low-Power Embedded System", IEEE Sensors Journal, 19(23): 11573–11582, 2019.
[16] Danica Fazekasova, "Evaluation of Soil Quality Parameters Development in Terms of Sustainable Land Use", In Sime Curkovic (Ed.), Sustainable Development - Authoritative and Leading Edge Content for Environmental Management, IntechOpen, USA.
[17] Tonismar dos S. Pereira, Adroaldo D. Robaina, Marcia X. Peiter, Rogerio R. Torres and Jhosefe Bruning, "The Use of Artificial Intelligence for Estimating Soil Resistance to Penetration", Journal of Brazilian Association of Agricultural Engineering, Engenharia Agrícola, 38: 142–148.
[18] Ralph J. McCracken and Robert B. Cate, "Artificial Intelligence, Cognitive Science, and Measurement Theory Applied in Soil Classification", Soil Science Society of America Journal, 50(1), 1986.

[19] Mohamed A. Shahin, "State-of-the-Art Review of Some Artificial Intelligence Applications in Pile Foundations", Geoscience Frontiers, 7: 33–44, 2016.

[20] https://www.ibm.com/blogs/research/2018/09/agropad/

[21] https://www.iotforall.com/ibm-research-agropad-iot

[22] Fulu Tao, Masayuki Yokozawa and Zhao Zhang, "Modelling the Impacts of Weather and Climate Variability on Crop Productivity Over a Large Area: A New Process-Based Model Development, Optimization, and Uncertainties Analysis", Agricultural and Forest Meteorology, 149: 831–850, 2009.

[23] https://interestingengineering.com/ai-might-be-the-future-for-weather-forecasting

[24] http://www.fao.org/e-agriculture/news/harnessing-power-ai-transform-agriculture

[25] Manpreet Kaur, Heena Gulati and Harish Kundra, "Data Mining in Agriculture on Crop Price Prediction: Techniques and Applications", International Journal of Computer Applications, 99(12): 1–3, August 2014.

[26] Yuehjen E. Shao and Jun-Ting Dai, "Integrated Feature Selection of ARIMA with Computational Intelligence Approaches for Food Crop Price Prediction", Hindawi Complexity, July 2018: 1–17, 2018.

[27] Lovish Madan, Ankur Sharma and Praneet Khandelwal, "Price Forecasting & Anomaly Detection for Agricultural Commodities in India", COMPASS '19, July 3–5, 2019.

[28] https://iapps2010.me/2018/12/19/weed-management-with-robotics-and-ai/

[29] http://agrinavia.com/artificial-intelligence-to-reduce-the-use-of-herbicides/

[30] Hea Choon Ngo, Ummi Raba'ah Hashim, Yong Wee Sek, Yogan Jaya Kumar and Wan Sing Ke, "Weeds Detection in Agricultural Fields Using Convolutional Neural Network", International Journal of Innovative Technology and Exploring Engineering, 8(11): 292–296, September 2019. (IJITEE) ISSN: 2278-3075.

[31] Aitkenhead Matthew, I.A. Dalgetty, Christopher Mullins, Allan James Stuart McDonald and Norval James Colin Strachan, "Weed and crop discrimination using image analysis and artificial intelligence methods", Computers and Electronics in Agriculture, 39(3): 157–171, 2003.

[32] https://iapps2010.me/2018/12/19/weed-management-with-robotics-and-ai/

[33] Razali, Zulkifli Nasution and Rahmawaty, "Optimization Model on the Use of Agriculture Land in the Catchment Area of Lake Toba", International Journal of Scientific & Technology Research, 3(11): 1–5, November 2014.

[34] https://www.researchgate.net/publication/335582861_Artificial_Intelligence_in_Agriculture_An_Emerging_Era_of_Research

[35] Durai Raj Vincent, N. Deepa, Dhivya Elavarasan, Kathiravan Srinivasan, Sajjad Hussain Chauhdary, and Celestine Iwendi, "Sensors Driven AI-Based Agriculture Recommendation Model for Assessing Land Suitability", Sensors (Basel), 19(17): 1–16, 2019.

[36] https://play.google.com/store/apps/details?id=org.cabi.ofra&hl=en_IN

[37] http://fert.nic.in/sites/default/files/Indian%20Fertilizer%20SCENARIO-2014.pdf

[38] https://www.nrcs.usda.gov/Internet/FSE_DOCUMENTS/nrcs141p2_017781.pdf

[39] https://www.worldgovernmentsummit.org/api/publications/document?id=95df8ac4-e97c-6578-b2f8-ff0000a7ddb6

[40] https://www.oliverwyman.com/our-expertise/insights/2018/feb/agriculture-4-0--the-future-of-farming-technology.html

[41] https://analyticsindiamag.com/top-ai-powered-projects-in-indian-agriculture-sector-2019/

11 Artificial Intelligence-Based Ubiquitous Smart Learning Educational Environments

S. Anuradha

Operations Manager, Perpetual Systems, Coimbatore, India

CONTENTS

11.1 INTRODUCTION

The innovation and applications of new technologies have taken the educational institutions into a new dimension. Usage of technologies in teaching and learning is inevitable and the institutions not opting for technologies are out of the box in the present context. The educational institutions need to develop a smart learning environment so that the students can study in any place at any time. Ubiquitous computing is a new technology that utilizes a large number of cooperative small nodes with computing and/or communication capabilities such as handheld terminals, smart mobile phones, and sensor network nodes, etc. (Sakamura and Koshizuka, 2005). Initial research was carried out in e-learning. From e-learning, the researchers have moved to m-learning. m-learning enables learners to use mobile devices. With the advent of smartphones, a new era of learning, namely smart learning, is introduced. Ubiquitous learning in the latest version of smart learning allows the learners to connect to the content server at any time from any place by using smart devices. The shift in the e-learning paradigm is presented in Figure 11.1.

This paper proposes a smart learning environment framework. This framework is used with the AI models. As the environment is ubiquitous, the learner is free from accessing the content from anywhere and anytime by using any of the smart

DOI: 10.1201/9781003175865-11

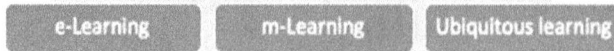

FIGURE 11.1 Shift in e-learning.

devices. The usage patterns are captured in the new environment and are stored in the data warehouse server. Supervised machine learning algorithms are then applied to this data set to understand more interesting and meaningful learning patterns. The machine learning models can use many techniques such as Linear Discriminant Analysis, KNN, Naïve Bayes (Quinlan, 1993).

11.2   NEED AND CONSIDERING THE FOUNDATIONS

Chen et al. (2015) present a smart learning environment technology namely *Smart Classroom 2.0*. This is a speech-driven PowerPoint system with automatic voice recognition features to assist the teacher during the lecture. The key characteristics of smart learning and the main challenges to overcome when designing smart educational environments is presented by Gros (2016). The author presents the need to consider future users in the design process of the smart learning systems. Li and Zheng (2017) discuss the ideas of electronic school-bag (eSchoolbag). This tool provides instructors and students with a smart learning environment. The learning model is then analyzed for personalized and adaptive learning.

The current problems in the flipped classroom teaching are presented regarding a case study in a University in Northwest China (Li, 2018). This paper presents a post hoc analysis of a failed case with flipped classrooms and attempts to discuss, at a macroscopic level, problems with preconditions for the flipped classrooms that currently exist. The challenges and opportunities for active and hybrid learning for future education is discussed by Ebba (2016). The lifelong learning journey (Ebba, 2017) and promoting active and meaningful learning for digital learners (Ebba, 2018) are the good motivational chapters for a smart learning environment.

Spector (2014) explains a learning environment that convergence of advanced developments in smart learning environments. The author elaborates on the environment for multiple contexts. The author also evaluates the presented environment. Hoel and Mason (2018) present standards for smart education and a framework standard. The author constructs a reference model for smart education by considering a cognitive smart learning model and a smartness level model. Hwang (2014) presents the idea behind smart learning environments in the context of ubiquitous learning. The author also presents a framework to address the design and development considerations of a smart learning environment. The author discusses the technologies that support the ubiquitous smart learning environment. Price (2015) discusses the lessons learned in implementing smart learning environments under Intel education initiatives. This author examines contextual factors of effective ICT implementation for smart learning environments resulting from a review of exploratory research, evaluation data, and study reports of successful ICT use in schools around the world.

Renato et al. present smart learning environments for the 21st century. The author presents the evolution of technology-enhanced learning (from e-learning to smart learning). A research framework for smart education is presented by Zhu et al. (2016). This paper discusses a four-tier framework for smart pedagogies and 10 key features of a smart learning environment. This framework includes class-based differentiated instruction, group-based collaborative learning, individual-based personalized learning, and mass-based generative learning. Technological architecture is also presented. Chin and Chen present mobile learning support systems for the ubiquitous learning environment. The systems architecture and the content learning function is presented in the paper (Chin and Chen, 2013).

The role of ubiquitous learning is very essential in the field of education. It can be used to provide personalized services in the context-aware u-learning environment. Learners might feel distressed or confused while encountering problems in the u-learning environment. Under such circumstances, the ubiquitous learning system could actively provide timely hints or assistance if the contexts concerning human emotions or attitudes can be sensed (Hwang et al., 2009). Digital ubiquitous museum (Sakamura and Koshizuka, 2005) and the ubiquitous computing technologies and context-aware recommender systems for ubiquitous learning (Thiprak and Kurutach, 2015) provides the smart and ubiquitous learning environments in detail. Kleftodimos and Evangelidis (2016) present how to use open source technologies and open internet resources in developing interactive video-based learning. The learner activity data is analyzed for effective decision-making.

Giannakos et al. (2016) introduce smart learning analytics in video-based learning. The prospects and limitations of smart learning analytics were discussed in detail. The author also presents the research challenges in using smart learning analytics. Analytics in higher education and its benefits are presented in ECAR-Analytics Working Group (2015). The ability to accurately predict future outcomes using learning data-called predictive learning analytics–is of significant strategic value because it empowers stakeholders in the learning process with intelligence on which they can act as means to achieve more desirable outcomes.

Based on the above-stated context and justifications, this chapter proposes a new framework for ubiquitous learning. The new environment also presents the method to apply predictive analytics for improving smart learning.

11.3 FRAMEWORK FOR UBIQUITOUS SMART LEARNING

ISO/IEC 23988:2007 gives recommendations on the use of IT to deliver assessments to candidates and to record and score their responses. The ISO/IEC 23988:2007 (revised in 2014) standard is being considered to develop the new framework. The following points prescribed in the standard are considered (ISO, 2018):

- Providing evidence of the security of the assessment, which can be presented to regulatory and funding organizations

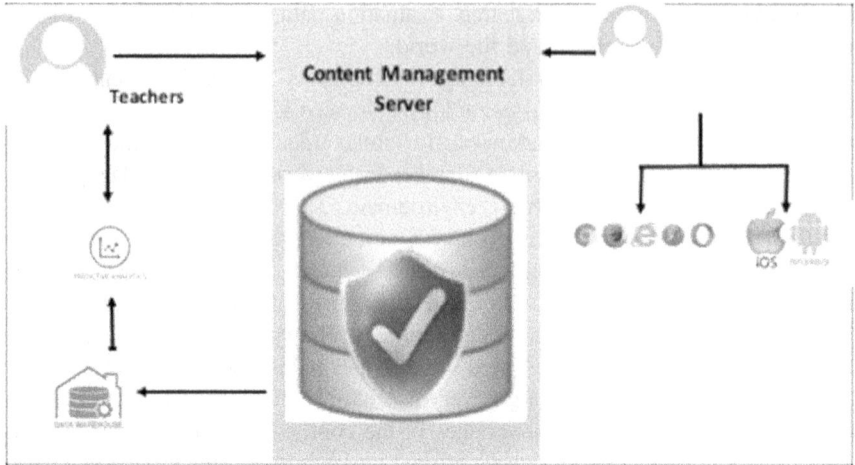

FIGURE 11.2   Framework for ubiquitous learning with predictive analytics.

- Establishing a consistent approach to the regulations for delivery, which should be of benefit to assessment centers who deal with more than one assessment distributer

The framework for ubiquitous smart learning is presented in Figure 11.2. The content management server contains the developed e-content of all the courses. The content may be in form of text, images, audio, or video clips. The security measures as prescribed in the ISO/IEC 23988:2007 standards will be considered to enhance data security in the content management server. These contents are supplied by the teacher and developed by the content developer. The teacher is supplied with a template for a lesson and prepares the content as stated in the learning outcomes in the courses.

The teacher provides the content, which includes text, audio, and video for the exercises. The content developer develops the e-content by using the standard tools. The content developer and the teacher work very closely to develop the content. The content management server runs in Windows/Linus platforms with Oracle/MS-SQL server in the database server.

As the environment is ubiquitous, the learners access the content not only from the classrooms but also from the home, library, or any other convenient locations. The learners can access through any browsers or smart devices of their choice. The content management server keeps track of all the learner behavior. The learning by the students can be synchronous or asynchronous. In the case of asynchronous learning, if the learner finds it difficult or takes more time on understanding a topic, the content management server acts smartly by way of communicating with the respective teachers. The interface available in the content management server coordinates the learner's behavior with the teacher. All the learners' navigational patterns are monitored and stored in the data warehouse server for predictive

TABLE 11.1
Data Warehouse Server Requirements

Component	Required
Operating system	A computer running a licensed version of Red Hat Enterprise Linux 7.3/ Windows 8 or higher
Virtual machine (VM)	This component can run in a virtual environment to implement virtualization
CPU	8–40 CPU cores
Memory	32 GB–2 TB RAM
Available disk space	200 GB–2 TB disk space
Database	Oracle 11g Enterprise Edition/MS-SWL Server 2012 or higher

analytics. The minimum expected configuration of the data warehouse server is provided in Table 11.1.

11.4 ROLE AND ADVANTAGE OF USING ARTIFICIAL INTELLIGENCE

The data stored in the data warehouse server are used for predictive analytics. Structured and semi-structured data is stored in the repository for further analysis as given in Figure 11.3. Initially, the stored data is pre-processed by an appropriate tool. Data cleaning, transformation, and reduction phases are considered in this stage. The cleaned data is given as input to a machine learning model (Witten et al., 2011). The artificial intelligence model may contain any data mining technique, machine learning, or artificial intelligence algorithm. The author of the classification rule mining technique (C4.5) in data mining for prediction. Classification rule mining techniques are the best techniques for prediction modeling and analysis.

The output produced as rules are then modeled and analyzed by any visualization techniques. The familiar visualization techniques such as Tableau, SAS, or R will be the best choice for this developed framework. The teacher then analyzes the generated results, and content developed to understand the good and bad practices or interesting navigational patterns. Based on the observation, the teacher and the content manager will further improve the contents.

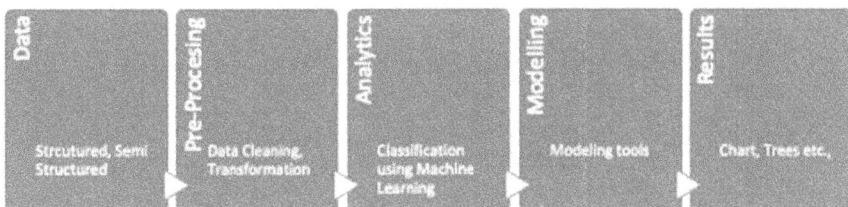

FIGURE 11.3 Main steps in machine learning.

11.4.1 Advantage of Artificial Intelligence

- Improves efficiency in course organization, delivery
- Boost confidence level to the students
- Detect the risks and plan for further modification/update
- Student/Learner/Teacher satisfaction
- Positioning of the department/university

Figure 11.4 represents the flow of information in the developed framework. The teacher interacts with the content developer for providing the needed content. The teacher provides the contents by considering the academic ethics and the pedagogy for the relevant course. The content manager looks into the pedagogy, technical resources, and design the interface for a lesson. The developed contents are then stores in the content management server. The learner accesses the content through any smart device from anywhere (ubiquitous). The navigational patterns and the other related data are captured and stored in the data repository for decision-making. This is the data warehouse server. The machine learning models are then applied to the data available in the data warehouse server. The results of the machine learning models are finally interpreted by the teacher for further improving the course content and delivery.

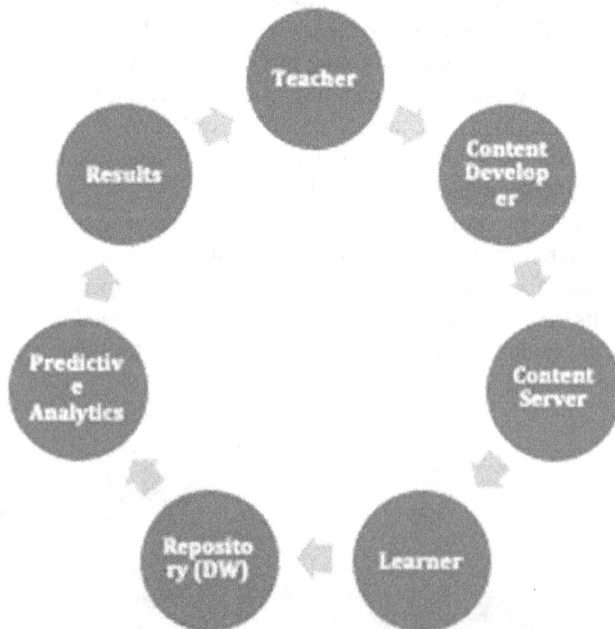

FIGURE 11.4   Flow of development and learning in a ubiquitous environment.

11.5   CONCLUSION

The developed framework provides a standard for implementing the ubiquitous smart learning environment by applying suitable predictive models. Using artificial intelligence models is the novel way of improving content management systems periodically. The proposed framework will enable ubiquitous learning. As the role of the Internet is very active in education, the proposed framework will bring a better way of education. The future direction of this paper is to study the flexibility and scalability issues in the framework.

REFERENCES

Chen C., Chang Y., Chien Y., Tijus and Chang C., (2015). Incorporating a smart classroom 2.0 Speech-Driven PowerPoint System (SDPPT) into university teaching, Smart Learning Environments, 2: 7.

Chin K., and Chen Y., (2013). A Mobile Learning Support System for Ubiquitous Learning Environments, 2nd International Conference on Integrated Information, Procedia - Social and Behavioral Sciences, 73: 14–21.

Ebba O., (2016). Challenges and opportunities for active and hybrid learning related to UNESCO, Handbook of Research on Active Learning and the Flipped Classroom Model in the Digital Age, Pages: 19.

Ebba O., (2017). Let the learners take the lead for their lifelong learning journey, Handbook of Research on Learner-Centered Pedagogy in Teacher Education and Professional Development, Pages: 22.

Ebba O., (2018). Promoting active and meaningful learning for digital learners, Handbook of Research on Mobile Technology, Constructivism, and Meaningful Learning, Pages: 22.

ECAR-Analytics Working Group (October 7, 2015). The Predictive Learning Analytics Revolution: Leveraging Learning Data for Student Success. ECAR Working Group Paper. Louisville, CO: ECAR.

Giannakos M. N., Demetrios G. Sampson and Kidziński L., (2016). Introduction to smart learning analytics: foundations and developments in video-based learning, Smart Learning Environments, 3: 12.

Gros B., (2016). The design of smart educational environments, Smart Learning Environments, 3: 15.

Hoel T., and Mason J., (2018). Standards for smart education – towards a development framework, Smart Learning Environments, 5: 3.

Hwang G., (2014). Definition, framework and research issues of smart learning environments — a context-aware ubiquitous learning perspective, Smart Learning Environments, 1: 4.

Hwang G., Wu T., and Chen Y., (2009). Ubiquitous Computing Technologies in Education. IGI Global.

ISO (2018). https://www.iso.org/standard/41840.html, 14 May 2020.

Kleftodimos A., and Evangelidis G., (2016). Using open source technologies and open internet resources for building an interactive video based learning environment that supports learning analytics, Smart Learning Environments, 3: 9.

Li S., and Zheng J., (2017). The effect of academic motivation on students' English learning achievement in the eSchoolbag-based learning environment, Smart Learning Environments, 4: 3.

Li Y., (2018). Current problems with the prerequisites for flipped classroom teaching — a case study in a university in Northwest China, Smart Learning Environments, 5: 2.

Price J. K. (2015). Transforming learning for the smart learning environment: lessons learned from the Intel Education Initiatives, Smart Learning Environments, 2: 16.

Quinlan J. R. (1993). C4.5: Programs for Machine Learning. Morgan Kaufmann Publishers.

Sakamura K., and Koshizuka N., (2005). Ubiquitous Computing Technologies for Ubiquitous Learning, IEEE International Workshop on Wireless and Mobile Technologies in Education.

Spector J. M., (2014). Conceptualizing the emerging field of smart learning environments, Smart Learning Environments, 1: 2.

Thiprak S., and Kurutach W., (2015). Ubiquitous Computing Technologies and Context Aware Recommender Systems for Ubiquitous Learning, IEEE, 2015.

Witten Ian H., Frank E., and Hall Mark A. (2011). Data Mining: Practical Machine Learning Tools and Techniques, 3rd Edition. San Francisco: Morgan Kaufmann. p. 191.

Zhu Z., Ming-Hua Yu and Peter Riezebos (2016). A research framework of smart education, Smart Learning Environments, 3: 4.

12 Artificial Intelligence in Assessment and Evaluation of Program Outcomes/Program Specific Outcomes

V. Saravanan[1] and D. Vinotha[2]
[1]Dean, Computer Studies, Dr. SNS Rajalakshmi College of Arts and Science, Coimbatore, India
[2]Assistant Professor in the Department of Computer Science and Engineering, School of Engineering and Technology, PRIST University, Thanjavore, India

CONTENTS

12.1 INTRODUCTION

Artificial intelligence (AI) is the need of the hour today: the media coverage and public discussion and usage about artificial intelligence are almost impossible to avoid [1]. AI has already been applied to education primarily in some tools that help develop skills and testing systems. Machine learning (ML) is the study of computer algorithms that improve automatically through experience [2]. It is seen as a subset of artificial intelligence. As AI educational solutions continue to mature, the hope is that AI can help fill needs gaps in learning and teaching and allow colleges and teachers to do more than ever before [3]. AI can drive efficiency, personalization, and streamline admin tasks to allow teachers the time and freedom to provide understanding and adaptability – uniquely human capabilities where machines would struggle [3,4]. AI can point out places where the course needs to improve. Assessment is defined as a process that identifies, collects, and prepares the data necessary for evaluation. Evaluation is defined as a process for interpreting the data generated through the assessment processes to determine how well the program outcomes/program specific outcome are being attained. Program Outcomes (PO) are the statements about competencies and expertise a graduate will possess after completion of the program. Program Specific Outcomes (PO) are the statements about a particular discipline graduate's competencies and expertise after completion of the program. Assessment and evaluation of POs/PSOs are very important for a higher education institution as the outcome results play a very important role in analyzing the various factors such as the usage of proper assessment tools, identification, and assignment of relevant courses to the teachers, etc. This paper is an attempt to use the artificial intelligence techniques in the data related POs/PSOs. A simple case analysis is considered for the analysis. The objectives of using artificial intelligence in the assessment and evaluation of POs/PSOs are to:

a. Review and provide innovative assessment tools.
b. Prepare strategies to introduce new assessment and evaluation tools as needed by the college authorities.
c. Enhance the learning capabilities of students at all levels.
d. Help students understand the ways to present and improve their soft and hard skills.
e. Encourage the students to learn about using artificial intelligence in many other applications with social impact.

12.2   ASSESSMENT AND EVALUATION

Assessment is defined as one or more processes that identify, collect, and prepare the data necessary for evaluation. Evaluation is defined as one or more processes for interpreting the data acquired through the assessment processes to determine how well the program outcomes/program specific outcome are being attained.

Assessment Process
  i. **Data Collection**
     a. The direct assessment is evidence of student learning. It is tangible and measurable and serves as evidence.
     b. Indirect assessment is indirect evidence that tends to be composed of proxy votes that students are probably continuously learning. An example

of indirect evidence is a survey asking students to provide feedback on what they have learned in a semester.

c. A course report is a piece of final evidence submitted by the teacher of an individual course. It contains the data collected of direct and indirect assessments, which were conducted during the semester. Information is gathered using several assessment tools at regular intervals. For example, an exit survey is a data collection tool that is used to collect information about final year students' opinions of PO/PSO achievement. It is offered at the end of each semester to all students when they apply for graduation.

ii. **Data Preparation:** Raw data is validated and transformed to make it ready for use in evaluation. For example, paper-based survey data is converted to an electronic format where necessary, and illegible, incomplete, erroneous, or duplicate submissions are discarded.

Evaluation Processes

i. **Data Interpretation:** Metrics are used to summarize data into points of interest. For example, survey responses on POs/PSOs' achievement are used to calculate weighted averages for POs/PSOs.

ii. **Attainment Evaluation:** Assessing the achievement of targets for POs/PSOs. For example, checking if the PO/PSO achievement from various data sources is above a set threshold.

iii. **Issue Analysis:** Where targets are not achieved, a deeper analysis is conducted to determine the possible causes. For example, reviewing faculty course review reports, speaking with faculty directly, or speaking with students can determine the underlying causes of poor achievement.

iv. **Improvement Plan:** An action plan is developed to remedy the identified issues.

Figure 12.1 summarizes data assessment and evaluation related to POs/PSOs. Artificial intelligence is used in the assessment process.

12.3 DATA SET ATTRIBUTES AND IMPLEMENTATION PLATFORM

The data set belongs to 150 courses that are considered for analysis. Python is used in the *Google colab* platform for implementation. The data set contains 6 attributes namely PO1, PO2, PO3, PSO1, PSO2, and Attainment. Table 12.1 presents the properties of the data set.

A snapshot is provided in Table 12.2 for better visualization to the users.

Attainment Level:

Three levels of outcome achievement at section or course level have been defined as provided in Table 12.3. For a section or whole course, the final judgment of the attainment of the student outcomes by all students enrolled in a course or a section is evaluated in the following Sections.

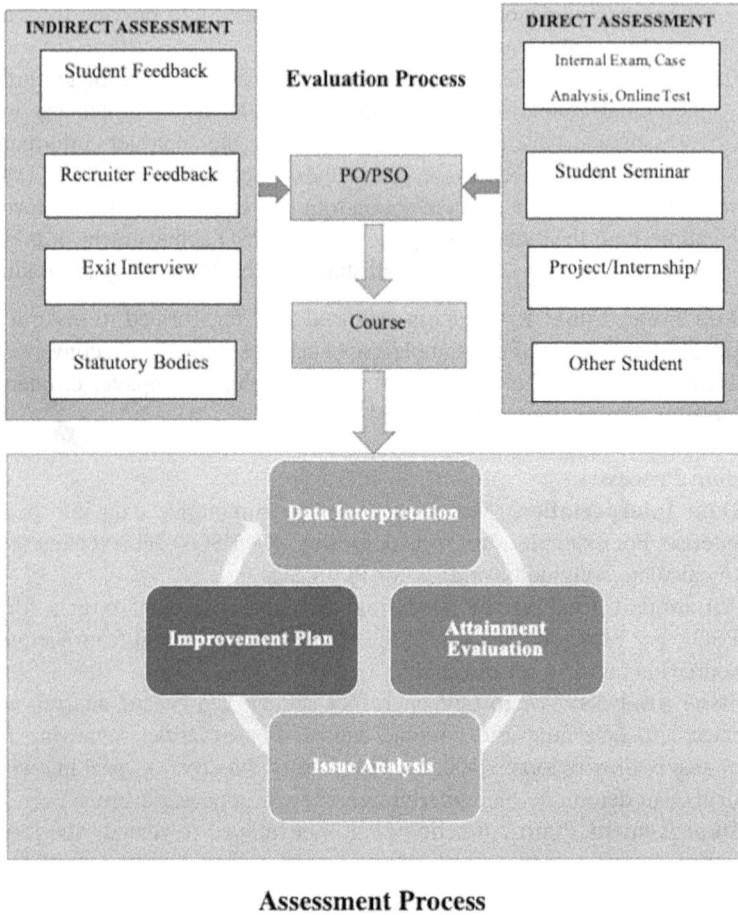

Assessment Process

FIGURE 12.1   Assessment and evaluation processes.

TABLE 12.1
Attributes of the Data Set

Dataset Characteristics:	Multivariate	Number of Instances:	150
Attribute Characteristics:	Integer	Number of Attributes:	7
Associated Tasks:	Classification	Missing Values?	Yes

12.4   EVALUATION USING MACHINE LEARNING MODELS

12.4.1   STATISTICAL SUMMARY

The summary of the data set is provided in Table 12.4. The table contains the data related to the number of rows, mean, the minimum value, and maximum value as well as some percentiles.

TABLE 12.2
Snapshot of the Data Set

PO1	PO2	PO3	PSO1	PSO2	Attainment
50	50	25	60	35	DNME
45	45	55	70	44	DNME
78	34	80	44	54	DNME
67	78	55	50	40	DNME
55	80	50	35	60	DNME
...					
55	60	76	65	56	PE
40	66	80	90	65	PE
66	76	68	76	65	PE
45	66	55	87	90	PE
55	56	90	77	87	PE
...					
77	65	89	89	87	EE
87	88	88	87	90	EE
78	90	77	67	98	EE
89	87	78	76	95	EE
87	77	80	90	87	EE

TABLE 12.3
Assessment of Attainment Level

Meets Expectations (ME)	Progressing Towards Expectations (PE)	Does Not Meet Expectations (DNME)
>=75% of the students who are achieving the satisfactory level or above	>=60% & <75% of the students who are achieving the satisfactory level or above	<60% of the students who are not achieving the satisfactory level or above

Table 12.5 presents the number of rows that belong to each table/worksheet in a data set. This can be viewed as an absolute count of the attribute "Attainment."

12.4.2 DATA VISUALIZATION

Multivariate plots are used in machine learning to better understand the relationships between attributes [5]. Multivariate plots are presented in Figure 12.2. The scatterplots of all pairs of attributes are presented in Figure 12.2.

TABLE 12.4
Statistical Summary

	PO1	PO2	PO3	PSO1	PSO2
Count	150.000000	150.000000	150.000000	150.000000	150.000000
Mean	69.366667	64.160000	64.626667	68.980000	70.126667
Std	15.030804	17.076252	16.641723	15.556121	16.748954
Min	34.000000	6.000000	5.000000	20.000000	35.000000
25%	56.000000	55.000000	55.000000	60.000000	56.000000
50%	67.000000	65.000000	67.000000	67.000000	67.000000
75%	78.000000	78.000000	77.000000	80.000000	87.000000
Max	98.000000	98.000000	98.000000	98.000000	98.000000

TABLE 12.5
Instance Count

Attainment	
DNME	50
EE	50
PE	50

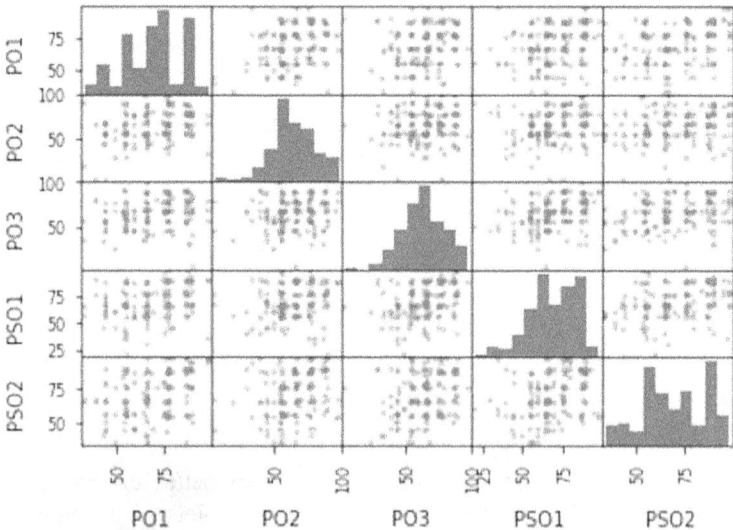

FIGURE 12.2 Multivariate plots.

These plots are helpful to show the structured relationships between input variables. The diagonal grouping of some pairs of attributes suggests a high correlation and a predictable relationship. Also, the attributes PO2, PO3, and PO4 are in Gaussian distribution and can be used for better model evaluation and prediction.

12.4.3   MODEL CREATION AND ESTIMATION

Create a Validation Data Set: Few rows of the data set will not be used and the algorithms will not consider these data to get an independent relation of how best and accurate the models might be in the given data set.

The loaded data set is split into two, 80% is used for training, and 20% will be used as a validation data set.

Test Harness: Stratified 10-fold cross-validation is used in this paper to estimate the model accuracy of the developed classifier. This splits the data set into 10 parts, train on nine and validate on one and repeat for all combinations of train-test splits.

12.4.4   BUILD MODELS

To know, which algorithm would be better for the chosen data set and what is the configuration to be used, the implementation test uses six different algorithms namely:

    i. Logistic Regression (LR)
    ii. Linear Discriminant Analysis (LDA)
    iii. K-Nearest Neighbors (KNN)
    iv. Classification and Regression Trees (CART)
    v. Gaussian Naïve Bayes (NB)
    vi. Support Vector Machines (SVM)

These are a good combination of a few linear (LR and LDA), few nonlinear (KNN, CART, NB, and SVM) algorithms.

12.4.5   SELECT BEST MODEL

Six models are generated and accuracy estimations for each model is calculates. The accurance of these models need to be as given in Table 12.6.

In the above case, we can see that it looks like Linear Discriminant Analysis (LDA) and K-Nearest Neighborhood (KNN) has the highest estimated accuracy score at 90%. A whisker plot of the model is generated as shown in Figure 12.3. We can see that the box and whisker plots are in the top of the range, with many evaluations achieving 90% accuracy and some evaluation down into the high 30% accuracies.

TABLE 12.6

Model Accuracy

Logistic Regression	0.650000 (0.062361)
Linear Discriminant Analysis	0.908333 (0.069222)
K-Nearest Neighbors	0.908333 (0.069222)
Classification and Regression Trees	0.733333 (0.161589)
Gaussian Naïve Bayes	0.891667 (0.075000)
Support Vector Machines	0.366667 (0.040825)

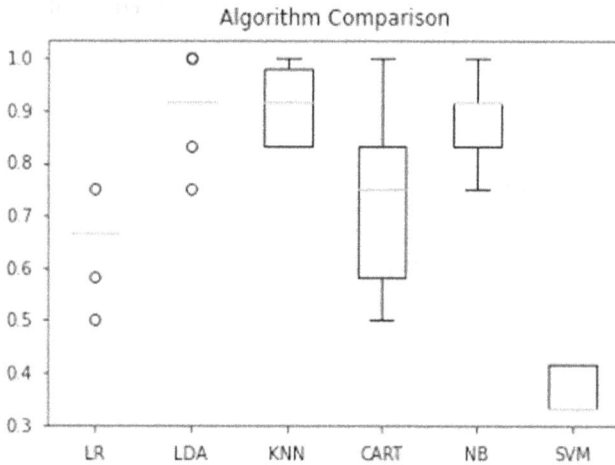

FIGURE 12.3 Box and whisker plots.

12.4.6 MAKE PREDICTIONS

Predictions are used to predict only the best classification model. From Table 12.6, it is very clear the LDA and KNN were considered as the most accurate models. We will use this model as our final model for our prediction. In the next stage, the accuracy of this model is tested against the validation set.

12.4.7 EVALUATE PREDICTIONS

The predictions are evaluated by comparing them to the expected results in the validation set (20%), and the classification accuracy is calculated. The confusion matrix and a classification report are generated at the end.

Confusion Matrix:

The confusion matrix is a table that is often used to describe the performance of a classification model on a set of test data for which the true values are known [3,5].

TABLE 12.7
Confusion Matrix

Confusion matrix		LDA				KNN		
		Predicted				Predicted		
	Actual	DNME	EE	PE	Actual	DNME	EE	PE
	DNME	11	0	0	DNME	11	0	0
	EE	0	6	0	EE	0	6	0
	PE	2	1	10	PE	3	0	10

The generated confusion matrix is provided in Table 12.7. We have 150 samples of which 50 DNMEs, 50 PEs, and 50 EEs. It is noticed that all the correct predictions are located in the diagonal of the matrix. The prediction errors can be easily located in the matric, as they will be represented by values outside the diagonal and the errors seem to be nominal.

The system has correctly predicted the following the case of LDA:

- 11 of the actual 50 DNMEs
- 6 of the actual 50 EEs and
- 10 of the actual 50 PEs, but in two cases it has predicted as DNMEs, and in one case it has predicted as EE.

The system has correctly predicted the following in case of KNN:

- 11 of the actual 50 DNMEs
- 6 of the actual 50 EEs,
- 10 of the actual 50 PEs, but in three cases it has predicted as DNMEs

Precision and Recall:

Precision is the fraction of cases where the algorithm correctly predicted class i out of all instances where the algorithm predicted i (correctly and incorrectly). Recall on the other hand is the fraction of cases where the algorithm correctly predicted i out of all of the cases which are labeled as i [1,3,5,6].

The classification report provides a breakdown of each data set by precision, recall, f1-score, and support showing excellent results. The precision and recall values of LDA and KNN are calculated and given in Table 12.8.

The classification report contains the precision value, recall, f1-score and support is provided in Table 12.9 for both the models LDA and KNN.

TABLE 12.8

Model Accuracy

	LDA	KNN
Precision	$Precision_{DNMEs}=11/(11+0+3)=11/14=0.79$ $Precision_{EEs}=6/(0+6+0)=6/6=1$ $Precision_{PEs}=10/(0+0+10)=10/10=1$	$Precision_{DNMEs}=11/(11+0+2)=11/13=0.85$ $Precision_{EEs}=6/(0+6+1)=6/7=0.86$ $Precision_{PEs}=10/(0+0+10)=10/11=1$
Recall	$Recall_{DNMEs}=11/(11+0+0)=11/11=1$ $Recall_{EEs}=6/(0+6+0)=6/6=1$ $Recall_{PEs}=10/(2+1+10)=10/13=0.77$	$Recall_{DNMEs}=11/(11+0+0)=11/11=1$ $Recall_{EEs}=6/(0+6+0)=6/6=1$ $Recall_{PEs}=10/(3+0+10)=10/13=0.77$

TABLE 12.9

Classification Report

Classification Report

LDA		Precision	Recall	f1-score	Support
	DNME	0.85	1.00	0.92	11
	EE	0.86	1.00	0.92	6
	PE	1.00	0.77	0.87	13
KNN		Precision	Recall	f1-score	Support
	DNME	0.79	1.00	0.88	11
	EE	1.00	1.00	1.00	6
	PE	1.00	0.77	0.87	13

12.5 OBSERVATIONS

From the precision, recall, and f1-score values it is observed as follows:

a. All three classes of variables namely DNME, PE, and EE are evenly distributed in the data set.

b. The precision for PE is 1 in both the prediction models and the precision for EE is 1 in the KNN model. This shows that the model has produced no false positives.

c. Also, it is noted that the precision values are larger in all cases, this indicates that the developed model clearly shows that the results are more relevant.

d. The recall is 1 for DNME and EE in both the models. This shows that the model has produces no false negatives.

e. As f1-score is the Harmonic meal of precision and recall and it is also maximum in most of the cases, this also proves that the developed model is true and can be applied to other similar data sets.

f. From the above observations, it is very clear that the assessment tools used to calculate the PO/PSO score are more appropriate.

12.6 CONCLUSION

Artificial intelligence (AI) in education needs to be further explored as the data available with the higher educational institutions. This paper attempts to use the supervised machine learning models for the prediction and evaluation of scores obtained from Program Outcomes (PO) and Program Specific Outcomes (PSOs). The machine learning model uses Linear Discriminant Analysis (LDA) and K-Nearest Neighborhood (KNN). Usage of further tools also will add more value to the results in the future.

REFERENCES

1. Precision-Recall (scikit-learn), The Relationship Between Precision-Recall and ROC Curves, A Probabilistic Interpretation of Precision, Recall and F-Score, with Implication for Evaluation, 2020.
2. https://www.technologyreview.com/2018/11/17/103781/what-is-machine-learning-we-drew-you-another-flowchart/, 01 Apr 2020.
3. https://www.forbes.com/sites/bernardmarr/2018/07/25/how-is-ai-used-in-education-real-world-examples-of-today-and-a-peek-into-the-future/#656c4353586e, 14 Apr 2020.
4. https://www.teachthought.com/the-future-of-learning/10-roles-for-artificial-intelligence-in-education/, 14 Apr 2020.
5. https://machinelearningmastery.com/machine-learning-in-python-step-by-step/, 14 Apr 2020.
6. https://pythonprogramming.net/machine-learning-tutorials/, 14 Apr 2020.

13 Artificial Intelligence-Based Assistive Technology

P. Subashini and M. Krishnaveni
Department of Computer Science, Avinashilingam Institute for Home Science and Higher Education for Women, Coimbatore, India

CONTENTS

13.1 INTRODUCTION

In recent days, it is clear that the increase in the importance of artificial intelligence (AI) is playing an important in business, finance, science, medicine, engineering, manufacturing, education, the military, law, and arts in making decisions under uncertainty. However, relatively only a few applications address the important problems of enhancing the quality of life for people with disabilities. The problems encountered with designing and developing general-purpose assistive devices are boundless. Today, assistive technology (AT) is not an option but a necessity and a right for special needs individuals. Today's advancement in AI systems closely

DOI: 10.1201/9781003175865-13

matches some of the special needs of differently-abled people. Speech recognition, speech generation, text understanding, language generation, limited-task manipulators, vision systems, and so on can be immensely useful to someone with severe physical limitations. Providing solutions for the constrained problems will make a big difference for the above-mentioned areas. Worldwide AI researchers have also contributed to the domain of assistive technology and in investigating new methods. It also consists of computer-user interfaces that allow people with different kinds of disabilities such as varying degrees of motor, hearing, or visual disabilities. The same type of AI techniques and principles that achieve flexibility in current applications should apply to tailoring devices for specialized needs. Research in this area needs to analyze earlier research on interface technology, as well as on AI methods, to come up with novel solutions that can be customized to the needs of specific individuals and adapt to changing needs. Few important features of the disability problems were reviewed where a substantial amount of AI research has been done relevant to the applications considered. For example, physical assist devices, vision-based recognition based on sign language, AI model for Brain-Computer Interface system, interface for analysis for speech-impaired people. To add more, embedded applied devices were developed under different categories of disabilities which are mentioned to be robust, portable, and cost-effective. This chapter is a collection of reviews under AT-based AI on many significant tasks that give a clear depiction of the research and the understanding of the real needs of special people who are in need of technological, which can integrate current AI technology.

13.2   OVERVIEW OF AI ON AT

In assistive technology (AT), there are many research laboratories and industries that have developed many remarkable lives by assisting equipment and technological devices for specially abled people for simpler and faster life. Few considered on a smaller scale such as visually controlled monitors, voice operators, and smartwatches. Today's world is forwarded in science and technology every minute and second where infrastructures are incorporating artificial intelligence into their settings to make AT much easier and approachable. Few applications and space where there is a scope for development in the assistive technology domain:

- Software for reading and writing difficulties such as frames, pens, light lamps.
- Individual handling situations like cooking, scheduling which requires talking watches, cooking utilization, etc.
- Restoring activity which can in form of accessible games and learning games that supports their education.
- Reading, writing, and presentation skill development independently.
- Navigation devices such as walking sticks, eye canes, mobility apps.
- Writing and learning through Braille's kind support.
- Home monitoring systems like Alexa, Google home created in support of artificial intelligence.

13.2.1 What Is Artificial Intelligence?

A synthetically generated Intelligence mode is the creation of a computer or a robot that functions like a human being. The primary objective principle is to make a robot or a machine, which can help in accomplishing something. Artificial intelligence can process individual information, accept any modifications, and put them together to solve many superior challenges without altering its elementary structure. In recent years, applications of artificial intelligence have become common and extensive. Successful applications are in business, manufacturing, science, medicine, engineering, finance, education, the military, law, and the arts. AI on these applications has shown the matter of saving time, increase throughput, reduce errors by reaching better solutions. The most important application of manhood addressed by AI is enhancing the quality of life for people with disabilities in developing assistive devices. The challenges with creating and constructing general-purpose assistive devices are encountered with the present capabilities of many AI systems that match some of the specialized needs of disabled people. For example, speech recognition, speech generation, text understanding, language generation, limited-task manipulators, vision systems, and so on. Today, AI researchers developed a high interest in technical knowledge in the domain of assistive technology for investigating new methods and techniques. Some concrete work includes eye cane, wheelchairs, textbooks readers, audio recordings for the blind. It also comprises computer interfaces that involve people with varying degrees of motor, hearing, or visual disabilities. The available AI methods and principles are applied in customizing devices for specially-abled people. AI's involvement in assistive technology is very interesting as the human-computer interface gives more opportunities to come with high-quality AI applications. Adding more large applications of AT requires only a portion of the problem to be solved, making the device fully intelligent. A very important issue with assistive applications is the cost of errors where systems developed must be reliable when end users use them in different situations. Some of the relevant AI research considered here are vision, movement, and robots, planners, speech and text recognition, decision making under uncertainty, troubleshooting systems, cognitive modeling, and intelligent interfaces. All the applications need strong engineering that is robust, compatible, and cost-effective. This chapter makes the reader understand how AI technology is progressive in making a significant difference in the likelihood of disabled people. The review done in this chapter addresses many important ideas and research problems to make understand the researchers about the need for differently-abled people and built new devices along with the objective of current AI technology. Some of the questions addressed in this chapter are

- How disabled people are limited in social partaking
- How Assistive technology helps and improves the quality of life and their independence
- The measures to ensure that people with disabilities have good access to the market products for their needs and requirements

- How AI is involved in a device the products that satisfy AT users' needs, characteristics, expectations, their interaction with the environment, and participation in society

13.2.2 How AI Is Changing the World

The quality of life for people with impairment goes way beyond the improvements to assistive technology. Every industry across the countries is using AI-driven technology is experiencing changes in Assistive technology products. AI plays a major role in electricity, transportation, and even water systems for applications such as electricity usage, traffic behavior, and even water consumption habits. These decrease the operational cost over systems that reduces loads and malfunction issues. Much more they also reduce the need for resources to operate the applications. Today's machines powered with AI are reducing the manpower around the companies which could make the uncertainty of jobs. On the other hand, service providers are using AI to analyze and understand customers' thoughts to improve their service and resolve customer issues much faster. Even though systems are in the impact of AI technology, it is still only the beginning.

13.2.3 How Can Artificial Intelligence Be Used in AT?

The advancement of Artificial Technology in robot development helps people with various disabilities in every scope of life. Home robots are in place that is customized for specially-abled for the betterment of their life. These robots have features such as emergency calls, controls electronic equipment, and food services accordingly. The advancement in technology should not be just a new educational technology or for real-time video games. It has to be useful for people with special needs to find innovative ways that put artificial intelligence to work with their current conditions. Due to the development in science and technology, the progress of AT is increasing in introducing new devices and platforms to help and create a better standard of living for disabled people. Few possible examples are given to understand an idea to integrate these two fields and differentiated them based on vision and voice areas. Here a, b, c, d, e indicates the vision areas and f towards voice-based application

a. Caretaker Robots
   An around-the-clock robot that never grows tired and makes mistakes is developed with artificial intelligence that carries great intelligence in the appointment, a medication, or even a meal. The development of technology and science globally has also met the needs of the elderly and mobility-impaired people. The application of these AI products plays a major role in healthcare to extend life hope, individuality, and therapies. This research focuses on interpersonal communication frameworks which will be very useful for understanding the long-term human-computer relational development. The healthcare industry lacks human-robot relationships which are considered to be a research effective place for the AI scientist to work.

b. Self-Assisted Wheelchair

The innovation in wheelchairs with huge maneuverability and navigational intelligence has brought great success in the life mobility of severely physically disabled people. Using a wheelchair in common environments is a problematic task for persons with hand impairments. Locomotion and localization are the major problems for blind people which finds to be a very deadly job. Few systems were developed to overcome their problems to have safe movements for them to accomplish necessary tasks. This system has robust hardware and software architecture with behavior-based control architecture. Scientists are working for people attacked with paralytics to walk on their own relieving the pressure from the wheelchair (Crisman and Cleary, 2006).

c. A Complete Vision for Blind People

The major difficulty of vision impaired people both partially and fully is to read and write. Artificial intelligence along with speech-to-text technology is more likely to the best invention for visually impaired people. Different needs that are satisfied by the above said technology are dictating the words on a screen, understanding the information from phone and other devices. Different AI-powered technologies are been developed for visual impairment to make their life experience easier. There are many products available in the market for non-verbal people such as Bright Sign, a machine learning tool that translates sign language into a voice that helps the users to communicate independently. There is much advanced computational linguistics available to help autistic people to improve their cognitive disabilities. There are also AI-based products like exoskeletons that help the visual impairment to explore the physical environment independently. Few other commonly available methods are object recognition, static environment understanding and visual conversation, and so on.

d. Assistive Technology for Housekeeping

The great difficulty that mobility-impaired faces everyday is to perform daily activities where the rest of the world does with ease and fine. Assistive technologies and devices are the best tools for them to have an easier life and remove challenges to enhance their physical capabilities. Assistive technology is very powerful with efficient motors and batteries which are very affordable and suitable for people. The state of the disabled people at home is not that easy without a caretaker and doctors. To clean their living space, the most popular device is the robotic vacuum cleaner works based on the traces which suck the dirt and dust. Few other devices that help are automated door openings, automated home monitoring systems, pot monitoring, pet monitoring, and so on. These are constructed with a reasonable budget and are very cost-effective in which the researchers have to continue to increase the involvement of artificial intelligence in the scope of the device.

e. AI-Driven Features in Standard PC and Notebook Software

Cutting-edge technologies like artificial intelligence can vest disability to partake more in every aspect of society. AI can empower everyone – not just individuals with disabilities – to achieve more. One app developed by

Microsoft called Binoculars that tackles color blindness. Color Binoculars help color-blind people to distinguish between colors in their everyday lives. It uses the camera that uses Color Binoculars to substitute most hard color combinations, like red and green, with combinations, like pink and green. This AI-based free app is very promising for low vision users to exhibit the world on learning text and objects.

   f. AI-Driven Language Translations – Atempo

The principles of AI and machine learning have been known for many years but it is not used much in the domain of AT. The AT field has the demand for an increase in computing capacity and speed and developments like the 'Internet of Things'. Conferring these potentials is always important in the development of AI which can prevent potential risks from becoming reality. An Austrian NGO has developed a capito app called Atempo, which is used to turn texts into easily understandable language. The mobile app is used to translate both printed and digital information from legal texts to demonstrate information and news concepts to annual reports. Machine learning is used to enable the developed automated translations which are cross-checked by representatives of the target group. The app supports five different levels of easily understandable languages.

13.3   A TRANSFORMATIVE IMPACT OF AI ON AT

The declaration from the World Health Organization (WHO) states that assistive technology is a product development domain to help, improve, and progress individual live hood. The devices are considered to be aids and tools for the hearing impaired, mobility devices such as wheelchairs, equipped eyeglasses, and prosthetic limbs, and a few on. These products have grown in terms of their capabilities, and adaptiveness. As its standard is improved and brings perceptible benefits for all users, these features have been converted into computers and mobile devices. Based on WHO's estimation, there are billions of people affected worldwide in some form of disability where assistive technology is a real potential gift for them. The real scenario states that out of 10 people only one gets the opportunity to access these life-changing devices. Beyond the risk of inability, the economic factor is also a major factor to be taken care and based on the market insights, assistive technologies are predicted to be worth over $26 billion in due of 2024.

   Integrating the most effective AI methods with assistive technologies will help to develop powerful features-based products for disabled people. This brings enormous progress in machine learning and optimization techniques to give the industries an opportunity to bring young scientists and developers to work on. Artificial intelligence improves the accessibility of special needs in the area such as employment, day-to-day life, and communication. In it, communication plays a major role due to the digital era. This AI-enabled tool allows every individual regardless of any disabilities. Early inventions are speech-to-text translation, captioning for visual, which is used for hearing and learning impairment people. Neural networks were introduced to enhance automatic speech recognition engines along with human requirements. The improvement done is producing fed back through machine learning technologies which help to improve accuracy. This is considered to be one of the most successful applications along with AI which is now used in various educational institutions, especially in higher education. AI-based enhanced dictation and captioning tools help disabilities to have effective learning manner. These technological augments will enable new possibilities for better training and involvement. When technology is evolved it leads to address the needs of all for all most all complex needs. Initially, the technologies are done only within the community which has now gone into the general population. The best of AI innovations are image recognition systems, speech-to-text translators, chatbots for environment understanding, and self-driving vehicles which are considered to be technological benefits to society. These types of products are sensed from the engineering perspective. The design of these types is more intuitive, feature-rich which finally reaches the required people. It is understood that if there is an improvement in the capabilities of assistive technology through AI it can reach all parts of the world where more people living with disabilities.

13.4   EXTENSIVE AT APPLICATIONS BASED ON AI

It is always important that disability society should be prepared to accept the essentiality of technologies to shape their lives. In it, artificial intelligence has high potential across the people. The reach of AI technologies should have adequate training and education to have an inclusive society. The key success for AI to be supportive for people with disabilities is the different dissemination done in part of conferences which has the lead of successful findings. The inclusion of AI is done precisely on the needs and the development of the diverse teams that include persons with disabilities. The organizations adopting AI in AT development have included recruitment and retainment of employees with disabilities to have an advantage on accessibility and inclusiveness. Policies and policy solutions should make sure that the technologies reach everyone in a society where accessibility should be the core part of all technological developments. The pace of development in artificial intelligence is very fast, and being aware of these developments is very important for the ability to engage in the discussions and ensure the developments are inclusive and accessible.

13.5   AI EXPERIENCE AND AT FOR DISABLED PEOPLE IN INDIA

India needs an AI strategy as the foundation framework which is to be utilized for the needs and objective of India and at the same, it should be very effective in leveraging AI developments to their fullest potential. The framework developed is an aggregation of the three distinct inter-related components: a) prospects and opportunity to improve the economic impact of India, b) goodwill a country that is for social development and complete growth, c) AI solution providers for 40% of the world across the globe for the economic improvement. In India, more than 90% of people with disabilities (PwDs) come from low-income households, with a majority of them having little to no access to the necessary assistive devices. With minimal chances of finding gainful employment, they are bound to stay acutely dependent on their families and are trapped in a vicious cycle of poverty. Ahmedabad-based start-ups, Torchit is trying to address this primary requirement of the visually impaired by providing a simple and affordable device. Saarthi is an assistive mobility device developed to act as a handheld smart cane with smart detection capabilities that assist visually disabled people in navigating obstacles in their physical environment. India includes different universities for providing solutions for assistive technologies and creating zones for people with disabilities to involve themselves for the betterment of their lives. Along with NGOs, professionals, special educators, the only way to reach disabled people is to produce good quality reasonable assistive devices. The projects designed based on AI should be in such a way that it brings actual transformation in people with disabilities on their thoughts both about themselves and society. India insists to have enough devices to be made readily available even in need of rural areas. To extend, all it is need is to see Mobility India in near future. Different initiatives were taken by India to form zones and nodal offices to be in a friendly manner for the people with a disability that brings mobility to India.

13.6   AI-POWERED TECHNOLOGY FOR AN INCLUSIVE WORLD

Here, the content is about some of the AI-powered Inclusive products developed and ongoing by Microsoft available to integrate the special people with the common man, and the product and its technology are categorized based on voice and vision areas.

13.6.1   APPLICATIONS BASED ON VISION AREAS

a. Making people aware of the environment
   UC Berkeley and Microsoft are building a mobile app for visually impaired people to partially and fully understand their surroundings based on sensors and cameras that provide captions and audio descriptions.
b. AI tool find career paths
   Leonard Cheshire's that uses Azure AI to develop a career guidance tool for job seekers with disabilities to know about jobs according to an individual's need for a person-centered career path. The assessment is done on their skills, goals, career paths and recommends the employer's results.
c. Image descriptor
   The University of Texas develops an accurate automatic image descriptor for blind or low vision person in partnership with Microsoft Research on AI to collect and use a wide-ranging of labeled data.
d. Training system for the blind through AI
   Education is an important aspect of young people who are blind or have low vision. It is improved using an Object Recognition for Blind Image Training which is done by the University of London and Microsoft with AI.
e. Exercise app for partially vision impaired people

An intelligent app is been initiated by the University of Iowa along with Microsoft for people blind or partially blind to independently walk nearly 400-meter track distance. It delivers real-time feedback when the person is veering from their lane and to make them stay on track.

13.6.2 APPLICATIONS BASED ON VOICE AREAS

a. Increasing reading fluency with AI
   In Microsoft, based on AI they have developed a reading fluency product called ReadAble Storiez which consists of STEM information that helps people with diverse learning.

b. Counting Zoo
   It is an immersive eReader that converts speech into a form of onscreen text that has the description of stories, video, and play with interfaces to occupy users.

c. Chatbots to support special need people
   Communication is a fundamental mode that proves equal access. This can be bought by AI technology to users no matter that the person is normal or with a disability. The Open University along with the support of Microsoft has created a chatbot to support people with disabilities. The admin source of the product will solve the difficulty faced during the independent living that occurs by the process.

d. Gamified speech therapy
   The major role of speech therapy is to understand the performance of the kids by the therapists which is always monotonous for kids as the therapists often have little data. A product called Verboso is developed to fill the gap by developing video games that are activated by speech therapy exercises which include clinical feedbacks to motivate the users.

e. Recognizing non-standard speech patterns
   Leveraging powerful new speech recognition technology supports spoken communication and increases independence for people with a speech disability. Voiceitt is a device developed for automatic speech recognition technology that understands non-standard speech patterns, real-time communication to provide the individual with a perfect recognizer. This integrates customizable speech recognition with mainstream voice technologies and devices enables environmental control through a universally assessable voice system. Some of the apps available are ACT Lab a storytelling app from images that improve communication, a visualizer that rhythms the music with a beat, an EVE that recognizes speech that generates captions, CAIR to recognize the words in spoken messages, Timlogo improves access to speech therapy, ReadRing, real-time converter of text-to-braille, and Helpicto that converts speech to pictograms.

f. Improving communication for ALS and MS patients
   Introducing AI capabilities on AT to create chatbots or data collection are reforming the value of technology in peculiar scenarios for disabled persons.

Pison is a technology that is used to develop a wrist-wearable neuromuscular sensing system that is hands-free, to progress communication skills for the person with neuromuscular disabilities.

g. Expanding inclusive hiring
An AI-powered chatbot that supports preparing for interviews that exist in cognitive disabilities in areas like manufacturing and the scientific research field by offering employment details.

h. Communication app for locked-in syndrome
Microsoft along with Tokyo Institute of Technology is creating a mobile app that consists of an interface to relate the features of the pictorial target and the responses.

i. Assistive navigation for all pedestrians
There is no specific navigation app for pedestrians as of now where iMerciv is developing a travel app named MapinHood. It includes machine learning concepts and crowdsourcing especially for inclusive people, they are providing personalized assistive navigation for all.

j. Warning system for epilepsy

A team of researchers is newly developing an intelligent and real-time brain signal processing system at the University of Sydney with the support of Microsoft for people affected with epilepsy. It is considered to be a smart seizure advisory system that delivers a timely warning about the occurrence of epileptic seizure strikes during their independent travel (Figure 13.1).

13.7   RESEARCH PERCEPTIVE OVER AI INFLUENCE ON AT

A significant amount of AI research is relevant to applications such as vision, locomotion, robotics, speech and text understanding, and intelligent interfaces. The information collected are well clear with the objective on the way of AI on AT meaningful challenges and for reader understanding the list is differentiate based on vision and voice applications.

13.7.1   VISION-BASED APPLICATIONS

a. Intelligent system controlled by mobile devices
This project is developed by a post-graduation student as a commercial remote-controlled device done through eagleeyes for wheelchair (Gips, 1998). It is a well-defined system for the drivers where they can receive information from a wheelchair and steer it with enough concentration. AI is implemented that plays a significant role in decision making in finding intersection points and to identify the turns open spaces. More work is done in improving the cross points and control methods. Therefore, the ultimate goal is to develop a wheelchair system that helps people with disabilities in an easy manner with no difficulties.

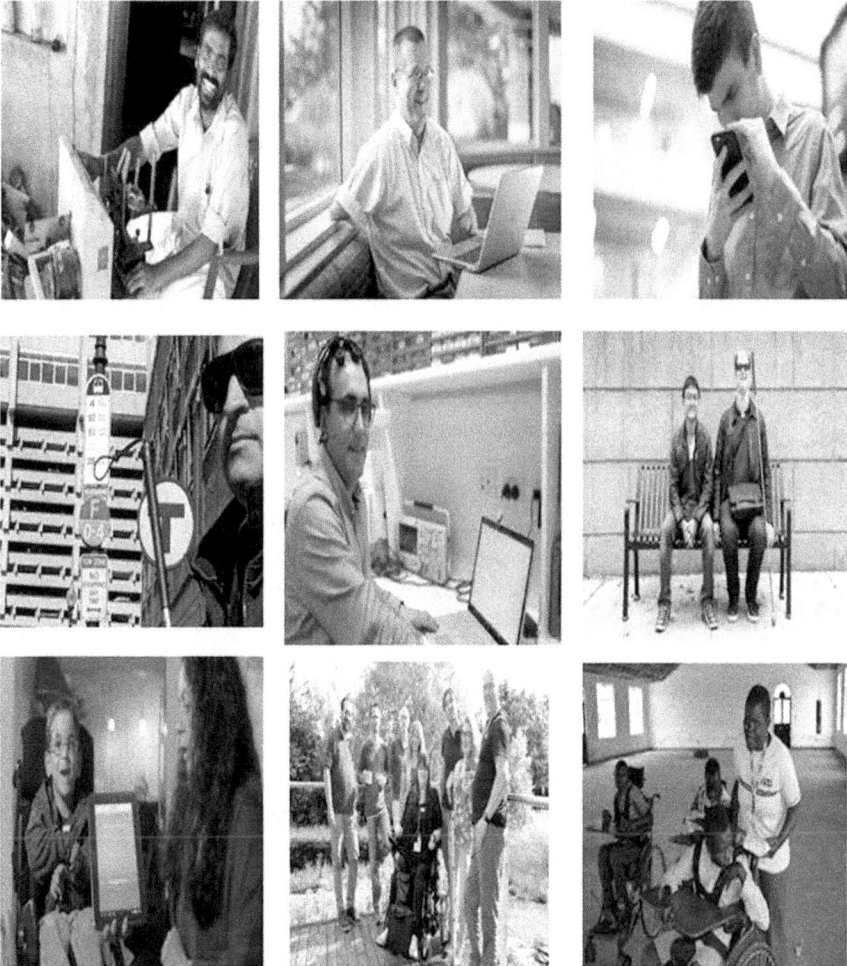

FIGURE 13.1 Beneficiaries of accessible systems featured by AI.

b. Saliency in human-computer interaction

It is considered that defining saliency is a substantial problem in AI. The problem is how to raid visual scenes or force strike is through artificial aid, often done by sensors. The context-dependency such as features that are predominate in one setup is different from others is a major challenge. There are many applications for human supervision that allows researchers to contribute to the integration of advanced technologies in complex domains that leads to operating autonomously. The work proposed can be limited to features such as colors, shapes and direction, and artificial agents which are considered as high level. This research provides scope to the application on areas of saliency in human-computer interaction, at high-level control.

c. Assistive robotics

Intelligent robotics is a study of how to develop machines to exhibit the qualities of people. This technology has greatly influenced the product development domain used by differently abled people who have lost certain basic lifestyles. Generally, disabilities are blind and speechless but the most difficult is the defect in the neural or information processing system of the brain that brings motor disability. Robotics technology blend of sensing, movement, and information processing has a huge scope for the development of a robotic system that assists the need of special people. Few listed applications where research contributions can be given are assisting people who are mobility impaired, helping a person to move from one place to another, to provide the person to have specific objects based on their desire from a remote location, automated operation, remote access of objects, a person to feed themselves, translating modalities and so on. The technical issue in getting these robotic systems to reach a useful level is how the users independently utilize the device. It is also known that robotic assistants and personal assistance have not reached disabled people Therefore, the goal is to make disabled people feel free in accessing robotic assistive technology effectively at a lower cost. The robotic issues allow opportunities for the industries and scientists to try for future work and development.

d. Assistive navigation

There is always a necessity to develop assistive aid that is capable of independent and semi-independent navigation in a lively world. This is addressed as the universal area to be focused on in developing intelligent navigation assistance to mobility-impaired people. The wheelchair users will get benefit only when a high-precision navigation methodology is implemented. These forms of proposed assistive navigation methodology can bring a noiseless, error-prone, high bandwidth control information system which leads its service to have specific navigation tasks.

e. Mobility aid for the infirm and elderly blind

Conventional mobility aids available for the blind are not that comfortable and they had great difficulty in using it. This is more complicated when there is a combination of both visual and mobility impairment which is very common in elderly people. PAM-AID is a support aid to provide physical support when walking and also to find obstacles. This project addresses the complexity in user interface design based on modular robot strategy. The modalities of certain issues such as user safety, reassurance, and information can be addressed using the research contributes to AI. The scope may be on user interface options, fusion in multisensor and control system. At present, the system work on speaker-dependent to prevent other people from voice to intrude. The high-level nature of voice commands and their low frequency is yet another challenge in the design of the control system. A shared control system will be the additional feature to determine the user's high-level goals that produce an action plan for the robot. This work is a long-term effort to integrate artificial intelligence and Robot Technology to meet the needs of the wider community.

f. Robotic Travel Aid

A Robotic Travel Aid (RoTA) is a development of motor equipment made up of a camera, sonar, tactile sensors, and a map database system (Gomi, 1992Gomi 1992). It is a visually impaired user assistance to present their location, landmarks, route, and orientation. This work describes the implementation of a guide for visually impaired people on roads and pathways. It is a small type of robot in form of a mobile that uses a wheelchair equipped as its under-carriage. In this project, solar power is used to identify walls and other obstacles that are not possible accurately for a vision system. To follow the routing system, a transportable digital map system is planned to integrate with a wheelchair which gives a follow-up of commands along with sign patterns and benchmarks. The digitalized map has a reply system through synthesized voice which indicates the place and building names when the user gives a command. Indeed, the system receives the mobility and direction information through the motion of the under-carriage. The success rate is considered to be between 92% and 94%. Meanwhile, accidents are identified through environmental change by a semi-automatic navigation system that infers the cause and intimate the user and also the next move using a synthesized voice. This project with high AI development activates the use of the user residual senses and makes the independence of life promoted.

13.7.2   VOICE-BASED APPLICATIONS

a. Intelligent Systems Interface and Language Issues for People with Disabilities

An intelligent eye-tracking system named as EagleEyes system which is developed as a physical interface to an Augmentative and Alternative Communication (AAC) system allows a user to control a computer through electrodes that could be placed on the head. The major challenge in this system is the use of relevant sensors, developing algorithms, improving accuracy based on various training methods. It also focuses on AAC devices which assimilates vision techniques to identify the sign language. The main objective of translating signs is done by an interface which the vision of the model is to be a recognition system as a wearable computer. This problem has a scope to combine several modalities such as spoken and gestural which can be in the form of a robot. To be more advanced in vision processing, HMM is included in order to identify and path the hands in the motion picture to interpret the observed sign. Different AI technologies can be included in order to provide an interface that enables a person who has physical disabilities to handle a formless environment. It is a combination of vision subsystems to identify object location, shape, and pose. The interface subsystem translates the spoken commands as well as the planning subsystem interprets the user commands.

b. Iconic Language Design for People with Significant Speech and Multiple Impairments

A specific type of visual language called Iconic languages is used for human-computer interface, visual programming, and human-human communication (Patricia et al., 1994). Its distinct features are accessing a database, manipulating forms, and image analysis and processing. An augmentative communication Chinese ideographs, the Mayan glyphs, and the Egyptian pictograms are utilized by Significant Speech and Multiple Impairments (SSMI) people. There is a system called Minspeak developed with a prescriptive model that has led to insight into the design of visual languages. This work extends its scope for multimedia environments where it provides scope for introducing AI to construct a robust system for AAC.

c. Dictionary for Computer Translation of American Sign Language

A dictionary to facilitate people with a Speech impairment is developed in America in which lexicon is a structure to deed American Sign Language (ASL) phonology to sign identification. This is to identify ASL's three-dimensional qualities and the method is promoted to encrypt only what is essential for sign identification using AI technology which makes the sign recognition problem controllable (McCoy, 1998). AI can be introduced to determine the significant sign boundaries which have additional formative and linguistic limitations so that a robust aid for identification can be build that reduce efforts.

d. Intelligent Language Feedback for Communication Users

An augmented communication device can provide speech synthesis in which the rate of communication is very slow. To improve the above, a natural language processing technique called compression-expansion can be used to expand uninflected content words and frame a well-formed sentence. It also requires accurate grammatical feedback which may be very beneficial in the learning process. The scope is to integrate AI to bring real-rules for a prototype application that uses the companion technique.

e. Japanese to Japanese Sign Language Automatic Translation system

The research work presents a prototype translation system called SYUWAN which translates Japanese into Japanese sign language (Tokuda and Okumura, 2006). One big challenge of the system is that it has only a few signs in a sign language dictionary when equated with Japanese dictionary. To provide a solution to this, AI techniques are applied to find a similar word from Japanese dictionary to substitute the word, if the original input word does not exist in a Japanese sign language dictionary. Therefore, it is expected to meet the accuracy of 82% in translating the words which can be analyzed morphological manner. A methodological approach should be implemented to automatically determine word sense which can be extended for future work. The complete research work focuses on the translation method of word-to-word correspondence for Coded Japanese (Figure 13.2).

f. Communication Interface on Conversational Schemata

Speech and motor impairments are the people who use augmentative and alternative communication (AAC) for storing and organizing words, phrases, and sentences so that it can be made accessible to them (Pennington and

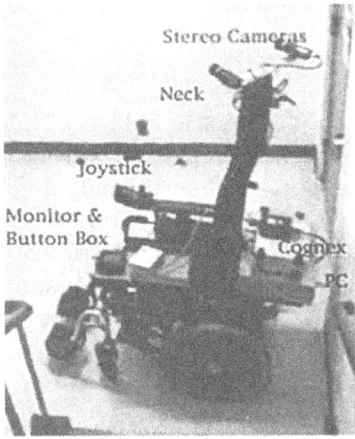

Assistive Robotics : Wheel chair   MT system for Sign Language

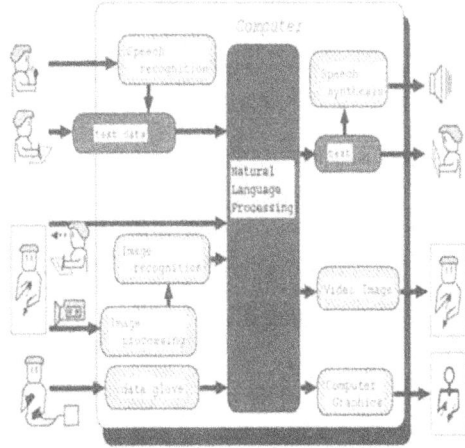

FIGURE 13.2   Examples over AI influence on AT.

McCoy, 2006Pennington 2006). The work enforced here is to use consistencies in an individual's conversational experiences to show that they can bring conversational context easily. To bring the above, a cognitive organization is done with a new interface and methodology for organizing and recovering sentences according to the appropriate context and sentences. By bringing AI for the objective, the interface will take less effort through conversations to facilitate the source of new schemas. In the future, the schematic text will be used by AAC users that improves the utilization of the interface.

g. Mediated Intelligent Teleoperation

Intelligence in a machine and human intervention are the characteristics of an assistive robotic system. The Multimodal User Supervised Interface and Intelligent Control (MMUSIC) project address the major issue of telemanipulation of day-to-day objects in an unstructured way. It also resolves a set of problems that telerobot can control with physical limits. It is done by integrating speech and gesture-driven human-machine interface along with a 3D vision system. This brings the opportunity to understand the unstructured world telemanipulation by people with physical disabilities that helps to improve time delay and lack of sensation along with coordination. The human-machine collaboration in a real-world environment will be introduced to bring a novel approach in the gesture-speech interface to makes realistic plans in an assistive domain.

13.8   AI IMPLEMENTATION ON ASSISTIVE TECHNOLOGIES – PRAGMATIC APPROACH

AI is defined as a system or a computer that is able to perform tasks similar to human intelligence. AI is generally powered by machine learning and recently by deep learning and basically by rule generation techniques. These basic techniques were implemented and tested in constructing robust research methodologies for developing assistive devices. Investigation and valuable publication were done to evaluate the findings. Some of the contributions done by the author's team were listed with an explanation which could be highly commendable for future researchers to understand the scope of the technology discussed over the chapter.

  a. Assertive framework for Tamil Sign Language Recognition System (voice area)

Sign language (SL) is the only communication mode considered to be a promising and prominent skill for hearing-impaired people. Sign language is said to be a method that has a well-structured gesture used for sharing information among their living society. Various sign language interpreters were developed and improved based on the recognition accuracy level using AI approaches such as machine learning techniques, Computational intelligence, and deep learning methods. Literature around the world suggests that there are many sign languages including British sign language, American sign language, Japanese sign language, Chinese sign language, and Indian sign language, leading to around 177 languages. Different computer-based methods were implemented in order to convert Sign language into voice or text to behave assign interpreters. The regional requirements are always a convivial development for every country and hence it is considered to have a unique sign language recognition system for Tamil Sign Language. It is understood that one of the common languages in India is the Tamil language which also holds a special dictionary for Tamil Sign Language (Subha Rajam and Balakrishnan, 2012; Subha Rajam 2012). The handshape data are gathered from different volunteers rather than just a single signer. The real-time Tamil Sign Language hand images which include 12 vowels, 1 Aayutha Ezhuthu, and 18 consonants are taken from 10 different people. In total, 130 images for vowels and 180 images for consonants are used (Krishnaveni et al., 2018). The figure shows few samples of the TSL hand gesture images from the database. Although India has Indian Sign Language (ISL), the need for a recognition tool for regional language is always there. Enough research and awareness are done on ISL and it has continuously evolved, but very few contributions have been done so far in the area of Tamil Sign Language (Figures 13.3 and 13.4).

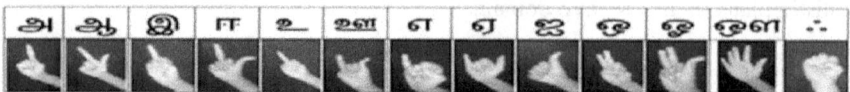

FIGURE 13.3   Manually generated Tamil vowels data set (12 uyir and 1 aayutha ezhuthukal).

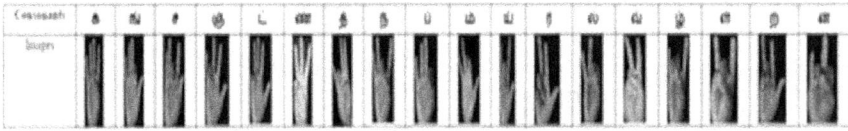

FIGURE 13.4 Manually generated Tamil consonants sign language data set.

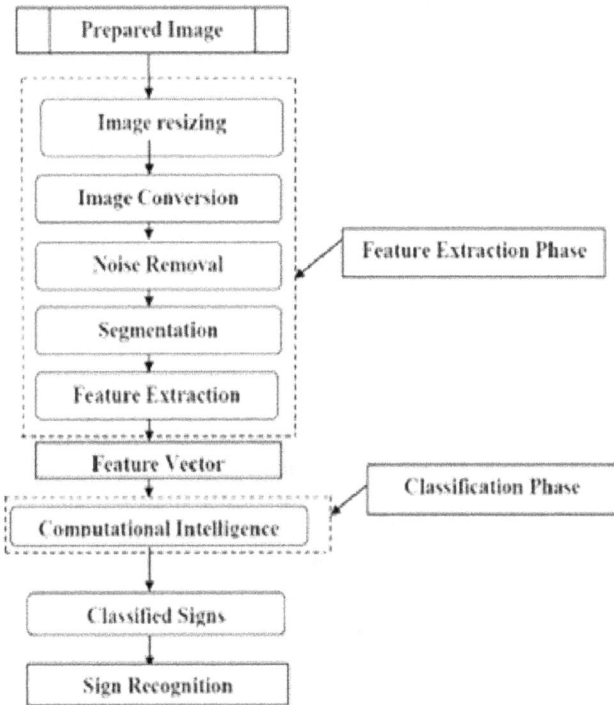

FIGURE 13.5 Steps involved in TSL recognition framework.

Tamil is an ancient language and also, it is a regional language in Tamil nadu state, India. A study on a statistical report of physically challenged children, during the past decade, reveals that there is a steady increase in the number. Henceforth, dissemination of sign language is needful to develop the linguistic skills of hearing-impaired people. Automated computational systems were developed to recognize gestures posted by humans through the implementation of image processing and computer vision applications, such as clipping and boundary tracing, fingertip detection, handshapes and movements, contour recognition, and contour matching. But the limitations identified in the non-selection of generalization and comprehensibility in feature extraction, feature analysis and selection, learning rules, and recognition in the computational model lead to the delivery of poor performance. Despite potential improvements, many research challenges are still existing which

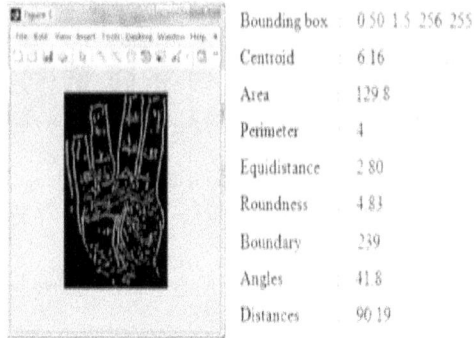

Bounding box	0 50 1 5 256 255
Centroid	6 16
Area	129 8
Perimeter	4
Equidistance	2 80
Roundness	4 83
Boundary	239
Angles	41 8
Distances	90 19

FIGURE 13.6   Screenshot for the results.

are necessary to explore. Figure 13.5 shows the framework designed for the TSL recognition system.

In this work, an optimized sign language recognition model is developed using computational intelligence techniques for noise removal, edge detection, classification, and recognition in which the goal is to motivate the regional-based hearing-impaired people. The potential contributions are (Figures 13.6 and 13.7):

1. In the preprocessing phase of the image processing stage, efficient removal of the Impulse Noise algorithm was introduced based on machine learning techniques for Tamil Sign Language Digital Images using PSO and SFO Based Weighted Median Filter.
2. Developed an optimized edge detector that enhances the localization accuracy of edge detection by introducing a hybrid optimization technique that finds optimal threshold value which is a combination of PSO with cellular organism inspired from fibroblast.
3. The structural features extraction is done based on region-based analysis on both boundary and interior pixels of an image in the digital images.
4. For accuracy improvement in classifying the Tamil Sign Language digital images is done using neural networks and optimization techniques.
5. The patterns are identified and categorized into distinct class labels by applying SOM network and the recognition accuracy of conventional SOM is highly improved, using computational methods with standard experimentation.

The constructed system, Automatic Tamil Sign Language Recognition (ATSLR) is a technological AI-based work disseminated here as a knowledge expansion that will be beneficial for researchers in machine vision application. This proposed framework will be very much useful for effective communication between the hearing-impaired people with normal people in learning Tamil language signs which are region-based. It has set a platform to develop an automatic Tamil Sign Language for an education and recognition platform for deaf students of India. The system can substantially provide services that can be used to correct, enable, maintain, or improve the

TSL letters	Correctly classified	Image	Misclassified	Wrongly recognized image	Wrongly recognized Letters
??	90	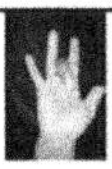	10	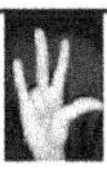	??
??	60	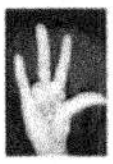	40	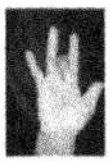	??
??	60	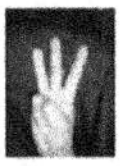	40	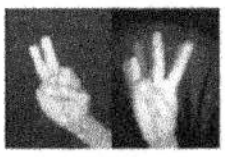	? , ??
??	70	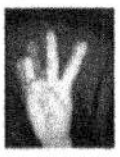	30	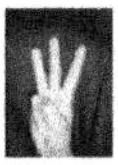	??
??	60	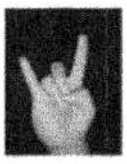	40	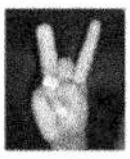	??
??	70	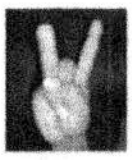	30	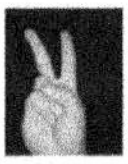	??
??	70	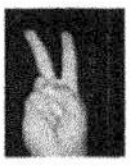	30	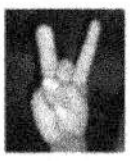	??
?	80	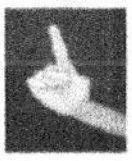	20	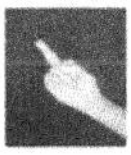	?
?	70	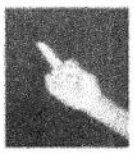	30	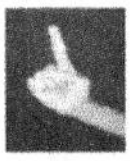	?
?	50	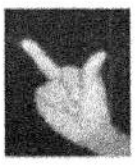	50	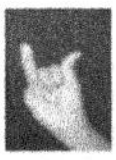	?
?	70	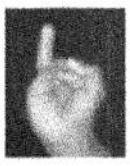	30	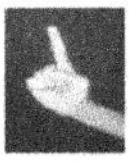	?
?	60	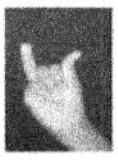	40	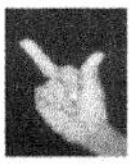	?
?	70	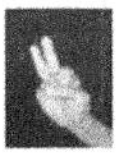	30	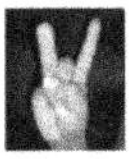	??

FIGURE 13.7 Classification output.

functional capabilities of individuals with disabilities in the primary/vocational/higher education of hearing-impaired students and people of India.

b. Reinforcement learning-based Intelligent cane (vision area)

In the mobility of a human, especially visually impaired people, safe movement and location identification are the two prime challenges faced without assistance. There is always a need for the most reliable, robust, intelligent assistive tool for the blind for object detection and obstacle avoidance which should be also inexpensive. The model is designed with a novel classical Q-learning (CQL) algorithm using Synergistic Fibroblast Optimization (SFO) to develop an intellectual walking stick prototype, for visually impaired people (Subashini et al., 2017). A most capable SFO algorithm is applied to significantly improve the learning ability of CQL for object detection, obstacle avoidance, and location identification in complex and dynamic environments (Subashini et al., 2019). The features used are providing effective decisions, voice messages, safety navigational directions, and interacting with the environment. The prototype developed will learn the obstacle avoidance experience with a large volume of real-time data instances collected in different real-world situations. An optimized learning structure is created using a derived control policy. The prototype demonstrates excellent generalization performance and precise results in object detection, location identification, and obstacle avoidance tasks effectively in ambiguous environments. Figure 13.8 shows the schematic representation of an intelligence walking stick prototype.

The implementation of the prototype is of two segments. Optimization of rule selection for knowledge representation is a task done in Arduino IDE and the optimization process is done by applying SFO to choose optimal rules which are updated in the Q-table value self-possessed of each state and possible actions (Subashini et al., 2017). The experimental platform setup is at Avinashilingam University, Tamilnadu and its aerial view map is given in Figure 13.9. The complete rules and their selection were done within the campus path map and this research work is a vision of contributing the intelligent walking stick beneficial to visually challenged people in the institution, which can be truly utilized by the blind students of the university in real-life situations. The well-developed device is more robust and of low cost, and easily adaptable to learn diverse sorts of environments as well as other different applications that will be greatly useful to blind people. Further research can focus on advanced AI to develop the prototype for outdoor environments and video processing frame by frame applications for object recognition. On the hardware side, optical fog sensor to detect the presence of foggy could be a better idea in the surrounding area.

c. Cognitive level analysis using BCI (voice area)

Communication disability is the main difficulty faced by fully non-speaking students in the education environment. Special education teachers without interpreters encounter a lot of challenges to realize non-speaking students learning ability, discover their learning barriers, and retrieve feedback during the teaching-learning process. The Census 2011 in India reported that 20.42 lakhs of children who belong to the age group of

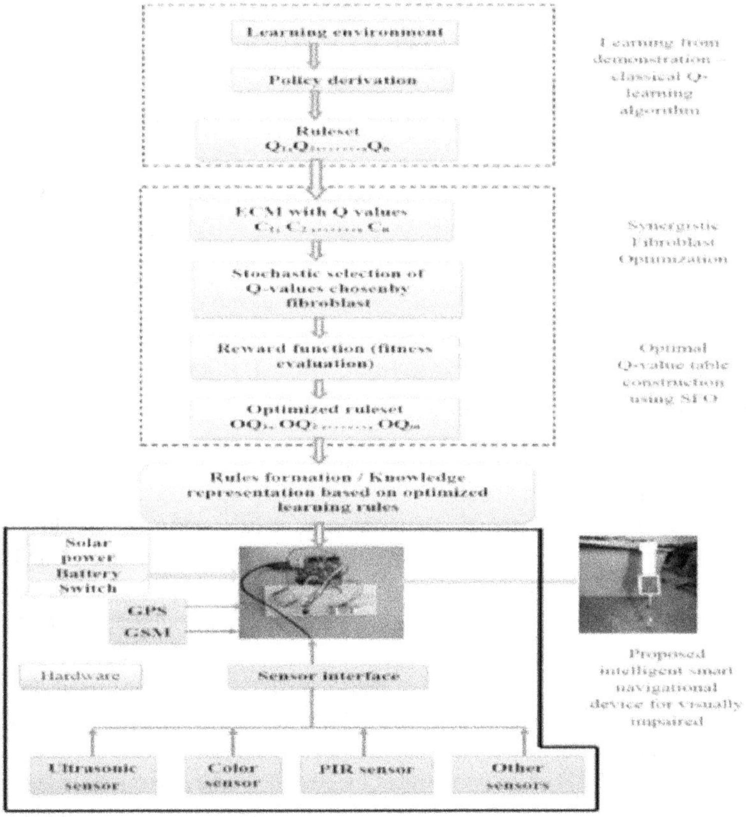

FIGURE 13.8 Schematic representation of an intelligence walking stick-proposed framework.

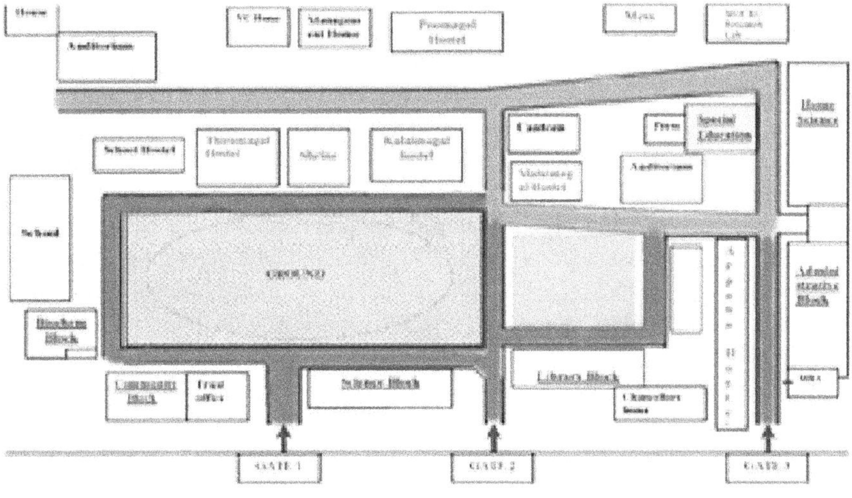

FIGURE 13.9 Aerial view of Avinashilingam University map, Coimbatore, Tamil Nadu.

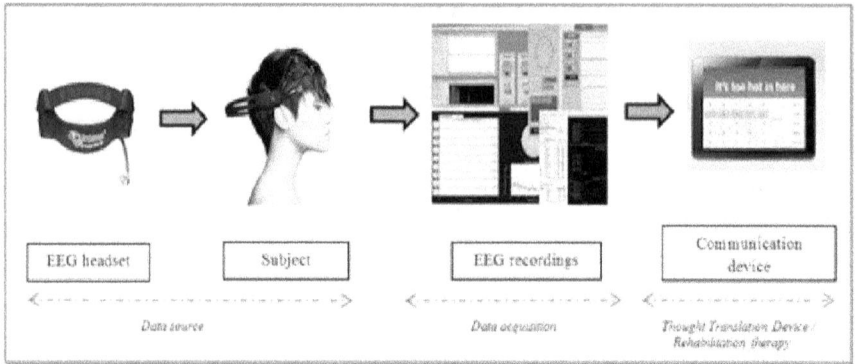

FIGURE 13.10   Flow diagram of EEG-based BCI system.

0–6 years are disabled (Krishnaveni et al., 2019). Among these, 5% of children are suffering from speech impairment. The proportion of disabled male children to total male children is higher than the corresponding proportion of total female children observed in the rural and urban areas in India. In particular, the investigation work concentrates on the regional language Tamil in which there is no evidence of research done. It is found out that modeling a Brain-Computer Interface (BCI) system provides alternative pathways to establish an effective message passing mechanism and deliver rehabilitation services for fully non-speaking students. BCI devices enable users to interact with the computer systems via electrophysiological signals captured from electrodes placed on the surface of the cerebral cortex of the brain. Many clinical studies confirmed that Electroencephalogram (EEG) based BCI system is considered the most appropriate non-invasive approach for cognitive assessment and rehabilitation practices. The architecture of EEG signal recordings-based BCI system is depicted in Figure 13.10.

In this work, the non-invasive approach is employed to acquire brain data (EEG recordings) by using electrodes that are fitted on the scalp of the brain. The objective of this research is to design and develop BCI-based Tamil character recognition system for non-speaking students, especially, vowels. Acquisition and analysis of EEG signals from the fully non-speaking students help special educators to formulate new teaching strategies/learning paradigms in order to improve the learning ability/skills and encourage equivalent participation of special children in community education (Figure 13.11).

An optimized BCI model is developed for preprocessing the acquired signal which leads to the classification of EEG signals for the recognition of Tamil language characters (அ and ஆ). Real-time EEG signals were collected from volunteers during the teaching-learning process by providing four different types of e-learning materials. The collected EEG signals were henceforth used to construct an optimal k-NN classifier and investigation of results indicates that machine learning algorithms have good performance and promising outcomes. The developed BCI model is advantageous to comprehend the non-speaking student's interest in pursuing the diverse sort of e-learning materials. The involvement of AI has greatly enhanced the recognition phase of the system.

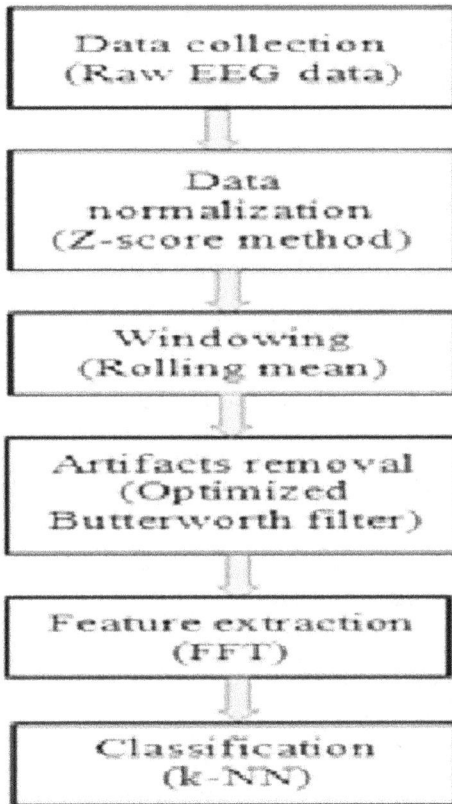

FIGURE 13.11 Process flow of SFO-based BCI model.

13.9 CONCLUSION

This chapter elaborates the solutions based on the interest of readers who wants to know about the advances of technology that can help disabled people to lead a better life. The focus here is to understand assistive technology and its devices that support differently abled people to extend their range of cognitive, sensory, or motor abilities. The mention of the above technology will somehow associate all over some point of the lives to help people to hear, speak, understand, or move about more easily. As people get older these wheelchairs would help to navigate around obstacles by themselves. Different workshops and conferences were carried out around the world to have informal affairs and extensive discussions, giving rise to several fruitful collaborations and fast associations in having artificial intelligence over assistive technology. One of the main objectives of this chapter is to have a significant amount of related work in diverse fields such as robotics, vision, planning, and natural language processing. It has complied with a collection of articles related to areas that are representing assistive technologies which will be helpful for future researchers to understand the great work carried in it. This technology has a unique aspect as a human is always part of the processing loop. Few scopes for the research are also addressed for the reader to work on similar problems and contribute by their findings based on this compendium.

REFERENCES

Crisman, J.D. and Cleary, M.E., 2006. Developing Intelligent Wheelchairs for the Handicapped. Assistive Technology and Artificial Intelligence, pp. 150–178.

Gips, J., 1998. On building intelligence into EagleEyes. Assistive Technology and Artificial Intelligence.

Gomi, T., 1992. Subsumption Robots and the Application of Intelligent Robots to the Service Industry. Applied AI Systems, Inc. Internal Report.

https://globalaccessibilitynews.com/2019/08/09/india-assistive-technology-for-all-2030-conference-focuses-in-infrastructure-assistive-devices/

https://newzhook.com/story/visually-impaired-assistive-technology-national-association-forthe-blind-beyond-eyes-accessibility-blind/

https://niti.gov.in/writereaddata/files/document_publication/NationalStrategy-for-AIDiscussion-Paper.pdf

https://www.microsoft.com/en-us/ai/ai-for-accessibility-projects?activetab=pivot1:primaryr2

Krishnaveni, M., Geethalakshmi, S.N., Subashini, P., Dhivyaprabha, T.T., Lakshmi, S., 2019. Optimized Backpropagation Neural Network Model for BrainComputer Interface System. In: IEEE International Smart Cities Conference. Casablanca: IEEE, pp. 1–6. E-ISBN: 978-1-7281-0846-9, USB ISBN: 978-1-7281-0845-2, Print on Demand (PoD) ISBN: 978-1-7281-0847-6, E-ISSN: 2687-8860, Print on Demand (PoD) ISSN: 2687-8852, DOI: 10.1109/ISC246665.2019.9071784.

Krishnaveni, M., Subashini, P., and Dhivyaprabha, T.T., 2018. An Assertive Framework for Automatic Tamil Sign Language Recognition System using Computational Intelligence. In: Hemanth, Jude, Balas, Valentina Emilia, eds, Springer Nature-Inspired Optimization Techniques For Image Processing Applications, Chapter 3, pp. 55–87. ISBN: 978-3-319-96002-9.

McCoy, K., 1998. Interface and Language Issues in Intelligent Systems for People with Disabilities. Assistive Technology and Artificial Intelligence, Applications in Robotics, User Interfaces, and Natural Language Processing. BOOK VL. 1458, DOI: 10.1007/BFb005596.

Patricia, A., Shi-Kuo, C., Giuseppe, P., and Bruce, B., 1994. Iconic language design for people with significant speech and multiple impairments. DOI: 10.1007/BFb0055967.

Pennington, C.A. and McCoy, K.F., 2006. Providing intelligent language feedback for augmentative communication users. Assistive Technology and Artificial Intelligence, pp. 59–72.

Subha Rajam, P. and Balakrishnan, G., 2012. Recognition of Tamil sign language alphabet using image processing to aid deaf-dumb people. *Elsevier Procedia Engineering*, 30, 861–868.

Subashini, P., Dhivyaprabha, T.T., Krishnaveni, M., Vedha Viyas, G., 2017. Synergistic Fibroblast Optimization Based Improved Reinforcement Learning For Intelligent Assistive Device. In: IEEE Symposium Series on Computational Intelligence. Hawaii: IEEE, pp. 2015–2022. ISBN: 978-1-5386-4058-6, DOI: 10.1109/SSCI.2017.8280942.

Subashini, P., Dhivyaprabha, T.T., Krishnaveni, M., and Vedha Viyas, G., 2019. Motility Factor-Based Optimized Q-learning Algorithm for Intelligent Walking Cane. *International Journal of Research and Analytical Reviews*, 6(1), 532–539. E-ISSN: 2348-1269, P-ISSN: 2349-5138.

Tokuda, M. and Okumura, M., 2006. Towards automatic translation from Japanese into Japanese sign language. Assistive Technology and Artificial Intelligence, pp. 97–108.

14 Machine Learning

Italia Joseph Maria[1] and T. Devi[2]
[1]Ph.D. Research Scholar, Department of Computer
Applications, Bharathiar University, Coimbatore, India
[2]Professor and Head, Department of Computer
Applications, Bharathiar University, Coimbatore, India

CONTENTS

DOI: 10.1201/9781003175865-14

OBJECTIVES

This chapter introduces machine learning in a simple way to novices in the area. It gives the reader an understanding of the importance of machine learning and the steps involved in making a machine learn. The chapter also provides an overall picture of the various forms of machine learning and the several algorithms that make machines behave like smart machines. It also deals with some problem areas where machine learning could be successfully used and introduces the various tools available for machine learning today. This chapter ends with a description of the various application areas where machine learning is used.

14.1   INTRODUCTION

The first thing one thinks of on a day when the sky is full of dark clouds and thunderstorms is that it is going to rain today. How does one ever know that it's going to rain? Just because, whenever one has seen the sky behaving the same, it has rained. This means that one has acquired a sort of knowledge over time, using experience that it will rain in situations similar to this where the sky was cloudy and rainstorms were on the outset.

Again, think of another situation where you have to travel to a city which you have never traveled to before. What would you do? You ask others about the route, get help from Google Maps, and somehow reach the destination. What happens if you need to travel to the same city another time? You don't go for getting help from others, though you may be using Maps. And what happens the third time? You may not need Maps, even. This means that humans learn from experience. The more experience you have, the more expert you will be.

Machine learning is nothing but, making machines learn, and that too, through experience. This is what this chapter will be discussing.

Machine learning. Or making machines learn.

How to make machines learn? In what all ways can a machine be of help to humans? How are learned machines helping humans? In what areas can you make use of these so-called learned machines? What are the tools to make a machine learn?

14.1.1   WHY SHOULD MACHINES LEARN?

Machines are made by humans to aid them in all walks of life, even from the time of Industry 1.0. Today too, in the wake of Industry 4.0, machines should be of help to humans. To be in sync with Industry 4.0, machines should be intelligent and smart, guessing what is needed next and coming to human's aid. If a person becomes an expert through continuous usage and experience, he is using the same method to make machines also learn. This means that machines are made to learn from experience, or, in other words, they are trained, again and again, to act according to situations.

Humans get tired and bored doing a single work multiple times, but a machine never. A machine can do the same work continuously without getting tired or getting bored. Suppose if you ask a human to recognize a person's movement in hundreds of people, he may get confused or distracted in some cases (Ramakrishnan, 2017). But a machine will not. Even long before machine learning, people were using machines to do the so-called repetitive and tiresome works. Now with machine learning, humans are training machines to think logically, make decisions, and get the works done.

Machines acquire intelligence when they are trained, and there are several ways in which they can be trained. Once they are trained the appropriate way, they can be of help to humans in numerous aspects (Vatsal, 2018). Machine learning consists of algorithms that make computers learn how to do the jobs that human beings do normally daily. Machine learning is now used in fields like spam systems, crime alerts, suspect recognition, plant improvement observation, crop enhancement, and other areas where humans cannot work sequentially, which shows how inevitable it is in daily life. machine learning is thus a big advantage for human beings where machines are trained to behave intelligently replacing humans. So that's why machine learning is becoming powerful in the world (Ramakrishnan, 2017).

14.1.2 THE IMPORTANCE OF MACHINE LEARNING

People will be familiar with the feed suggestions Facebook provides them with, or the product recommendations Amazon extends to them. This is just evidence of how machine learning is peeping into the world humans are living in. They deal with data and machines are using it. That is, a person deals with his/her everyday matters, and machine learning is bringing power out of the data that he/she is working on with. By accessing data and performing analysis on it using forecasts and classifications, machine learning allows computers to continuously learn and improve from experience (Chaudury, 2020).

Today, in the wake of Industry 4.0, machine learning is all the more important since wherever a person is and whatever he/she does, he/she can see machine learning there. There is not a single day today without weather predictions. Whenever a person opens YouTube, Amazon, or Netflix he/she see his/her home page customized based on his/her previous searches. If he/she goes a step ahead and ask Alexa, the virtual assistant developed by Amazon, to play his/her favorite music station, Alexa goes to the music station the person has played the most. If you provide more inputs to Alexa such as skipping a song, increasing the volume, or searching for particular artists, it will learn more, get trained, and provide more accurate results on the next interaction (Priyadharshini, 2020). That is how each time it comes in front of humans with personalized suggestions.

So, machine learning is everywhere around. Humans cannot live today avoiding its existence. Looking around, one can see that any technology that man has benefitted from, has something to do with machine learning (Vatsal, 2018).

14.2 WHAT IS MACHINE LEARNING?

Machine learning is all about making machines learn something and act accordingly. A machine which forecasts weather is made to learn a lot about weather from previous days. The machine is trained with weather data and made to learn how the weather was each day given the conditions. When the training or learning finishes or is considered to be sufficient, the machine is given weather conditions of the current day and it provides the weather forecast for the day. Taking data from two consecutive days, the machine will predict the weather for the next day. It is all about the learning the computer gets. Or the training that is given to the machine.

But, the big question is, how does this happen?

14.2.1 THE SIMPLE SIDE OF ML

Anyone who has at least a small foundation in computer science knows that machines are made to get the work done for people, by getting them programmed. If a person writes a program to add two numbers, the machine provides him/her with the sum of any two numbers which are provided to it as input. Meanwhile, if a person is writing a program to add a list of numbers, the only thing he/she needs to do is to write an appropriate program for it. Similar is the case for getting any repetitive, logical, complicated, or computation-intensive work done by the machine. There should be an appropriate program behind getting the task done.

But for tasks where a person uses his/her intelligence to discern and decide upon matters in real-time scenarios, he/she may not be able to write a program for it then and there. But, surely machines should be brought to his/her rescue. To make the decisions and to get the job done, you need to make the machines discern situations and behave as if humans would naturally do. How does it happen? It is here that machine learning comes into place.

In traditional programming, a person programs computers. Machine learning is allowing computers to write programs on their own. If programming is said to be the process of automation, then machine learning is more fun, it is automating the procedure of automation (Brownley, 2020). So instead of writing the code, data is fed to the algorithm, and the algorithm/machine builds the logic learning from the given data, which then enables the machine to behave in a learned manner [Figure 14.1].

You can consider machine learning like gardening or farming (Brownley, 2020). In the traditional approach, you provide nutrients as the data and plants as the program to produce seeds or flowers as the output. But in machine learning, you use nutrients as the data and the seeds that are output to produce a plant which is the program. This program will make the machines behave as learned machines. This is the reason why it is said, computers program themselves (Brownley, 2020).

14.2.2 THE TECHNICAL SIDE OF ML

If machine learning is so simple, what makes it a hot topic? How does it become the buzz word of the day?

Though it seems to be simple, coming to the other side of the coin, you can see that machine learning is a sub-part of artificial intelligence and comes under the domain of computer science. It has its roots in statistics, linear algebra, programming,

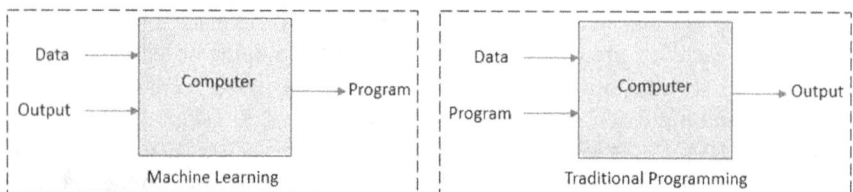

FIGURE 14.1   Traditional programming vs. machine learning.

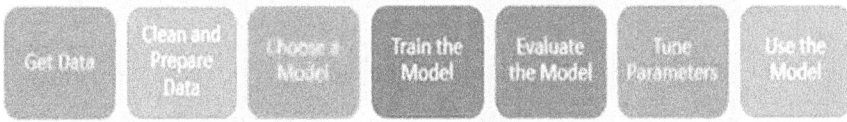

FIGURE 14.2 Steps in training a model.

data mining, and calculus and spreads its wings to Big Data, Data Analytics, Predictive Analytics, Cloud, and Internet of Things (IoT) to work wonders in the normal lifestyle of people.

But, how are machines trained? That is the topic of this section.

A learned machine that can answer any particular question is needed. This model of a question answering system is made by a procedure named training. This process aims to build an accurate model that answers questions correctly, for a majority of the instances. But to train a model, data has to be gathered on what need to train on. Once it is done, the rest follows (Bakshi, 2017). The detailed steps are given below (Figure 14.2).

14.2.2.1 Gathering Data

The first step required is data collection and one should remember that the amount of data and its quality will be determining the performance of the model. Once one knows exactly what his/her requirements are, go and get data to train the model. Though, it is real-time data or freely available open data sets related to his/her requirements, having them at one's fingertips is the first step.

14.2.2.2 Data Preparation

Once the data for training is collected, the next step is data preparation, where the data is loaded into an appropriate place and then cleaned for use in the training process. Here, since the order of data should not affect the process, the order is randomized after putting it all together (Bakshi, 2017).

Here, in this step, the data is cleaned. It involves finding out relationships among data features and eliminating redundant ones, getting rid of data imbalances or outliers, integrating data in a meaningful manner, and normalizing it.

Moreover, the data is split into three different categories (Figure 14.3).

1. **Training Data:** This sample of the data will comprise a majority of the data set and will be used to train the model. It is used to make sure the machine recognizes patterns in the data.
2. **Validation Data:** This sample of the data is used to validate the model while it is trained to ensure better efficiency and accuracy of the particular algorithm which is used to train the machine.

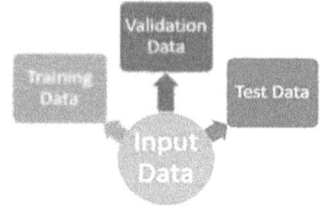

FIGURE 14.3   Input data divided into three types.

3. **Test Data:** This sample of the data is needed to evaluate the performance of the final model once it is built to see how well the machine can predict new answers based on its training.

14.2.2.3   Choose a Model

The third step is to choose a model which means, to choose an algorithm that will get one's work done. Based on the data and the problem at hand, the model may be capable of performing classification, prediction, recommendation, or any such job one wants the machine to perform for him/her. Choose the appropriate model for your data and requirements.

14.2.2.4   Training

Once the first three steps are completed, the next step is training where the ability of the model to predict is incrementally improved using the data. This step comprises the majority part of machine learning (Bakshi, 2017). In some ways, this is like someone learning to drive for the first time. On his/her first drive, one will surely be confused about how the pedals will work, how the knobs will turn, and how the switches will behave. But, with constant practice with trial and error corrections, one will, at last, be a licensed confident driver. And later, at the end of a year, one certainly becomes skilled. Driving a vehicle and reacting to the situations around will surely bring a change in one's skills of driving (Yufeng, 2017).

To explain it with an example, take the model of regression. $y = mx + b$, where, x is the input value, m is the slope of that line, b is the y-intercept, and y is the value of the line at the position x, is the formula for a straight line. Here, the values that have to be adjusted, or 'trained', or, will affect the position of the line, are only m and b, because x and y are the input and output values. The prediction is made accurate by changing the values of m and b.

You may find many m's in machine learning because there can be many features. The collection of these m values is usually formed into a matrix, which is termed the weight matrix, and b is organized together and called biases. The training procedure comprises giving the weight matrix and the biases some random initial values and trying to predict the output with those values. Though it will perform very poorly first, you can compare your model's predictions with the expected output and adjust the values of the weight matrix and the biases such that correct predictions will be obtained (Yufeng, 2017). Continuing this procedure is the process of training the model.

14.2.2.5   Evaluation

You can check whether the model is good enough once training is complete. This is the time when that data set you reserved earlier comes into play (Bakshi, 2017). This data which was kept aside is meant to represent how the model will perform in the real world. It helps to tune the model too (Mayo, 2018). There are many measures on which you can evaluate the model. Accuracy, prediction and recall, squared error, likelihood, posterior probability, cost, margin, entropy k-L divergence are some measures that can be used to evaluate the model (Brownley, 2020).

14.2.2.6   Parameter Tuning

The next step of tuning the parameters is used to improve the model further, once the evaluation is over. There will be some parameters that will be indirectly assumed during the training. The learning rate which tells how far the line should be shifted during each step is another parameter that is included, based on the information obtained from the previous training step. How accurate the training model will be and what may be the duration of training depend on these values (Bakshi, 2017). In the case of regression, the learning rate is defined by the change in the shift of the line during each step, based on the previous training step (Yufeng, 2017).

During the training process, some parameters were implicitly assumed and it is here that these assumptions are tested and other values are tried (Yufeng, 2017). Training the model again and again by adjusting or changing these hyperparameters is referred to as tuning the parameters. The data set, model, and training influence the tuning of these parameters (Bakshi, 2017). Once you change the values of these hyperparameters and train the model to perform better and better, you get a model of reasonable performance (Yufeng, 2017). In some cases, the model could give better accuracy when the training data set is run through the model multiple times (Yufeng, 2017). Simple model hyperparameters can include learning rate, initialization values, number of training steps, and distribution among others (Mayo, 2018).

14.2.2.7   Using the Model

This is the final step where the model is used to get answers to your questions. That means, it is here that you use the model to predict or classify or recommend or do whatever the model was meant for.

14.2.3   Summing Up

Machine learning is all about building a model and using that model in situations where it was intended for. By learning, it means that the machine is building some logic of its own. Learning can be used to model algorithms to find relationships, detect patterns, understand complex problems, and make decisions. Finally, it is the quality, diversity, and volume of one's training data that determines how good one's machine learning models are (Agarwal, 2017).

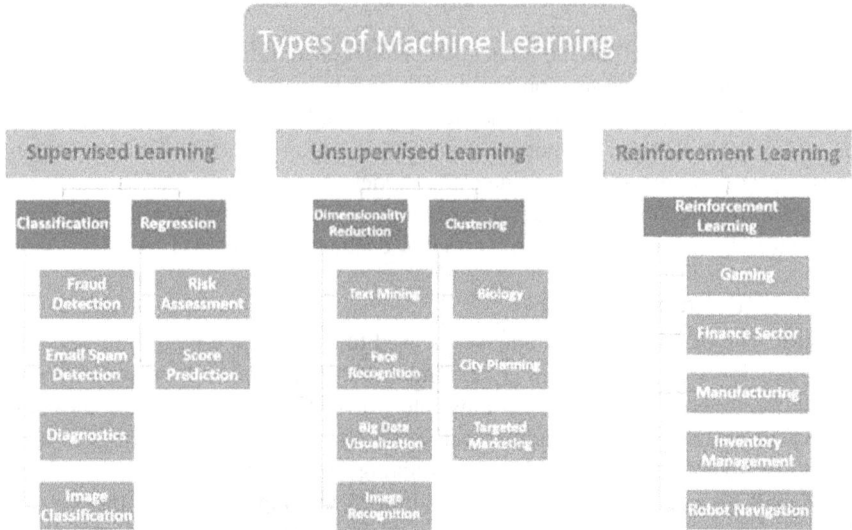

FIGURE 14.4 Types of machine learning.

14.3 TYPES OF MACHINE LEARNING

The three different ways in which you can train models for machine learning to achieve different qualities are supervised learning, unsupervised learning, and reinforcement learning (Figure 14.4). These different algorithms vary in their approach, the type of data they input, the type of data they output, and the type of task or problem that they are intended to solve (Wikipedia Inc., 2020c).

14.3.1 SUPERVISED LEARNING

This is a kind of machine learning where what the machine should do is first told to it. It can learn from previous examples, just like a teacher or supervisor is instructing him and giving directions. The model that is built will be trained on an adequate amount of input data, but the data at hand will have the output also with it. For example, if one is are building a model that should predict the wind speed at a particular time, the training data set will contain a lot of parameters that affect the speed of the wind, like, temperature, pressure, relative humidity, and wind direction. Once the machine is trained on this data it will be able to accurately predict wind speed at any time, given the temperature, pressure, relative humidity, and wind direction at that time (Guru99 Team, 2020b).

This learning is termed supervised training because the data had already input data and output data and it was trained likewise. In this method, during the training phase the machines are learning in what all conditions are the corresponding outputs produced and so when validation data is given, if the machine makes mistakes, the training is continued to bring out better performance minimizing errors and later during evaluation it should behave as a good model. It is the same as teaching your

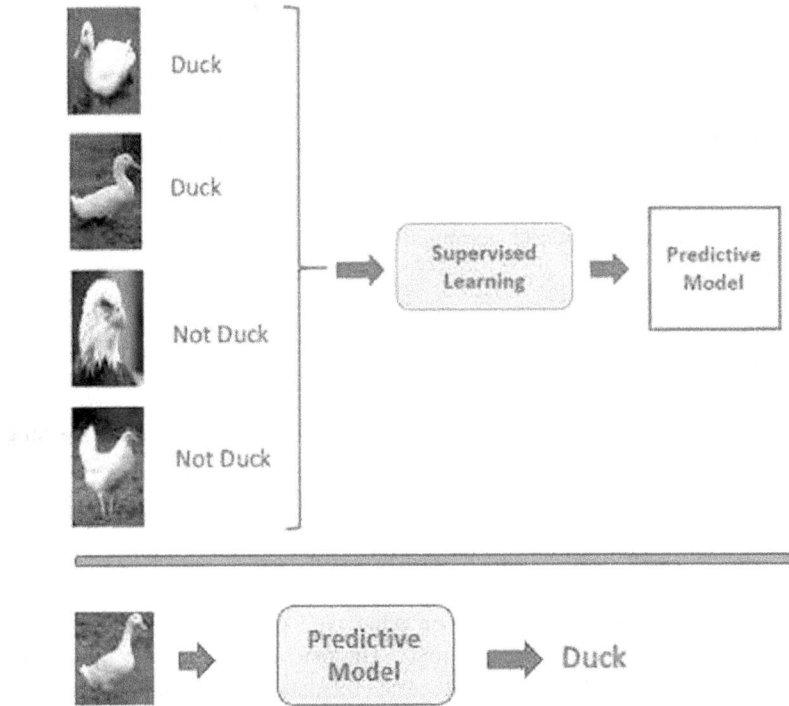

FIGURE 14.5 Supervised learning.

child to differentiate between a duck and other birds or animals while the child is still a toddler and correcting him each time he makes mistakes. Finally, there will be a time when the child never mistakes a duck for a hen or vice versa [Figure 14.5]. This is the rationale behind supervised machine learning. Train the machine with labeled data and build up a perfect model.

How supervised learning works: Supervised learning algorithms comprise a target/result variable (or dependent variable) which has to be predicted when a set of predictors (independent variables) are given. Using them, a function that can map inputs to the required outputs can be generated. This procedure continues till the model has a required level of accuracy on the training data (Ray, 2017).

Examples for Supervised Learning: Decision Tree, Random Forest, Linear Regression, Logistic Regression, etc. (Ray, 2017).

Challenges in Supervised Algorithms (Guru99 Team, 2020b)
- Can produce inaccurate results due to insignificant input features present in the training data
- Challenging data preparation and pre-processing
- Impossible, unlikely, and incomplete values in input training data can affect the accuracy

- Applying a brute-force approach to select the right features (input variables) to train the model in the absence of an expert can produce inaccurate (Guru99 Team, 2020b).

Advantages of Supervised Algorithms (Guru99 Team, 2020b):
- Data from the previous experience can be used
- Using experience, you can optimize performance criteria
- Various types of real-world computation problems can be solved (Guru99 Team, 2020b).

Disadvantages of Supervised Algorithms (Guru99 Team, 2020b)
- Good examples from each class should be collected while training the model
- Classification of big data is a real challenge
- A lot of computation time is needed for training in supervised learning (Guru99 Team, 2020b).

14.3.2 Unsupervised Learning

As the name indicates, here the learning is unsupervised. There is no teacher or supervisor present to direct the model on what type of output to produce. The training data will have inputs, but no outputs. The machine is trained to find some sort of patterns within the data and to categorize the data likewise. It is the same as the child seeing many cats and dogs and without the help of anyone being able to correctly distinguish some as cats and some as dogs by the passage of time. And one a fine morning, when a neighbor walks in with a new pet dog the child will be undoubtedly identifying it as a dog (Guru99 Team, 2020c).

In unsupervised learning, the machine is given huge chunks of data and is trained to find certain kinds of patterns in the data, and based on those patterns the machine accomplishes certain tasks. It works somewhat similar to a human brain, how humans learn behavior patterns of people and then learn whom to trust and whom to not. Here the data by which you learn is life experience (Vatsal, 2018). Unsupervised learning algorithms find patterns and group objects accordingly. Given images of animals, the model will be able to classify them into different groups based on some underlying patterns (Figure 14.6).

How Unsupervised Learning Works: Here, the input data contains no target or outcome variable to estimate or predict. It is used for customer segmentation in various fields by clustering the population into different groups (Ray, 2017). Primarily dealing with unlabeled data, the model works on its own to discover patterns. Taking some input data, these algorithms find structure in the data, like clustering them or grouping the data points. Therefore, these algorithms are said to learn from unlabeled test data, classified or categorized, and try to identify similarities in the data and based on whether such similarities are absent or present in each new data they react or provide outputs (Data Core Systems, 2018).

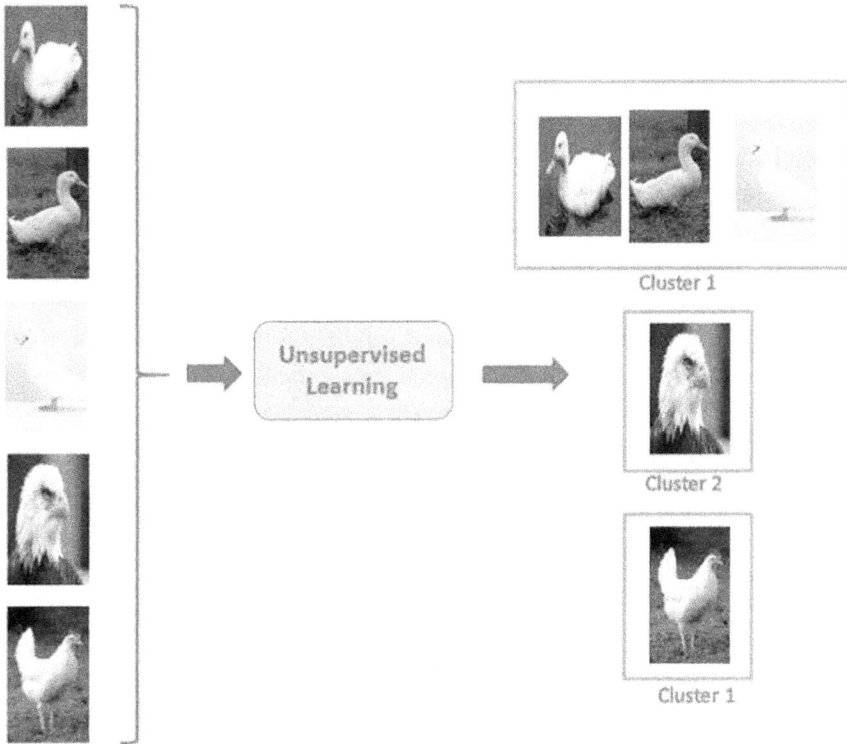

FIGURE 14.6   Unsupervised learning.

Examples for Unsupervised Algorithms: Apriori algorithm and K-means (Ray, 2017).

Advantages of Unsupervised Algorithms (Guru99 Team, 2020c)
- Used for finding all kinds of unknown patterns in data.
- Helps to find features that are useful for categorization.
- Since the data is taken from real-time, input data to be analyzed are labeled in the presence of learners.
- Unlabeled data is easier to obtain from a computer than labeled data, which needs manual intervention (Guru99 Team, 2020c).

Disadvantages of Unsupervised Algorithms (Guru99 Team, 2020c)
- Data sorting may not be precise, since the input data used in unsupervised learning is unlabeled and unknown
- The accuracy of the results is less because the input data is unknown and unlabeled. The machine may have to do this by itself
- Consumes the time of the user since he has to interpret and label the classes (Guru99 Team, 2020c).

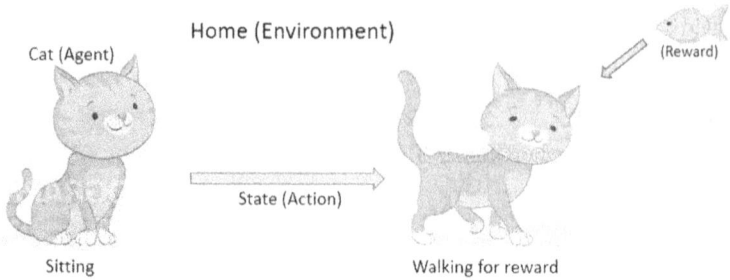

FIGURE 14.7 Reinforcement learning.

14.3.3 REINFORCEMENT LEARNING

In this learning the machine is left in a situation where something is happening and there is a reward if the machine does what you want and there is a punishment if the machine does what you don't want and based on it you instruct the machine to maximize the reward and eventually, the machine learns how to do the thing which you want it to do (Guru99 Team, 2020a). Taking the example of a child itself, imagine what happens if the child feels attracted to fire and puts his hands in it. Anyone near the child, be it his mother or neighbor will threaten or scold or even beat the child for doing so. And if you want the child to have some nutritious food, you may offer sweets to the child if he haves food willingly. Eventually, due to the reward and the punishment, the child learns what to do and what not to.

To cite another simple example to understand reinforcement learning, whenever a cat disturbs you, you beat and make it run away from you, and when it is loving and obeying you may reward it with fish pieces or likewise (Figure 14.7). As time passes, the cat will understand the situations where it will be rewarded and act accordingly.

A computer and camera within a self-driving car interacting with the road and other cars and learning how to navigate a city is another example of reinforcement training (Gupta, 2019). Again, if you want to develop a program to play chess, you simply program your model with the rules of chess. Then the model is allowed to play thousands of games and thus trained to decide which moves to make given a certain configuration. You can reward it when it wins or punish it when it loses, so it 'learns' which moves are 'good' and which are 'bad'. All the moves it makes are 'learned' through training (Singh, 2020).

How Reinforcement Learning Works: Any machine can be given the training to make precise decisions using these algorithms. The machine is given an environment where using trial and error it trains itself continually. This machine tries to learn using the best possible knowledge to make precise business decisions by learning from past experience (Ray, 2017). These algorithms don't need any information about an exact mathematical model but are used when exact models do not work correctly or give feasible results. These reinforcement learning algorithms find applications in self-driving vehicles or in gaming, where the machine learns to play a game where the opponent will be a human.

Examples of Reinforcement Learning: Markov Decision Process (Ray, 2017), Q Learning (Guru99 Team, 2020a)

Why use Reinforcement Learning Algorithms? (Guru99 Team, 2020a)
- Helps to find situations where actions are needed
- Aids to find out which action gives the maximum possible reward over the longer run
- Provides a reward function to the learning agent
- Permits you to find out the best way of getting bigger rewards (Guru99 Team, 2020a)

Reinforcement Learning Applications (Guru99 Team, 2020a)
- Automating industry using robots
- Business strategy planning
- Gaming machines
- Robot motion control and aircraft control (Guru99 Team, 2020a)

When Is Reinforcement Learning Algorithms Not Used? (Guru99 Team, 2020a)
- When the problem can be solved with a supervised learning algorithm
- These algorithms are computationally intensive and take a lot of time (Guru99 Team, 2020a)

14.4   MACHINE LEARNING ALGORITHMS

This section provides a list of commonly used machine learning algorithms. They include linear regression, logistic regression, decision tree, Support Vector Machines (SVM), Naïve Bayes, K-Nearest Neighbor, K-Means, Random Forest, Dimensionality Reduction Algorithms, and Gradient Boosting algorithms.

14.4.1   LINEAR REGRESSION

This is a type of problem where one variable is an independent variable and the other one is a dependent variable. The dependent variable changes in accordance with the independent variable either in a positive or negative manner. This is a supervised machine learning algorithm where the input data set will contain both the independent and dependent variables. The machine during its training finds the relationship between both the variables and builds the model. Here there is a linear relationship among the variables, which can be modeled using a straight line (Figure 14.8). Once the linear regression model is ready, whenever a known independent value is provided to the machine, it is able to predict the value of the unknown dependent variable.

To cite a simple example, if the data set consists of heights and weights of people, the model will during its training learn the relationship between height and weight of persons and later after training, when the model is given the height of a person, it would be able to predict the weight of that individual.

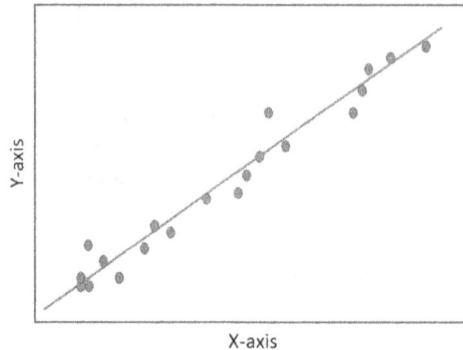

FIGURE 14.8   Linear regression.

There are two different types of linear regression, simple linear regression, and multiple linear regression. The first one will have only one independent variable, whereas, the latter will have more than one independent variable. Simple examples are:

- Predicting the electricity bill for each month depends on how much electricity was used each month in the past.
- The student administrator can predict a student's performance depending on how many hours the student use for his studies.

14.4.2 LOGISTIC REGRESSION

This is a supervised learning algorithm that forecasts the probability of the occurrence of an event. Mathematically, this is a multiple linear regression function where the dependant variable is a binary variable, which means, it is used to find discrete values like 0 or 1, true or false, and yes or no, depending on a set of independent variables. Here, the model built is a logit function to which the input data is fit and it outputs values between 0 and 1 since the output will always be a probability [Figure 14.9].

To make it clearer, suppose you are given a problem to solve. There are only two possible outcomes for the task before you, either you will solve it or, will fail in solving it. But, suppose you are given a series of puzzles, what would be the output? This is where logistic regression comes to your rescue and gives you the chance of your success or failure, which will be a probability value between 0 and 1.

Some real-time scenarios where logistic regression can be used are:

- To find how the probability of having lung cancer changes for each cigarette pack that is smoked per day and every extra pound a person is overweight
- How does body weight, age, calorie intake, and fat intake affect the chance of having a heart attack?

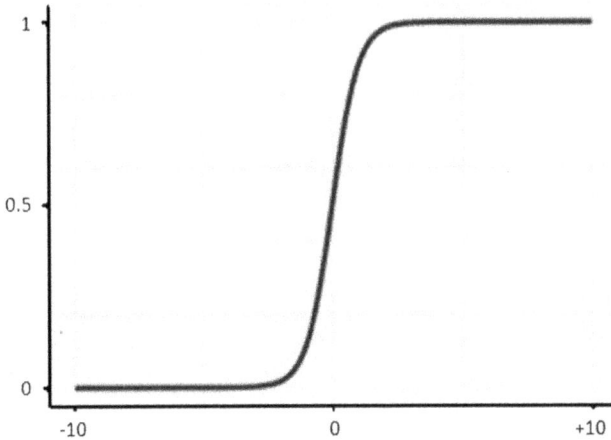

FIGURE 14.9 Logistic regression.

14.4.3 DECISION TREE

This is a supervised machine learning algorithm that is mainly used for solving classification problems (Saurabh, 2018). Classification algorithms classify or categorize data into different classes or different homogeneous populations. It is applicable for both continuous and categorical dependant variables. A decision tree algorithm uses a tree representation to solve the problem of classification. In this tree, each class label is represented by leaf nodes and internal nodes of the tree stand for the attributes of the problem set. Certain statistical methods such as information gain, gini index, or gain ratio will be used for ordering attributes as root or internal nodes of the tree.

To cite an example, one can create a model, or, a classifier, as it is called in this case, to filter out spam emails from regular emails. The model will be fed with regular emails labeled as 'regular' and spam emails labeled as 'spam'. The model will learn to filter spam from regular emails from the characteristics of spam emails, and later will be able to filter out spam email when it encounters new emails. Here, the target classes or, the output of the classifier are the labeled classes, 'spam' and 'regular'.

To cite another example, suppose you want a model to decide what to do each day. The model can be built with known data of the various things you do, such as, 'stay in', 'go running', 'go to movies' and 'go to the beach', which are the class labels or target classes. From the figure, it is clear that class labels are the leaf nodes of the tree. The input parameters are the root and other internal nodes and their corresponding values become branches for each corresponding node (Figure 14.10). Once the model is built and new data is fed into it, the model will be able to predict what will be the task for that particular day.

Classification can be binary classification, where the classifier classifies the input data only to two output classes, or can be multivariate where any number of target

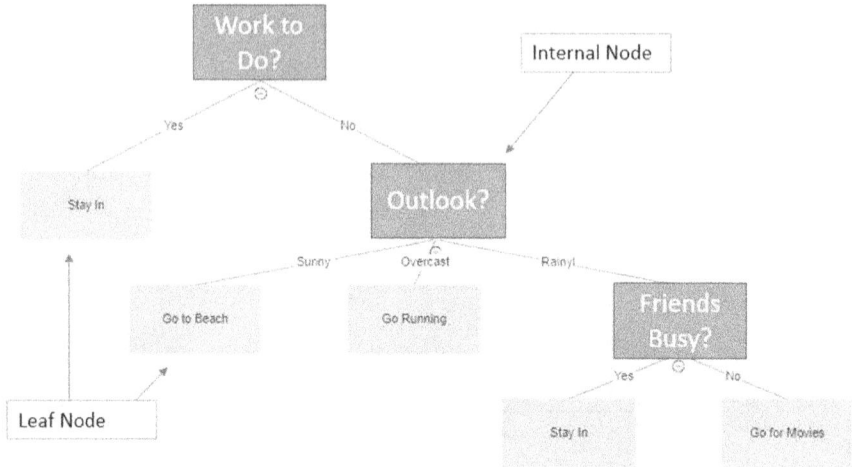

FIGURE 14.10 Decision tree.

classes can be produced. A decision tree is a multivariate classifier. It is a supervised classifier since the input data contains labeled classes.

14.4.4 SUPPORT VECTOR MACHINE (SVM)

SVM is a supervised machine learning algorithm that is used for two-group classification, thus making it a binary classifier. This classifier is able to perform classification, regression, and even outlier detection. The linear SVM classifier draws a straight line between two classes (Figure 14.11). The data points will be classified as on which side of the line they fall. All the data points that fall on one side comprise one class and all points falling on the other side constitute the second (Maklin, 2019). The points on each side close to the straight line or hyperplane are called the support vectors.

To cite a simple example, face detection algorithms are mostly SVMs. Whenever you open people's pictures on Facebook, you see squares drawn on faces. The technology that works behind this is SVM. The training data will consist of images, which are nxn pixels, labeled as 'face' and 'non-face'. The model learns by extracting features from both types of pixels and thus will learn to differentiate or classify 'face' and 'non-face' and draw a square boundary around faces (DataFlair Team, 2018b).

The SVM classifier in simple terms is a straight line drawn on a two-dimensional space, but in real-life applications, a hyperplane will be drawn in n-dimensional space (Figure 14.11). In a two-dimensional space, the two coordinates are called support vectors and so in an n-dimensional space, you have n support vectors. Real-life applications include face detection, handwriting recognition, image classification, and bioinformatics (DataFlair Team, 2018b).

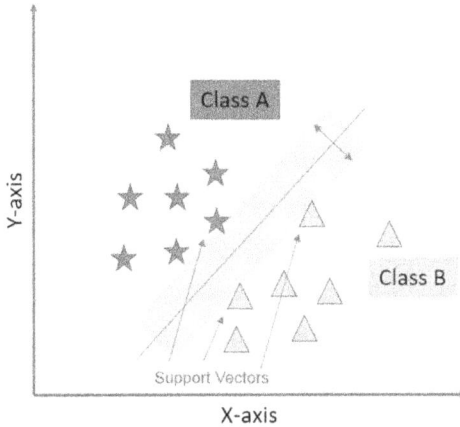

FIGURE 14.11 A simple SVM classifier.

14.4.5 NAÏVE BAYES

This is also a supervised algorithm that belongs to a class of conditional probability classifiers that are based on the Bayes Theorem. Bayes Theorem describes the probability of a feature, based on prior knowledge of conditions that might be related to that feature (Stecanella, 2017). Moreover, it assumes independence of assumptions between the features. In simple terms, a Naïve Bayes classifier assumes that if a particular feature is present in a class it is not related to the presence of any other feature.

To cite an example, suppose that the probability of a person having cancer is somehow related to his age, using Bayes' theorem this feature of age can be used to more efficiently predict the probability of cancer than when the age was not known (Wikipedia Inc., 2020a). For example, an apple is round, red, and about 3 inches in diameter. If it is seen that these features are related or dependent on each other, a Naïve Bayes classifier will use all these features and use them to find the probability that fruit is apple indeed (Ray, 2017).

This classifier is simple, fast, accurate, and reliable (Stecanella, 2017). The Naïve Bayesian model is useful for big data sets and easy to build. Though it is simple, Naïve Bayes is seen to be superior to many other powerful classification methods (Ray, 2017). Some applications of the **Naïve Bayes** algorithm include face recognition, medical diagnosis, categorizing news, sentiment analysis, email spam detection, natural language processing, digit recognition, and weather prediction (Sagar, 2018).

14.4.6 K-NEAREST NEIGHBOR (K-NN)

This is an algorithm that is very simple and stores all obtainable data and classifies new data by a majority vote of its k neighbors. The k neighbors of an object are measured using a distance function and the object is assigned to the class which is

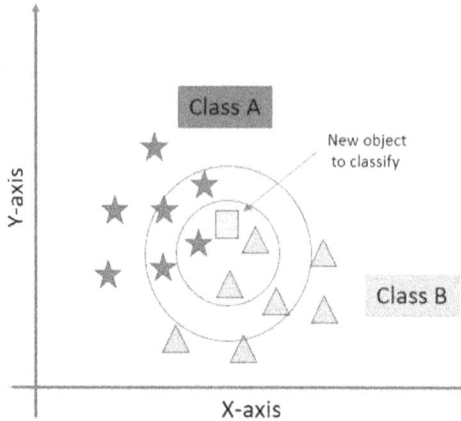

FIGURE 14.12   A simple K-NN classifier.

most popular amongst its k-nearest neighbors. The distance functions used can be Euclidean, Minkowski, Manhattan, or Hamming distance. The first of these three functions are used for continuous functions and the last one, Hamming distance is used for categorical variables (Ray, 2017). In the figure given (Figure 14.12), the unknown object will be assigned to class B, if k=3, and will be assigned to class A if k=7.

To cite an example, to gain information about a person whom you don't know, you will try to get some information from his close friends you find out and the spaces he moves in and obtains information about him/her (Ray, 2017). Based on the knowledge you get about people it is easy for you to categorize people into cheerful ones, jovial ones, intellectual ones, arrogant ones, and the like.

K-Nearest Neighbor has many uses in data mining and machine learning. One particular use is in anomaly detection. K-Nearest Neighbor can be used on airplanes to warn pilots and air traffic if something is going wrong on an airplane in ways that the human brain cannot compute or understand. It can be used in biological health monitoring to notify technicians if anything is going wrong (Dhiman, 2017).

14.4.7   K-MEANS

This is an unsupervised machine learning algorithm coming under the category of clustering algorithms. Clustering is the procedure of combining a set of objects so that objects of the same group are more related to each other than to objects of other groups (Wikipedia Inc., 2020b). Here, data points inside a cluster are similar to each other and dissimilar to peer groups (Ray, 2017). When a group of n objects is given, the algorithm divides the group into k sub-groups. Each of the divided groups has a similar basis where the distance of each data point in them is directly related to their mean values (DataFlair Team, 2019a), and hence the name k-means (Figure 14.13).

To cite a simple example, if the model is given data about different types of dogs without telling that it is data about dogs, the algorithm will partition the input data into different categories of dog breeds. This is done by finding similarities in the

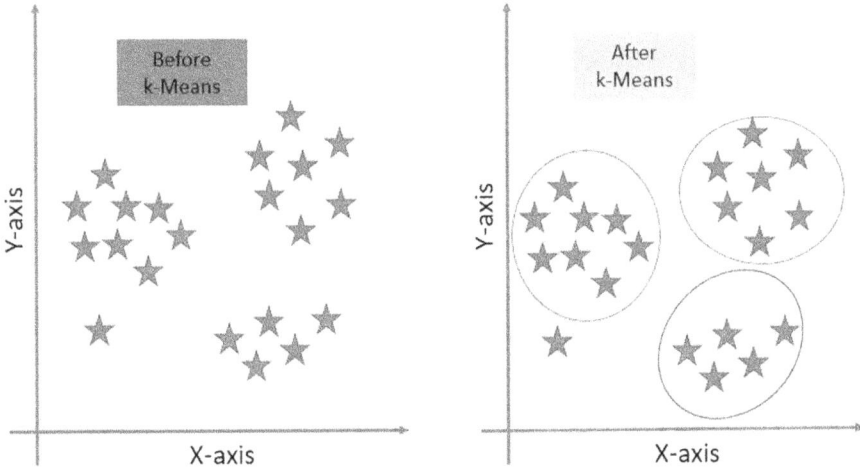

FIGURE 14.13 K-means clustering.

training data and clustering them likewise. Similarities are found by using some distance measures.

K-Means has a wide variety of applications in diverse fields like bioinformatics, data compression, pattern recognition, information retrieval, image analysis, and computer graphics (Wikipedia Inc., 2020b).

14.4.8 RANDOM FOREST

The name of this algorithm is a trademarked term which is a collection of decision trees. Here, you have a collection of decision trees which gives it the term 'forest' in its name. Based on input values to categorize a new object, each tree provides a classification and you can tell that the tree is voting for that particular class. At last, the classification having the majority of votes than all other trees in the forest is chosen by the forest (Ray, 2017). The average of all the trees is taken to make the final prediction or classification (Figure 14.14). Since, they use a collection of results they are referred to as ensemble techniques (Hatalis, 2019).

To cite an example, if you are planning for a trip and would like to choose a place you haven't visited yet what would you do? You would do some online search, read some reviews about travel blogs or get an opinion from friends (Navlani, 2018) for recommendations of places favorite to them and each friend will be suggesting some places. From all the places searched or suggested, you will vote them and at last, select a particular place that ranks the top. Getting individual recommendations is similar to building decision trees and the voting procedure to select the best constitutes the random forest algorithm (Navlani, 2018).

Random forests have a multitude of applications such as feature selection, image classification, and building recommendation engines. It can be used to identify fraudulent activity, classify loyal loan applicants, and predict diseases (Navlani, 2018).

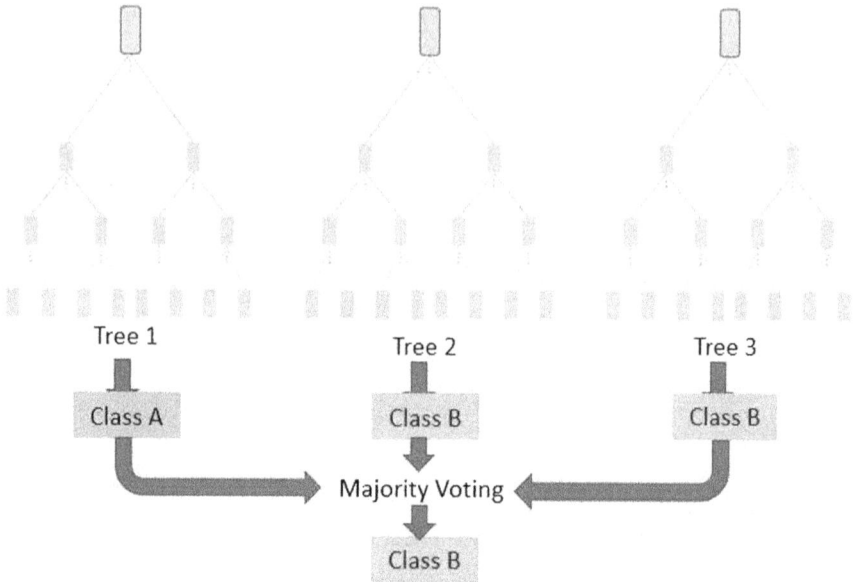

FIGURE 14.14 Random forest.

14.4.9 DIMENSIONALITY REDUCTION ALGORITHMS

In real-life applications of machine learning, the data collected to be fed as input to the algorithms will have numerous features. When the number of features becomes high, it will be difficult to envision the training set for working on it. The majority of the times, many of these features are related, and so repeated. In those scenarios, dimensionality reduction algorithms are used to reduce the features and select appropriate ones (DataFlair Team, 2018c).

There are mainly two types of dimensionality reduction algorithms, namely, feature selection and feature extraction. Feature selection algorithms find a small subset of the original set of variables and feature extraction algorithms reduce data in high dimensional spaces to lower-dimensional spaces (DataFlair Team, 2018c).

Dimensionality reduction can be either linear or non-linear, based on the approach used. The different types of algorithms used for dimensionality reduction include Principal Components Analysis (PCA), Generalized Discriminant Analysis (GDA), and Linear Discriminant Analysis (LDA) (DataFlair Team, 2018c).

14.4.10 GRADIENT BOOSTING ALGORITHMS

Gradient boosting is said to be one of the most powerful methods for building predictive models. It is a machine learning technique for regression problems and classification problems that builds a prediction model as an ensemble of not so strong prediction models. There are two ways to boost the accuracy of a predictive model; either by doing feature engineering or by using boosting algorithms straight away (DataFlair Team, 2018a).

The idea of whether a weak learner can be modified to become better is the basis for the idea of boosting (Brownley, 2019a). Gradient boosting algorithms comprise three elements:

- A loss function that can be optimized
- A weak learner so that predictions can be made
- To minimize the loss function, an additive model so that weak learners can be added (DataFlair Team, 2018a)

There are many boosting algorithms like Gradient Boosting, XGBoost, AdaBoost, LightGBM, CatBoost, and Gentle Boost (DataFlair Team, 2018a).

14.5   TOOLS AVAILABLE FOR MACHINE LEARNING

As technology is developing, the tools that can be used for developing machine learning applications are myriad. From the conception of an idea to the deployment, choosing the correct tool for the correct job is crucial for the success of any machine learning application. Tools required for the development of a machine learning application include programming languages, databases, frameworks, and deployment tools.

14.5.1   PROGRAMMING LANGUAGES

Machine learning is still a developing area that is growing, and various programming languages dominate the development domain. Here is a list of programming languages that are used by developers to build projects with machine learning.

14.5.1.1   Python

Having various tools in its toolset, Python is a language that is stable and flexible (Gupta, 2020). As a popular and powerful interpreted language, Python can be used for both research and development and developing machine learning applications (Brownley, 2019b). Python has a rich set of libraries catering to the needs of any discipline, which makes it the primary toolkit for any developer. The Python ecosystem is very much suitable for AI-based projects. Python is a simple language and with a big community and a lot of tools, it allows developers to build architectures that almost perfect when used to build business-driven applications (Beklemysheva, 2020). Some other benefits of Python are:

- Simple and consistent
- Flexible
- Rich set of libraries and frameworks
- Readable
- Platform independence

14.5.1.2   R

R is known to be a statistical programming language that is generally applied when you need to analyze and manipulate data. It has packages such as Class, Tm, Gmodels, and

RODBC that are usually used for building machine learning applications. They permit developers to implement machine learning algorithms without much struggle and let them quickly deploy business logic. Created by statisticians to meet their needs, this language gives you deep statistical analysis when you are manipulating data from an IoT device or performing financial analysis (Beklemysheva, 2020).

14.5.1.3 Scala

Scala is used for big data applications. It has good concurrency support, which enables it to process large volumes of data. Scala runs together with Hadoop, which is an open-source distributed processing framework managing data processing and bog data storage running in clustered systems. Moreover, it is easy to maintain Scala (Beklemysheva, 2020).

14.5.1.4 Julia

Julia can provide high-performance computing solutions and analysis. Its syntax is similar to Python and is created to manipulate numerical computing tasks. Deep Learning too is supported by Julia, via the TensorFlow.jl wrapper and the Mocha framework (Beklemysheva, 2020).

14.5.1.5 Java

Java is a programming language that is portable, maintainable, object-oriented, and transparent. Supported by numerous libraries such as WEKA and Rapidminer, it is very popular for natural search algorithms, language processing, and neural networks. You can quickly build large-scale systems with excellent performance using Java (Beklemysheva, 2020).

14.5.2 Frameworks

There are libraries or tools which permit developers to make machine learning models quickly, not going deep into the complexities of the background algorithms. Such interfaces are called machine learning frameworks (Sayantini, 2020). They help machine learning developers to build machine learning models in accurate, transparent, and crisp ways and are used to deliver already built and optimized components to aid in model building and other jobs (Jack, 2020).

14.5.2.1 Tensor Flow

For a variety of jobs, tensor flow is an exceptional open-source library for database programming. It provides support for regressions, classifications, and complex tasks and algorithms like neural networks. It is a flexible and portable framework useful in research and development operations (Jack, 2020). For data flow graphs that use numerical computing too, it serves as an open-source software library (Sayantini, 2020).

14.5.2.2 PyTorch

Pytorch is a machine learning library and a framework for scientific computing. Associated with it is a scripting language interface from the Lua programming user interface. PyTorch is used by major companies like Facebook, IBM, Yandex, and

Idiap Research Institute (Jack, 2020). PyTorch aims to have the utmost flexibility and to be fast in building your scientific algorithms together with an extremely simple process (Sayantini, 2020).

14.5.2.3   Spark ML Library

This is the machine learning library of Apache Spark. This library aims to make practical machine learning expandable and easy (Sayantini, 2020). For data scientists familiar with R & Python this is a cluster-computing framework that offers simple APIs. It is scalable and enables you to run machine learning code on both small and big machines (Jack, 2020).

14.5.2.4   CAFFE (Convolutional Architecture for Fast Feature Embedding)

Convolutional Architecture for Fast Feature Embedding (CAFFE) is a tool for deep learning and a very efficient machine learning framework. It is the latest framework for deep neural networks and supports GPU training for sample data (Jack, 2020), and the utmost priority while developing it was articulation, speed, and measured quality (Sayantini, 2020).

14.5.2.5   scikit-learn

This is a strong Python library for coding machine learning programs and is explicitly used for creating models. It is a very efficient tool for classification, regression, clustering, and statistical modeling (Jack, 2020). It can be recommended for both supervised and unsupervised learning problems (Sayantini, 2020).

14.5.2.6   Amazon Machine Learning

Amazon's machine learning framework, Amazon machine learning is a collection of tools and wizards to create highly sophisticated, intelligent, and high-end applications without tinkering with code (Jack, 2020). It provides visualization tools that enable you to create machine learning models without having to know the complexities of machine learning algorithms and technology (Sayantini, 2020).

14.5.3   DATABASES

A database management system is one of the most important components in machine learning applications. With this system, it is easy to sort and gain good insights from huge volumes of data (Chaudury, 2020). Below listed are some of the top databases used in machine learning projects.

14.5.3.1   MySQL

Powered by Oracle, MySQL is the most user-friendly and common open-source relational database management system (RDBMS). Big successful organizations like Facebook, Twitter, YouTube, and others use this database (Chaudury, 2020).

14.5.3.2   PostgreSQL

This is a powerful, open-source object-relational database system that uses the SQL language and extends it combined with many features that securely manage and keep the most complex data workloads. The goal of this DBMS is to aid developers in building applications, help administrators in protecting data integrity, and building environments that are fault-tolerant (Chaudury, 2020).

14.5.3.3 MongoDB

This is a document-based, distributed, general-purpose, database which is designed for expert application developers. Being a document database, mainly it uses JSON-like documents to keep data. It gives support for aggregations and is useful for graph search, geo-based search, and text search (Chaudury, 2020).

14.5.3.4 MLDB

The machine learning database is an open-source system that can solve problems in machine learning involving big data. It can be used right for collecting and storing data, analyzing it, training models, and finally for deployment too (Chaudury, 2020).

14.5.3.5 Spark with Hadoop HDFS

While working with machine learning projects, one will have to deal with large amounts of unstructured data. Normal relational database management systems may not suffice in terms of quantity, data structure, and database performance when it has to run big data. Spark with HDFS (Hadoop Distributed File System) is the right database solution in these scenarios (Powar, 2018). HADOOP is the primary data storage system used by Hadoop applications.

14.5.3.6 Apache Cassandra

This is a highly expandable and open-source NoSQL DBMS that is developed to handle large amounts of data quickly. Netflix, Reddit, Instagram, and GitHub use this database (Chaudury, 2020).

14.5.3.7 Microsoft SQL Server

Microsoft SQL Server is an RDBMS (relational database management system). It queries across relational, non-relational, structured, and unstructured data to gain insights from them (Chaudury, 2020).

14.5.4 DEPLOYMENT TOOLS

All of the activities that comprise a software system available for use, is given the name software deployment. The general deployment process comprises of various interrelated activities with ample transitions amongst them (Wikipedia Inc., 2020d). Following are some of the tools available for deploying machine learning projects.

14.5.4.1 Github

Github has its own features and offers the distributed version control and source code management (SCM) functionality of Git. It provides access control and several collaboration features such as feature requests, task management, bug tracking, and wikis for every project (Xiao, 2020).

14.5.4.2 PyCharm Community Edition

This is an integrated development environment (IDE), which consists of code analysis, a graphical debugger, an integrated unit tester, and integration with version control systems. It supports web development too (Xiao, 2020).

14.5.4.3 Pytest

This is a tool that is simple and easy, and at the same time, supports complex functional testing for libraries and applications. It avoids wastage of time from manual testing. In cases where you need to test each time you change the code, it is nice that it is automated with Pytest (Xiao, 2020).

14.5.4.4 CircleCi

This is a continuous integration and deployment tool which creates an automated testing workflow ensuring code quality and is used while working with large teams (Xiao, 2020).

14.5.4.5 Heroku

Whenever you need web hosting, you can go for this tool. This is a cloud platform that helps developers in building, running, and operating applications. Automatic deployment is possible when it is integrated with CircleCI and Github (Xiao, 2020).

14.5.4.6 MLFlow

Developed to work with any machine learning algorithm or library MLFlow can manage the whole lifecycle, with experimentation, reproducibility, and deployment of ML models (Rizvi, 2019).

14.6 APPLICATION AREAS OF MACHINE LEARNING

Everywhere you can see machine learning now it is finding applications in almost all walks of life, even when you may not be understanding that it is at work. As a branch of AI, these algorithms or, these learned machines tend to behave very similarly to the human brain. Below given are some applications that you see in your everyday life.

14.6.1 EVERYDAY LIFE

Learned machines are a part of everyday life today. It may be in the form of virtual personal assistants, may be helping you in having a very personalized shopping experience or by giving you weather forecasts. Another service that you avail everyday by the advancement in machine learning is the services provided by Google. Be it Google search, Gmail, Maps, or Calendar, machine learning is in the background.

14.6.1.1 Virtual Personal Assistants

Today you can see virtual personal assistants in the form of Siri, Alexa, or Google Assistant. They assist in finding information when asked over voice, just as their name suggests. The only thing is that they should be activated and anyone can ask, 'What is my schedule for today?', 'What and when are the flights to New York from California', or such questions. Recalling your related searches and queries, the personal assistant you have will answer you by collecting information (Daffodil Software, 2017).

These personal assistants function due to the speech recognition and face detection algorithms built into them. For speech recognition, with the utterance from a user, machine learning algorithms are capable of finding out the user who made the specific request. Such a program enables a machine to understand that request and try to grant that request (Brownley, 2018). Again, if one is given a digital photo album consisting of hundreds of digital photographs, he/she can find out those photos that include a given person just because of face detection algorithms, which are really machine learning algorithms. Such a program will allow a machine to systematically organize photos by person (Brownley, 2018). In the case of digit recognition, if envelopes with handwritten zip codes are given, there are machine learning algorithms that can correctly recognize the digit for each character that is handwritten. With such a program, a computer can read and understand handwritten zip codes from any place and sort envelopes geographically (Brownley, 2018).

14.6.1.2   Personalized Shopping

If you have shopped for a product online at any time, you might have seen emails and online advertisements and recommendations popping out of sites and apps that you open for products matching your interests. This refined shopping experience is certainly due to the machine learning algorithms doing the magic in the background. Each time the product recommendations are made based on the pattern you have related to your website browsing, app purchase, items liked or added, preferences of a brand, and other things (Daffodil Software, 2017).

14.6.1.3   Weather Forecasts

Today, weather forecasting provides near to perfect predictions, thanks to machine learning. It can also be used to compare previous weather forecasts and observations. Machine learning also helps in giving more accurate predictions and these weather models can be responsible for prediction inaccuracies too. Apart from better accurate forecasts, machine learning can also be used to improve immediate weather prediction, called nowcasting, which provides minute-by-minute precipitation forecasts (Ganshin, 2019).

14.6.1.4   Google Services

Google is the next-door friend in everyone's everyday life. There are machine learning algorithms behind almost every Google service and provides a very personalized and valuable experience to customers. It is already embedded in Google services like Gmail, Search, Maps, YouTube, and Photos (DataFlair Team, 2019b). The classification of your emails into primary, social, and promotional categories, the 'smart replies' and 'smart compose' features, and that too in even non-English languages are applications of machine learning. The suggestions provided for words typed in the Google search bar are based on recommendations from past searches, recent trends, and/or the present location. Google Assistant, Google translate, Google music, and other Google services also rely on machine learning algorithms.

14.6.1.5 Spam Detection

Machine learning algorithms can be used for identifying emails that are spam or not, given access to email in an inbox. This program will eventually move all spam emails to the spam folder and leave all non-spam emails in the inbox. This example might be very familiar to all of you (Brownley, 2018).

14.6.1.6 Credit Card Fraud Detection

If a customer's monthly transactions of credit card are given, machine learning algorithms can be used to find out those transactions that were done by the customer and the transactions that were not done by him. This program could refund fraudulent transactions (Brownley, 2018).

14.6.2 HEALTHCARE

The healthcare industry is an area where machine learning has got a variety of use cases. From streamlining the administration of hospitals to mapping and treating infectious diseases and personalizing medical treatments machine learning comes to aid. It has an important role in many healthcare domains, which includes the innovation of new medical procedures, manipulation of data taken from patient records, and the treatment of fatal diseases. Below given are five areas where machine learning can be applied in healthcare (Thomas, 2019).

14.6.2.1 Personalized Medicine/Treatment

Today, doctors can provide personalized or customized treatment to individuals according to their specific needs since huge data is available as genetic information and electronic health records. This huge volume of data is used to mine insights from them to provide individual healthcare to patients. These insights will help to suggest personalized combinations, and thus predict the disease risk with the help of machine learning technologies (DataFlair Team, 2019e).

14.6.2.2 Medical Imaging and Diagnostics

Traditionally, physical irregularities were inspected using X-ray and CT scan, but today with the exponential increase in diseases, more sophisticated techniques are required. Using such techniques even microscopic deformities in the scanned images of patients can be found out and as a result, which enables doctors to conduct an appropriate diagnosis (DataFlair Team, 2019e). Breast cancer is another use case where the speed and accuracy of diagnosis can be increased and tumors can be differentiated (Thomas, 2019).

14.6.2.3 Identification of Diseases and Diagnosis

With a multitude of disease types, today it is difficult to diagnose diseases manually. Systems using machine learning algorithms are highly beneficial in finding out the disease of a patient monitoring his health and suggesting essential steps that are to be taken to prevent the disease. Even minor and major diseases like cancer can be identified even in the early stages using this. Machine learning enabled systems can address the critical needs of patients and provide information that provides quicker and more precise diagnosis, personalized treatment, and more accurate results (DataFlair Team, 2019e).

14.6.2.4 Drug Discovery and Development

It is a very expensive and prolonged process to discover or manufacture a new drug because there are a variety of compounds that are made to the test and at last only one will be found to be successful. Today sophisticated machine learning algorithms can stimulate this process. You may have seen machine learning algorithms being used in developing technologies for cancer treatment and personalizing drug combinations for patients (DataFlair Team, 2019e). It can also be used for developing drugs so that patients can be cured faster and at a low cost (Thomas, 2019).

14.6.2.5 Smart Health Records

To an extent, machines have made the process of data entry easy due to technological advancements. But, still, there are tasks to be automated. Maintenance of updated health records everyday is tiring as well as consuming a lot of time. Machine learning can help in the maintenance of health records saving time, money, and effort. Machine learning has been utilized to analyze oncology data, and thus provide insights that allow oncologists, pharmaceutical companies, merchants, and providers to practice precision medicine and health. It can also be used to better match patients with doctors (DataFlair Team, 2019e).

14.6.2.6 Treatment and Prediction of Disease

There are a variety of machine learning techniques that are utilized in monitoring and predicting diseases both, severe and small. Scientists have access to huge volumes of data collected from satellites, social media platforms, websites, and these machine learning techniques collaborate with this information to help in detecting the disease early, pinpointing therapy requirements, and highlighting opportunities for clinical trials (DataFlair Team, 2019e). Machine learning can be employed for mapping diseases and treatments in oncology, neurology, and other rare conditions (Thomas, 2019).

14.6.3 AGRICULTURE

The key role in increasing the global economy of any country is agriculture. The cultivation and production of crops have become ever more important due to the increase in population (Techno Stacks, 2018). In the agriculture sector, machine learning techniques can improve the productivity and quality of the crops. In a variety of agricultural sectors, farmers have been exploiting machine learning models and innovations made by them. Creating a business network among farmers using machine learning and analytic tools can drive the results of data on pricing. In many places, robots have started managing the crops and monitoring them and again, sensors are used for data collection related to crops. According to research if machine learning is used in agriculture, then the agriculture sector will witness a big boost in the coming years (Techno Stacks, 2018). Below given are some areas where machine learning can be applied in agriculture.

14.6.3.1 Crop Management

Crop management encompasses a variety of tasks such as yield prediction, matching of crop supply with demand, disease detection, detection and discrimination of weeds, detection and classification of crop quality, prediction and classification of geographical origin for crops, and identification and classification of plant species (Liakos, 2018). All these areas are under study and research and getting automated with machine learning. Taking the advantage of new technologies in agriculture, farmers can find productive ways to save their crops and also protect them from weeds. Companies are developing automation tools and robots to achieve this (Techno Stacks, 2018).

14.6.3.2 Livestock Management

There are two sub-categories for the livestock category which are animal welfare and livestock production. The first category deals with the health and well-being of domestic animals, with machine learning algorithms helping in the monitoring of animal behavior so that animal diseases can be detected early. On the other hand, livestock production deals with problems in the production system, where machine learning applications can be used to accurately estimate economic balances for the producers depending on production line monitoring (Liakos, 2018).

14.6.3.3 Plant Breeding

Plant breeding requires checking for a specific trait regularly. Plant breeders try to identify the factors which will help to use water more efficiently, using nutrients, and also adapting to the climate changes or any diseases. The right gene has to be found out by scientists if the plant needs to give the desired result. Machine learning techniques are already capable of finding the correct sequence of genes (Techno Stacks, 2018).

14.6.3.4 Soil Management

This section is concerned with machine learning applications on the prediction and classification of properties of soil, such as the estimating of condition, temperature, and moisture content for drying soil. Most often it very expensive and requires a lot of time to measure soil properties. Hence an effective solution that will be reliable and economic for estimating soil properties accurately can be obtained with the use of computational analysis based on machine learning techniques (Liakos, 2018).

14.6.3.5 Agriculture Robot

Today, even in the agricultural field, many companies are designing and building robots to handle the essential tasks related to agriculture. These agricultural robots can be used to automate slow, dull, and repetitive tasks for farmers, thus permitting them to focus more on improving overall yield production. There are innovative and creative ways in which robots are implemented in the agricultural sector like utilizing drones, autonomous tractors, robotic arms, and robots (Robotics, 2017).

14.6.4 Transportation

By its complexity and real-world impact, transportation is an excellent area to develop new machine learning methodologies. Already driverless cars are on the roads at least in developed countries. Again, while you are on the roads, you need predictions about the next moment traffic both in normal commuting and in stress scenarios. Moreover, video surveillance systems are installed everywhere on roads to monitor and improve transportation services. Online transportation services are another area where machine learning is finding applications.

14.6.4.1 Driverless Cars

The potential applications of machine learning in autonomous cars include evaluation of driver condition or driving scenario classification through data fusion from different external and internal sensors (Ravindra, 2017). Machine learning algorithms when used in the self-driving car can continuously render the surrounding environment and predict possible changes that can happen to those surroundings (Gupta, 2019). The main task of machine learning algorithms in an autonomous car will be a continuous rendering of the surrounding environment and forecasting the changes that can happen to these surroundings. These tasks are subdivided into tasks like detection of an object, object localization, and prediction of movement (Ravindra, 2017).

14.6.4.2 Predictions While Commuting

The transport system as you know it today is a dynamic one. The traffic predictions you receive while you are traveling are using GPS navigation services. While using GPS navigation services, for managing traffic, your current locations and velocities will be saved at a central server and this data will then be used to build a map of the current traffic. This is useful in predicting the traffic, performing congestion analysis, and thus preventing traffic (Daffodil Software, 2017). Machine learning is also used in stress scenarios such as special events, incidents, breakdowns, and road works which need good predictions.

14.6.4.3 Video Surveillance

Nowadays, there are a lot of video surveillance systems that track live activity on roads, ATMs, shops, malls, junctions, and many more. These systems track unusual behavior from the video captured and provide alerts which in turn will prevent accidents. Moreover, if such reported activities are found to be true, they can be used to improve the surveillance service itself (Daffodil Software, 2017).

14.6.4.4 Transportation Services

Sometimes it may be very difficult to model and predict the travel patterns. In such cases, it is challenging to deal with transportation problems. Hence, artificial intelligence is deemed to be useful for transportation systems to overcome the barriers of greater demand for traveling, carbon dioxide emissions, safety concerns, and environmental degradation (Abduljabbar, 2019). Even in the case of booking an online cab for transportation, you can see the app estimating the time when the cab reaches you and predicting the fare which is another application of machine learning (Daffodil Software, 2017).

14.6.4.5 Interactive Journey

Today, passengers can make purchases, check statuses and schedules, find nearby stations and attractions, and much more during their travel using mobile applications. The main features of these applications, such as notification systems, location tracking, and suggestion features are powered by machine learning algorithms. These applications will have in their background rich data sets that continually adjust and improve over time (Data Core Systems, 2018).

Again, machine learning can help in using powerful features such as updates about train status and current location, parking assistance, alerts for equipment malfunction or maintenance, targeted messaging and notifications sent to users, an alarm indicating arrival at destination and nearby ATMs, hotels, restaurants, and the like.

14.6.5 EDUCATION

Education is an area where machine learning can be applied to provide a form of personalized learning to each student so that each of them gets a personal experience in their period of study. Machine learning algorithms guide the students at their own pace, enabling them to make their own decisions thus having their personal learning experience (DataFlair Team, 2019c).

14.6.5.1 Customized Learning Experience

Adaptive learning is analyzing the performance of a student in real-time and modifying the curriculum and the methods for teaching based on that data. Thus a personalized engagement is achieved by adapting the individual for a better education. The software is customized so that the students come to know which learning paths are suitable for them. Suggestions and other learning methodologies will be obtained from such software itself (DataFlair Team, 2019c).

14.6.5.2 Increasing Efficiency of Education

Providing quality content and having an organized curriculum is of top priority in any educational platform. This may lead to dividing the work among all and co-operating in everything understanding the potential of each. Moreover, it helps to find out which work is suited for the teacher and which curriculum is best for the student (DataFlair Team, 2019c). It will make learning happier and make everyone comfortable with education, and also gets students to love participation in learning, which will in turn increase the efficiency of education. Educators will also be benefitted from this because they too will learn new methods of classroom management and scheduling. Thus they will be free to focus on tasks that machines cannot do and so require a human touch (DataFlair Team, 2019c).

14.6.5.3   Predictive Analytics

Knowing the attitude and mindset of students is very essential in education. This is what predictive analytics has to do in education. It enables a student to take decisions on his own and make conclusions about future matters. It can even tell which students will perform nicely in the forthcoming class tests and other exams and who will perform poorly. This enables both parents and teachers to remain alert and take necessary actions. This can help a student to work more on his weak subjects and score more next time (DataFlair Team, 2019c).

14.6.5.4   Personalized Learning

Personalized learning is the best use case of machine learning in education. It is a process that can be customized and individual interests can be given due priority. Here each student guides his learning. Having their own pace in learning, students can choose what to learn, when to learn, and how to learn. The subjects that they are interested in can be chosen and the curriculum, patterns, and standards also can be chosen individually by the student. Moreover, he is free to choose his teacher too (DataFlair Team, 2019c).

14.6.6   Urbanization

Recently urbanization has emerged as a rising trend in most countries. Globally, 55% of the world's population lives in urban areas. When urbanization takes over, there will be more demand for housing, infrastructures, and industrial and commercial uses.

14.6.6.1   Automatic Classification of Buildings
and Structures

In urban areas and settlements, basic maps of existing buildings should be generated by city planners and leaders. Machine learning can come to their help in this scenario. This an in turn helps them in estimating population size, neighborhood density, and provides access to resources, and acts as a base across which to extrapolate household-level information (Barragán, 2019).

14.6.6.2   Urban Population Modeling

The population distribution in an urban area can be modeled as a spatiotemporal regression problem using machine learning, which obtains the binary urban footprint from the population distribution through a binary classifier plus a temporal correction for existing urban regions. It can estimate the urban footprint in color from its previous value, as well as from past and current values of the binary urban footprint using certain algorithms. Combined with the population data of any city in the world, this model can provide approximate growth predictions of any city in the world.

14.6.6.3 Other Applications

There are a variety of areas where machine learning can be used for urbanization. Visualization of urban-growth patterns, road network extraction, building detection, and water resource extraction are some among them. Spatial analysis of urban landscape changes, 3D analysis of the urban landscape, land cover, and land use classification also are areas where machine learning techniques can be applied.

14.6.7 SOCIAL MEDIA SERVICES

Today social media is very powerful and getting information and maintaining it is not an easy task. Machine learning helps in automating data, collecting, maintaining, and manipulating it without the need for human intervention. Below given are some specific areas where machine learning is applied in social media services.

14.6.7.1 Personalized Feeds

Every day you can see your news feeds getting more and more personalized, YouTube showing you videos matching your interests, or Amazon providing advertisements targeting you. It is the application of machine learning when Facebook provides you with friend suggestions and asks you to tag friends by recognizing them when you upload their photos (Daffodil Software, 2017).

14.6.7.2 Email Spam and Malware Filtering

You are not even aware of some emails addressed to you going to the spam folder. These spam filters are continuously updated too, thanks to machine learning. Again, your computers getting protected from malware is another application of machine learning (Daffodil Software, 2017).

14.6.7.3 Online Customer Support

Most websites today have chatbots to interact with customers instead of customer support representatives. The purpose of these bots is to extract information from websites and present it to the customers, inviting them to a one-to-one conversation. Meanwhile, as time passes by these bots tend to understand the user queries better and serve users with more accurate answers. This is achievable due to the machine learning algorithms working behind these bots (Daffodil Software, 2017).

14.6.7.4 Search Engine Result Refining

Every time you pose a query to Google, you can see your results getting refined. It is done by the machine learning algorithms Google and other search engines use. These algorithms watch how you respond to query results presented every time. If the topmost links the search engine provides are opened by the user, it assumes that the displayed results were correct and it learns likewise. Again, if none of the top links are opened, it assumes that the results it gave are incorrect and learns likewise. This in turn will help the model to perform better in future searches (Daffodil Software, 2017).

14.6.8 FINANCIAL WORLD

Machine learning has a lot of use cases in the financial arena. From online fraud detection to providing robots for advice and monitoring there are a lot of applications where machine learning can be used in banks. In a time when most financial affairs are done online, these machine learning algorithms can monitor web activities, identify risks, make correct predictions, and thus help people in the financial domain.

14.6.8.1 Online Fraud Detection

With most of the banking transactions becoming online, machine learning algorithms are at the forefront to monitor them. They help in finding out fraudulent behavior with high accuracy and identifies any distrustful account transactions. For example, money laundering can be prevented by the usage of these algorithms, as is used by Paypal. Millions of transactions between the bank and the customers are compared by the company to differentiate between authentic and not authentic transactions using machine learning algorithms. These algorithms require only a split second to evaluate a transaction. This helps in preventing the crime online, instead of detecting it and reporting it later for action to be taken (DataFlair Team, 2019d).

14.6.8.2 Robo-Advisory

The financial domain today makes use of robo-advisors in most places. There are basically two use cases for machine learning in the financial domain, which are portfolio management and recommendation of financial products. The first one is an online service in the field of wealth management which uses algorithms and statistics to allocate, manage and optimize the clients' assets, and where the user has to enter their current financial assets and goals. Today, many online insurance services use these advisors to recommend customized and calibrated insurance plans, which is the second use case (DataFlair Team, 2019d).

14.6.8.3 Customer Service

Most financial institutions may want to achieve their targets and get maximum profit, but by exploiting the customer, which is a problem today. Biases can be reduced in this field by the use of virtual assistants. Here, chatbots can be enabled to learn and change their approach based on the behavior patterns of customers, which can be achieved by employing machine learning algorithms. Chatbots are today so sophisticated that instead of just answering queries, they can help a user by addressing his query like a normal human being does (DataFlair Team, 2019d).

14.6.8.4 Risk Management

The financial sector is a domain that involves high risks, and hence setting high premiums is also essential. Machine learning helps in both, to identify risks and to set high premiums. When previous data with historical patterns and current trends are available, machine learning algorithms can help insurance companies to improve their profits. These algorithms can also handle any type of risk related to protecting money in all forms like, loans, health, mortgage, or life insurance (DataFlair Team, 2019d).

14.6.8.5 Marketing Strategy

With Predictive Analytics in marketing, machine learning is helping finance and banking domain people. Machine learning algorithms can be used to monitor web activity properly and user trends and patterns of mobile usage also can be identified. Analyzing advertising campaigns can also be done. Again, with these machine learning algorithms, one can obtain accurate predictions that enable the evolution of a marketing strategy.

14.6.8.6 Network Security

One major challenge in the banking sector was to identify modern sophisticated cyber-attacks and the presence of computer viruses and worms. The global financial data must be kept secure at any cost, which can be implemented by machine learning algorithms. This is possible because of the powerful analysis of intelligent patterns and capabilities of big data (DataFlair Team, 2019d).

14.7 CONCLUSION

Unlike the traditional way of explicit programming, machine learning is a subset of artificial intelligence that provides systems the ability to learn and improve from experience automatically. The focus is to implement programs that can access data and use them to learn for themselves. This learning makes machines more and more smart and useful in real-life scenarios. What is the need for machines to learn is discussed along with the procedure for training the machines to become learned machines. The various methods of machine learning and the different machine learning algorithms are discussed in a simple manner for a novice to understand. Moreover, some tools available for developing machine learning algorithms are discussed and finally, popular applications of machine learning are also discussed.

REFERENCES

Abduljabbar, R. et al., 2019. Applications of artificial intelligence in transport: An overview, sustainability, *MDPI*, 11(1), 1–24.
Agarwal, V., 2017. What is a training data set & test data set in machine learning? What are the rules for selecting them? https://quora.com/What-is-a-training-data-set-test-data-set-in-machine-learning-What-are-the-rules-for-selecting-them [Accessed 23 March 2020]
Bakshi, K., 2017. The seven steps of machine learning, https://techleer.com/articles/379-the-seven-steps-of-machine-learning/ [Accessed March 20, 2020]
Barragán, P.Z. et al., 2019. Urban machine learning model: Automatic classification of buildings and structures, https://blogs.iadb.org/ciudades-sostenibles/en/urban-machine-learning-automatic-classification-of-buildings-and-structures/
Beklemysheva, A., 2020. Why use Python for AI and machine learning? https://steelkiwi.com/blog/python-for-ai-and-machine-learning/ [Accessed March 20, 2020]
Brownley, J., 2018. Practical machine learning problems, https://machinelearningmastery.com/practical-machine-learning-problems/ [Accessed April 15, 2020]

Brownley, J., 2019a. A gentle introduction to the gradient boosting algorithm for machine learning, https://machinelearningmastery.com/gentle-introduction-gradient-boosting-algorithm-machine-learning/ [Accessed March 23, 2020]

Brownley, J., 2019b. Your first machine learning project in Python step-by-step, https://machinelearningmastery.com/machine-learning-in-python-step-by-step/ [Accessed March 24, 2020]

Brownley, J., 2020. Basic concepts in machine learning, https://machinelearningmastery.com/basic-concepts-in-machine-learning/ [Accessed March 24, 2020]

Chaudury, A., 2020. Top databases used in machine learning projects, https://analyticsindiamag.com/top-databases-used-in-machine-learning-projects/ [Accessed March 24, 2020]

Daffodil Software, 2017. Applications of machine learning from day-to-day life, https://medium.com/app-affairs/9-applications-of-machine-learning-from-day-to-day-life-112a47a429d0 [Accessed March 25, 2020]

Data Core Systems, 2018. 6 ways machine learning can transform the transportation industry, https://datacoresystems.com/insights/6-ways-machine-learning-can-transform-transportation-industry [Accessed March 27, 2020]

DataFlair Team, 2018a. Gradient boosting algorithm – Working and improvements, https://data-flair.training/blogs/gradient-boosting-algorithm/ [Accessed March 25, 2020]

DataFlair Team, 2018b. Real-Life applications of SVM, https://data-flair.training/blogs/applications-of-svm/ [Accessed March 24, 2020]

DataFlair Team, 2018c. What is dimensionality reduction? https://data-flair.training/blogs/dimensionality-reduction-tutorial [Accessed March 25, 2020]

DataFlair Team, 2019a. 11 Top machine learning algorithms used by data scientists, https://data-flair.training/blogs/machine-learning-algorithms/ [Accessed March 25, 2020]

DataFlair Team, 2019b. How Google uses machine learning to revolutionise the Internet world? https://data-flair.training/blogs/how-google-uses-machine-learning/ [Accessed March 27, 2020]

DataFlair Team, 2019c. How is machine learning enhancing the future of education? https://data-flair.training/blogs/machine-learning-in-education/ [Accessed March 25, 2020]

DataFlair Team, 2019d. Machine learning in finance – 15 applications for data science aspirants, https://data-flair.training/blogs/machine-learning-in-finance/ [Accessed March 25, 2020]

DataFlair Team, 2019e. Machine learning in healthcare – Unlocking the full potential!, https://data-flair.training/blogs/machine-learning-in-healthcare/ [Accessed March 25, 2020]

Dhiman, A., 2017. What is the k-nearest neighbour algorithm? What type of problems can be solved by this algorithm? What type of math is required? https://quora.com/What-is-the-k-Nearest-Neighbour-algorithm-What-type-of-problems-can-be-solved-by-this-algorithm-What-type-of-math-is-required?q=k-nearest%20neighbou [Accessed March 25, 2020]

Ganshin, A., 2019. Advancing weather forecasting with machine learning, https://itproportal.com/features/advancing-weather-forecasting-with-machine-learning/ [Accessed March 24, 2020]

Gupta, A., 2019. Machine learning algorithms in autonomous driving, https://iiot-world.com/machine-learning/machine-learning-algorithms-in-autonomous-driving/ [Accessed March 25, 2020]

Gupta, N., 2020. Why is Python used for machine learning? https://hackernoon.com/why-python-used-for-machine-learning-u13f922ug [Accessed March 26, 2020]

Guru99 Team, 2020a. Reinforcement learning: What is, algorithms, applications, example, https://guru99.com/reinforcement-learning-tutorial.html [Accessed March 26, 2020]

Guru99 Team, 2020b. Supervised machine learning: What is, algorithms, example, https://guru99.com/supervised-machine-learning.html [Accessed March 26, 2020]

Guru99 Team, 2020c. Unsupervised machine learning: What is, algorithms, example, https://guru99.com/unsupervised-machine-learning.html [Accessed March 23, 2020]

Hatalis, K., 2019. Random forests (algorithm), https://quora.com/topic/Random-Forests-algorithm?q=random%20forest [Accessed March 25, 2020]

Jack, 2020. Top 10 machine learninglearning frameworks, https://hackernoon.com/top-10-machine-learning-frameworks-for-2019-h6120305j [Accessed March 25, 2020]

Liakos, K.G. et al., 2018. Machine learning in agriculture: A review, *Sensors*, 18, 2674.

Maklin, C., 2019. Support vector machine Python example, https://towardsdatascience.com/support-vector-machine-python-example-d67d9b63f1c8 [Accessed March 27, 2020]

Mayo, M., 2018. Frameworks for approaching the machine learning process, https://kdnuggets.com/2018/05/general-approaches-machine-learning-process.html [Accessed March 27, 2020]

Navlani, A., 2018. Understanding random forests classifiers in Python, https://datacamp.com/community/tutorials/random-forests-classifier-python [Accessed March 26, 2020]

Powar, S., 2018. Which database is best for machine learning? https://quora.com/Which-database-is-best-for-machine-learning [Accessed March 23, 2020]

Priyadharshini, 2020. What is machine learning and how does it work, https://simplilearn.com/what-is-machine-learning-and-why-it-matters-article [Accessed April 15, 2020]

Ramakrishnan, N., 2017. How does machine learning work? https://quora.com/Why-is-machine-learning-being-given-so-much-importance [Accessed April 14, 2020]

Ravindra, S., 2017. The machine learning algorithms used in self-driving cars, https://kdnuggets.com/2017/06/machine-learning-algorithms-used-self-driving-cars.html [Accessed March 29, 2020]

Ray, S., 2017. Commonly used machine learning algorithms (with Python and R Codes), https://analyticsvidhya.com/blog/2017/09/common-machine-learning-algorithms/ [Accessed March 28, 2020]

Rizvi, M.S., 2019. 21 Must-know open source tools for machine learning you probably aren't using, https://analyticsvidhya.com/blog/2019/07/21-open-source-machine-learning-tools/ [Accessed March 29, 2020].

Robotics, 2017. Robotics in agriculture: types and applications, https://www.automate.org/blogs/robotics-in-agriculture-types-and-applications [Accessed April 16, 2020]

Sagar, N., 2018. In what real world applications is Naive Bayes classifier used? https://quora.com/In-what-real-world-applications-is-Naive-Bayes-classifier-used [Accessed March 30, 2020]

Saurabh, 2018. Types of machine learning algorithms and their use, http://www.volrum.com/2018/09/30/types-of-machine-learning-algorithms-and-their-use/ [Accessed April 20, 2020]

Sayantini, 2020. Top 10 machine learninglearning frameworks you need to know, https://edureka.co/blog/top-10-machine-learning-frameworks/ [Accessed March 30, 2020]

Singh, A., 2020. How does machine learning work? https://quora.com/How-does-machine-learning-work [Accessed March 30, 2020]

Stecanella, B., 2017. A practical explanation of a Naive Bayes classifier, https://monkeylearn.com/blog/practical-explanation-naive-bayes-classifier/ [Accessed April 15, 2020]

Techno Stacks, 2018. Role of machine learning in modern age agriculture, https://technostacks.com/blog/machine-learning-in-agriculture/ [Accessed April 16, 2020]

Thomas, M., 2019. 15 Examples of machine learning in health care that are revolutionizing medicine, https://builtin.com/artificial-intelligence/machine-learning-healthcare [Accessed April 17, 2020]

Vatsal, A., 2018. What is machine learning for? https://quora.com/What-is-machine-learning-for [Accessed April 14, 2020]

Wikipedia Inc., 2020a. Bayes' theorem, https://en.wikipedia.org/wiki/Bayes%27_theorem [Accessed April 18, 2020]

Wikipedia Inc., 2020b. Cluster analysis, https://en.wikipedia.org/wiki/Cluster_analysis [Accessed April 9, 2020]

Wikipedia Inc., 2020c. Machine learning, https://en.wikipedia.org/wiki/Machine_learning [Accessed April 26, 2020]

Wikipedia Inc., 2020d. Software deployment, https://en.wikipedia.org/wiki/Software_deployment [Accessed April 16, 2020]

Xiao, I., 2020. The most useful machine learning tools of 2020, https://kdnuggets.com/2020/03/most-useful-machine-learning-tools-2020.html [Accessed April 18, 2020]

Yufeng, G., 2017. The 7 steps of machine learning, https://towardsdatascience.com/the-7-steps-of-machine-learning-2877d7e5548e [Accessed April 5, 2020]

15 Machine Learning in Human Resource Management

M. Punithavalli

Professor, Department of Computer Applications,
Bharathiar University, Coimbatore, India

CONTENTS

DOI: 10.1201/9781003175865-15

OBJECTIVES

    a. Exposure to HRM
    b. Concepts of Machine Learning
    c. Application of ML in HRM
    d. Typical Case Studies

15.1 INTRODUCTION

In the present era of modernization, any industry or organization is on the lookout for improved floor performance for better productivity. HRM should be in a way that it is prepared for dealing with all the effects of change in the work atmosphere. It depicts how globalization is implied and to handle a diverse workforce with continuous skill and improvement measures and reengineering for HR personnel. HR is increasingly receiving attention as a critical strategic partner in functioning in the organization to maximize the employee's performance while providing the appropriate welfare measures for them. Machine learning is the science of getting the computer to "learn and act" like humans improving learning by amassing and analyzing actual interactions. Machine learning has made an enormous contribution in every domain in recent years owing to the massive technological development with great impact on the world's business and specifically how human resources are managed and revolutionizing stunningly.

15.2 HOW MACHINE LEARNING HELPS HUMAN RESOURCE MANAGEMENT

Since HR management is primarily focused on dealing with humans, the management becomes very critical and also challenging due to the dynamic behavior of mankind (Matyunina, 2019). No two individuals can be similar in their

    a. Mental strength

b. Sentiments
c. Thinking ability
d. Behavior

Further, because of mass psychology, their group behavior is different from varied influences and hence the management personal have to tackle them carefully. Human resource management is how the people are managed in an organization with a humankind approach and it is termed as a system that concentrates on Human development on one side and the efficient management of the personnel on the other so that the employees do not compromise the human values. It is also the process in which employees are managed in an organization in a well-equipped manner. The essentiality of HRM is the people management from a macro perspective through collective relationship management between the employers and employees. Machine learning schedules the functions of HR, such as staff recruitments, training, performance appraisals, streamlining workforce, reducing staff turnover, personalized training, and other HR tasks.

15.3 MACHINE LEARNING CONCEPTS

Machine learning is a study on the computer algorithms which can self-learn with data. The essential focus is to develop computer algorithms that access the data for self-learning. These are closely identical to that of computational statistics, where the focus is kept on predictive outcomes through systems. It is a system where artificial intelligence is applied to enable the system to learn it by themselves and to self-improve through the experience in the absence of special programming (Varghese, 2018; Varghese 2018).

ML methods are broadly classified into three categories namely, supervised, unsupervised, and reinforcement learning. In supervised learning, the more frequent data are labeled to intimate which model is to be taken by the data for performing. It is just like the learning dog scenario where the goals are achieved once the right tracks are identified. A practical example is when we click on the "PLAY" button in the NETFLIX: Here were are instructing the algorithm to find and operate through similar programs. Unsupervised learning on the other side does not have the data labeled. The system looks for any of the models that are found. This is akin to letting a person control many objects and finally classify the same which has similar characteristics. These are not often used owing to the lack of obvious applications but has a great impact in the security domain.

Reinforcement learning is the combination of the aforesaid learning methods. The important difference between the supervised and unsupervised methods is that the former is performed using the ground reality or in other terms, there is a decent knowledge of the expected output. The latter performs learning without prior knowledge of the expected output and learns from the different outputs themselves.

15.3.1 SUPERVISED LEARNING

These are methods where the algorithm learns from the data which are used as input and then use this knowledge for classifying new observations. The data set here will be usually of the bi-class type like that of identifying whether a human is "a male or a female," classifying whether an "email is a spam or a genuine" and classification of degrees like distinction, first class, second class, or third class.

Some of the types of classification techniques used in machine learning are given below:

a. Naive Bayes Classifier
b. K-Nearest Neighbor
c. Support Vector Machines (SVM)
d. Regressions
e. Decision Trees
f. Random Forest
g. Neural Networks

15.3.1.1 Naïve Bayes Classifier (Generative Learning Model)

NB classifiers are based on probability and use the Bayes theorem which assumes that the predictors are independent. These assume that the existence of a specific feature inside a class is not related to the existence of any other feature. As shown in Figure 15.1, it converts the data set into a frequency table and finds the probability. Then the NB equation calculates the probability of every class. The class that has the maximum probability is considered as the output of the prediction.

15.3.1.2 K-Nearest Neighbor

This method assumes that similar items that exist will be close to each other. This algorithm takes a group of labeled points and uses them in the learning process as to how the other data points can be labeled. For the new data point to be labeled, it takes the already labeled points and which are closer to the new point. The degree of closeness is normally expressed in terms of the non-similarity function. Once the process is iterated with "K" no of close neighbors, the label of the closest item is assigned to the new label. Figure 15.2 shows similar data points exist close to each other.

It uses the geometric distance to decide its nearest neighbor. This is because when the input is in the form of text, there will not be clarity on how the items are depicted in a geometrical manner making the distance calculation impossible.

15.3.1.3 Support Vector Machine (SVM)

These classifiers work in small data sets but are more powerful and also stronger when used in model development. From Figure 15.3, the identification of correct hyperplanes (A, B, C) that classifies a star and the circle is how a typical SVM works.

15.3.1.4 Logistic Regression (Predictive Learning Model)

The logistic regression analysis is to predict when the dependent variable is binary. These are used for the data description and also for explaining the relationship among one dependent binary variable with that of one or more independent variables. It is a statistical approach of data analysis where there is more than one independent variable that can determine the outcome. The outcomes are normally

Weather	Play
Sunny	No
Overcast	Yes
Rainy	Yes
Sunny	Yes
Sunny	Yes
Overcast	Yes
Rainy	No
Rainy	No
Sunny	Yes
Rainy	Yes
Sunny	No
Overcast	Yes
Overcast	Yes
Rainy	No

Frequency Table

Weather	No	Yes
Overcast		4
Rainy	3	2
Sunny	2	3
Grand Total	5	9

Likelihood table

Weather	No	Yes		
Overcast		4	=4/14	0.29
Rainy	3	2	=5/14	0.36
Sunny	2	3	=5/14	0.36
All	=5/14	=9/14		
	0.36	0.64		

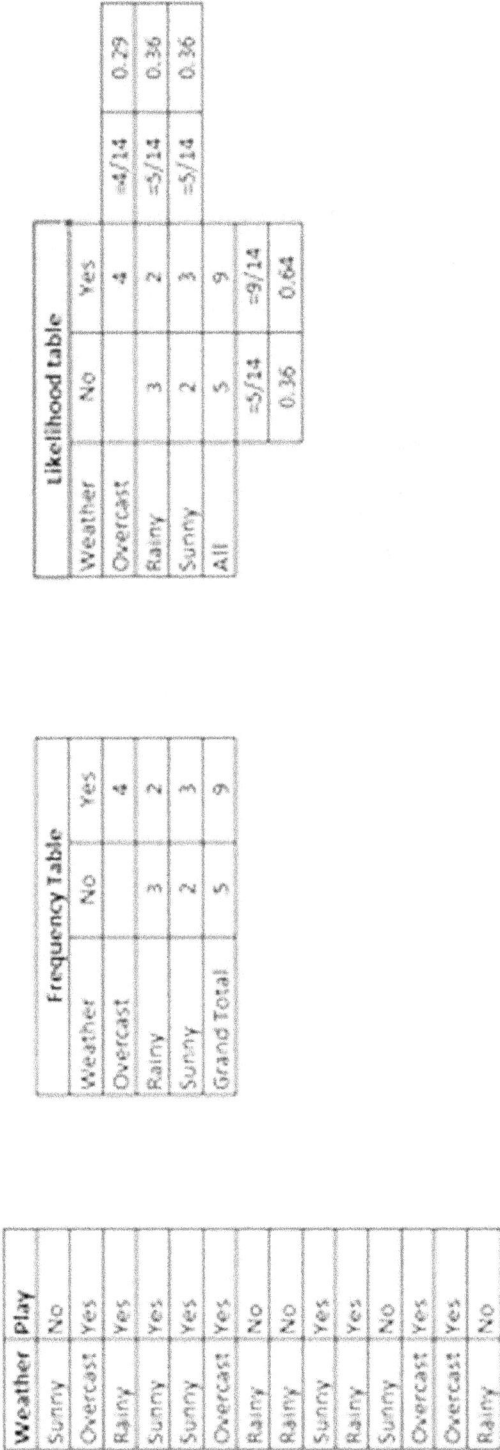

FIGURE 15.1 Naïve Bayes classifier.

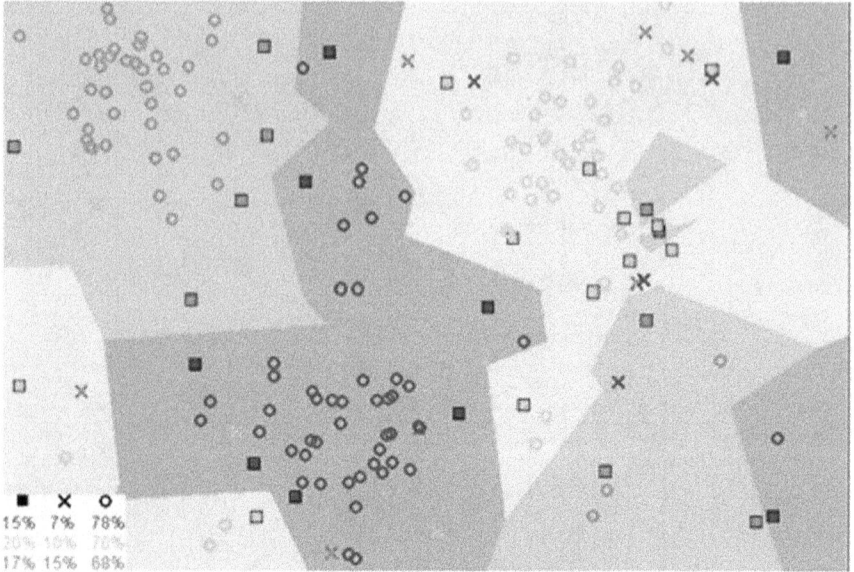

FIGURE 15.2 KNN.

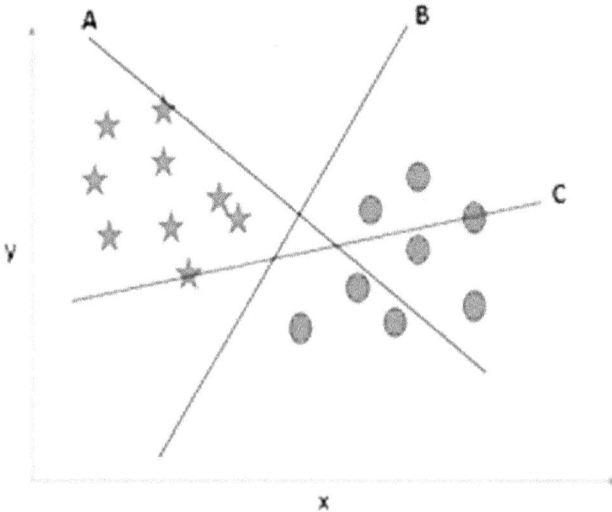

FIGURE 15.3 SVM classification.

measured using the binary variable where there are two outcomes predicted. It uses the log(sigmoid) function to find the relationship among variables shown in Figure 15.4. The log (sigmoid) functions are S-shaped curves that can take any real number and map that to a value between 0 and 1 but can never take the upper and

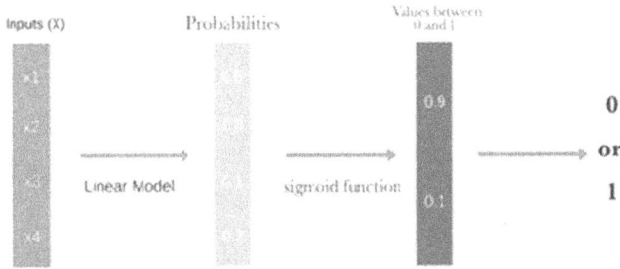

FIGURE 15.4 Logistic regression.

lower limit values. For example, whether the customer will buy the product or not based on the dependent features age, salary, marital status, gender, etc.

15.3.1.5 Decision Trees

These help in building models for classification or regression in the tree format. The data set here is broken into smaller subsets and at the same time, an associative decision tree is also parallel constructed. The final output will be a tree with deciding nodes and leaf nodes. A deciding node can have two or multiple branches along with a leaf which represents either a classification or a decision. The top decision node would be a tree that represents the best predictors which are termed as "ROOT." These models can efficiently handle both the categorical well as numerical data. Figure 15.5 shows explain that in industries based on the employee's nature of the job, his capability, and the need for training mode of training is decided whether online or offline.

15.3.1.6 Random Forest

These are also termed random decision trees and are supposed to the ensemble method of learning towards classification and other tasks and they operate by developing multiple decision trees during the time of training and to output the class in case of classification or output the mean value of prediction in case of regression techniques which shows in Figure 15.6. This method is used to correct the decision trees' nature of overfitting during the training of the data set.

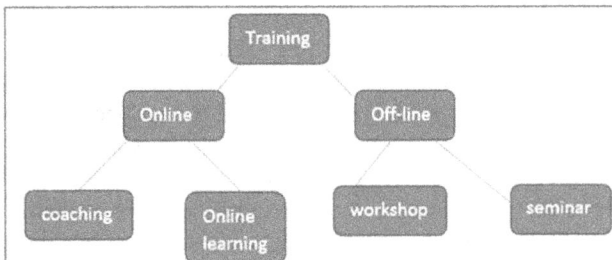

FIGURE 15.5 Decision trees.

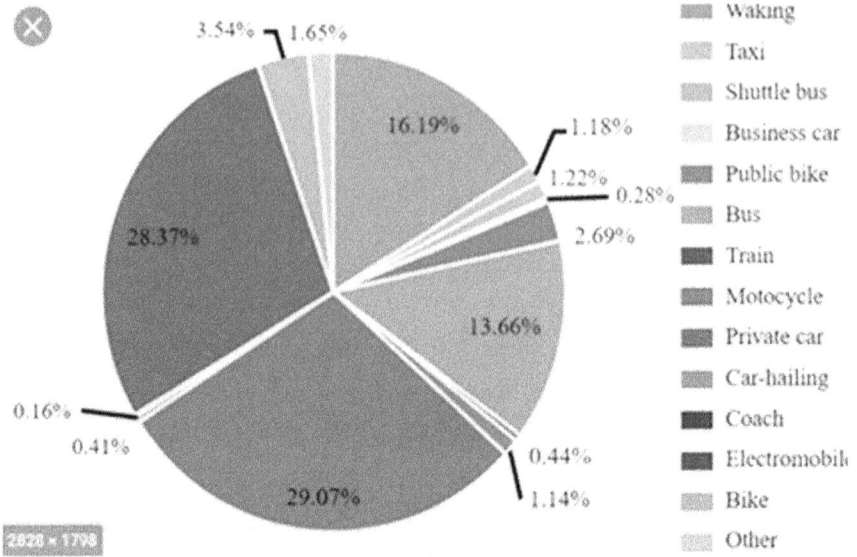

FIGURE 15.6 Random forest.

Neural Network Model

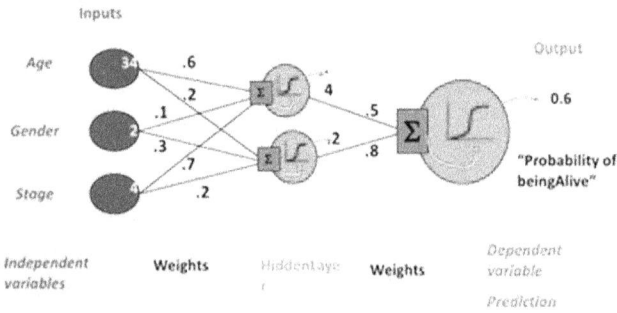

FIGURE 15.7 NN model.

A neural network has several units arranged in different layers that convert the input to an output vector showed in Figure 15.7. Each of the units takes up the input and then applies a function on it and then passes on the output to the following layer. Generically, these networks are termed feed-forward networks. Here, a unit starts with feeding the output to all the other units of the subsequent layers with no feedback on the previous layer. Weights are then applied to every signal that passes from one point to the other and it is these weights that were applied to the signals that pass from a single unit to another which are tuned during the training for adaption of a neural network for the specific problem.

15.3.2 Unsupervised Learning

These are ML techniques where there is not a significant need for a supervised model. Instead, the model works on the own for discovering the information. It deals with unlabeled data. These are used when the process of data processing is complex when compared to the supervised method. Although the supervised method is more unpredictable compared to that of other learning methods, unsupervised learning identifies all the possible models. It also helps to identify the features which can be used for the categorization. Cluster analysis or clustering is unsupervised learning. Grouping of objects of a similar kind is called clustering (Hitka et al., 2017).

15.3.2.1 Exclusive (Partitioning)

In this method of clustering, data are clustered in a way that one data set can be present in one cluster alone; e.g., K-Means (Figure 15.8).

In this type of clustering, all the data are clusters. The iterated union is between any two nearest clusters by reducing the number of clusters.

Example: Hierarchical clustering (Figure 15.9)

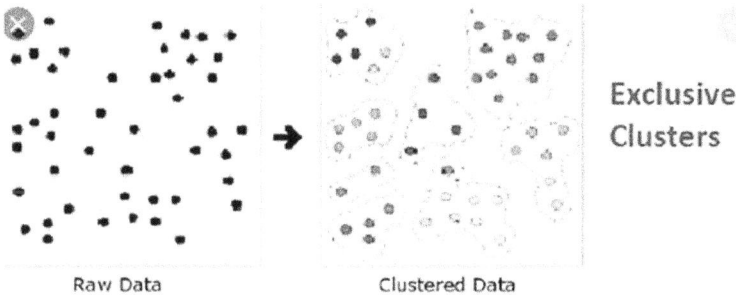

FIGURE 15.8 Exclusive.

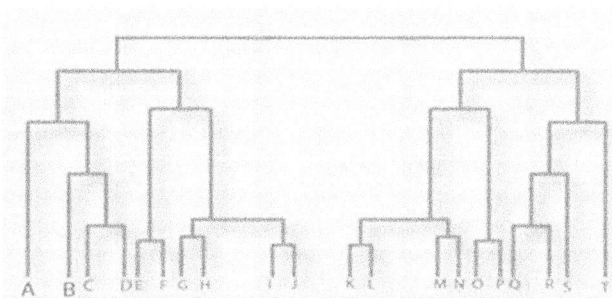

FIGURE 15.9 Agglomerative.

Overlapping clusters

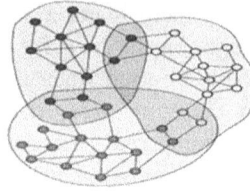

FIGURE 15.10 Overlapping.

15.3.2.2 Overlapping

In this method, fuzzy sets are made to be used for clustering the data. Every point might belongs to two or more clusters with individual degrees of memberships (Figure 15.10).

15.3.3 REINFORCEMENT LEARNING

This learning is all about decision making sequentially. In simple words, it works like the other two methods are combined. Here, the output depends on the state in which the present input and the next input depend on the previous output. This kind of learning is semi-supervised and it is a technique for allowing the agent to take actions and interact with the environment to maximize the total rewards. As shown in Figure 15.11, it considers feedback for processing.

15.4 APPLICATIONS OF MACHINE LEARNING IN HRM

Machine learning begins with the automated process in recruitment, training, performance appraisal of employees, attrition, etc. Organizational leaders and human resource executives have strong faith in machine learning for HR functions (Faggella, 2019).

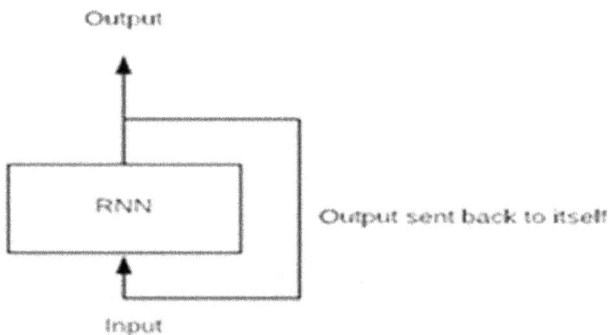

FIGURE 15.11 Working principle of reinforcement learning.

HRM is responsible for

a. Managing job recruitment, selection, and promotion
b. Developing and overseeing employee benefits and wellness programs
c. Developing, promoting, and enforcing personnel policies
d. Promoting employee career development and job training
e. Providing orientation programs for new hires
f. Guiding disciplinary actions
g. Serving as the primary contact for work-site injuries or accidents

Almost all tasks of HRM like recruitment, training, appraisal, and welfare are using machine learning concepts (Tomassen, 2016). HRM is termed the organizational process that deals with manpower, which includes hiring, performance monitoring, safety, wellness, compensation, and training. Human resource management is a strategic approach in achieving organizational goals while caring for the working life of employees in an ethical and socially responsible manner.

Internally, machine learning can greatly assist the HR function. Many traditional activities like "Talent Acquisition" and "Employee Engagement" can be greatly improved by using machine learning. Machine learning can help quickly sift through thousands of job applications and shortlist candidates who have the credentials that are most likely to achieve success at the company. This also helps HR managers have access to continual insights into how their employees feel about their work and how engaged they are; a definite improvement over comparing engagement surveys.

Although the developments in terms of computational power and large space servers in the last decade have made it possible for systems to analyze data and make helpful predictions, its adoption within companies has been relatively slow. Talent restrictions, along with skepticism of newer technology and inadequate management of data some of the reasons that stop organizations from reaping the benefits of machine learning. But if one was to move ahead of such problems, the potential benefits would be significant. By developing talent in-house and streamlining data collection and management, companies can improve their decision making. The following sections describe it briefly (Latheef, 2017).

15.4.1 Recruitment

Recruitment is the process of identification, attraction, interviewing, and onboarding employees. Machine learning in the recruitment process is to completely automate the job matching process efficiently. Corporate companies receive thousands of resumes with lots of varied parameters of qualification, experience, skill sets, etc., for a specified number of vacancies. This enormous amount of data continuously being received cannot be manually handled by the HR department. The solution to this problem is using machine learning that is perfect for consistently accepting, storing, and processing such voluminous data with the appropriate software. This recruitment process is performed with machine learning with lesser time and the solutions are more transparent and unbiased.

15.4.2 APPLICANT TRACKING AND ASSESSMENT

Corporate companies that receive high volumes of applications apply machine learning technique for applicant tracking and assessment. The machine learning tools are used in tracking the applicant's itinerary until the interview process thus enabling the HR department to thoroughly assess the track part and performance of the applicants. It also helps in receiving feedbacks quickly. Machine learning tools are also available to enable the companies to enumerate appropriate fit scores for talent, digital screening, and online interview results. This helps the HR professions to arrive at decisions quickly. In choosing the best talent in practice the ML tool is not solely applied. However, the HR personal insights are also used with questions such as 1. How can the applicant's trait be converted as a business deliverable? 2. What is the focus of hiring? and 3. How the predictions can be made in a non-biased way?

15.4.3 ATTRACTING TALENT

Talent attraction happens before the process of hiring and also seen as an upswing in the domain of Machine learning. Black, who is the senior director of organizational development in Glint, has recognized LinkedIn as one of the companies which used simple ML methods in job recommendations. Many other job search portal creates interactive maps that were based on the user data obtained from search histories, visited links, connections, and other posts. PhenomPeople is one of the examples of a suite that uses ML algorithms to help talent academies through various social media applications and other job portals. The process is one step ahead of just being keyword search mechanisms.

15.4.4 ATTRITION DETECTION

Identifying and recruiting is the top talent among the important function of HR (Karabey, 2019). Employee attrition in an organization is being hotly debated in recent years. Retaining the resource person depends more than just an HR department but also very important for the prediction of the attrition rate. Machine learning with all its software can generate interesting patterns that can give valuable insights on these factors allowing the HR for dealing with attritions more effectively. ML technology has been tested and it gives better results with time to enable the management to plan before they face skill gaps. Getting the exact grounds on the decision of an employee to stay or leave a company is the tough part for HR to identify. Identifying the risk of attrition requires an advanced pattern analysis method in an array of variables. If the process of attrition detection is done manually, the conclusions will be very drastic and hence there is a need for machine learning methods to make the HR personnel save time in analyzing the data as the ML does it in no time. Advances in natural language processing can process a large volume of data that are normally unstructured and ML algorithms can also be used to detect the emotional activities. Black, describes the "Prototypicality" methods can bring out the individual comments which represent the sum of all others opinion that allows the companies to get an inclusive but certainly a digestible pulse on the processes and particular issues. One example of ML in HR management is JPMorgan, a financial institution where algorithms were used for analyzing the employee's behavior before any inquiry and disciplinary action.

15.4.5 MACHINE LEARNING TECHNOLOGIES TO OPTIMIZE STAFFING

Machine learning tools are used to

  a. Identify potential employees
  b. Identify the overloaded employees
  c. Identify resource usage and low valued activities
  d. Identify inefficient manpower and to terminate them

The data collection on the work distribution can be analyzed by tracking total time spent on the office and tracking the work hours smartly through scanning of employee passes. After analyzing every employee's workload, models can be built for performance analysis of the employees in various criteria. This allows a change in the work schedule of the manpower, for instance, increasing the number of sales representatives during an influx and also abandon the resource if required. And importantly, it helps for identifying the manpower who are less productive and who do not bring expected benefits.

15.4.6 TALENT MANAGEMENT

Machine learning helps the employees to determine what kind of specific skills are developed by an employee. For every employee, data to be collected continuously for the tasks performed, additional educational qualifications acquired, and any other improvement an employee has shown. The ML algorithms conclude the expected development from an employee at the competency level and so that the HR department can initiate programs that train the employees. In the year 2018, technology helped 27% of its employees get a promotion or a new job. Also, based on the ML methods, proposals for promotion and advancement in career can be given. To do this, IBM has launched a virtual trainer that was created by the employees themselves. The virtual assistants generate the personalized career guidance recommendation for a person based on the big data analytics of the performance indications. The system also predicts the time required for a particular employee to get the promotion if he continues to be at the same pace of knowledge and talent acquisition.

15.4.7 INDIVIDUAL SKILL MANAGEMENT

Machine learning shows its potential in building the individual's skill management and development. While there is room for significant growth in this area, there are platforms that can give a calibrated procedure in the absence of human trainers. It saves time and provides an opportunity for many other people to grow in their careers and be engaged. The workday is an example of one such company that built a personalized recommendation for employees based on the company's need and the market trend. Machine learning is applied to assess an employee's performance with their traits such as depth of knowledge in his field, learning ability, and updates in the advancements. Also, to decide his caliber as excellent, good, or to be improved and if has to improve, what sort of training is needed can also be decided using ML approaches. Machine learning helps in analyzing and concluding, and also it makes sense with enormous amounts of varying data.

15.4.8 CHATBOX FOR FAQs OF EMPLOYEES

The Chabot gives ongoing responses to a scope of HR questions, including, "Are we off on Ambedkar Jayanti?" or "What are my health advantages?" Chatbots are fit for responding to any question and answer set that can be put away in a database. They can likewise be intended to elevate advantages to representatives proactively they may not yet think about. "Hello Nabeel, have you attempted our meditation class that we are offering in your structure today at 3:00 pm?" Snap here to book yourself consequently. You've been trying sincerely and you merit it. There is also a chance to follow representative issues utilizing continuous examination and afterward applying assessment investigations to address these issues. Suppose that most workers are approaching inquiries concerning late installments for movement repayments. This information can show something in the framework isn't working accurately. Before things become an out and out issue, HR pioneers can reveal the issue and convey a solution. Granted, there will be questions chatbots can't reply to yet. However, the open door is here to give AI to a wide range of HR-related inquiries that may be coming into your HR service center.

15.4.9 CLUSTERING FOR STRATEGIC MANAGEMENT OF HRM

The clustering concept can be used group the employees two or three. So that similar character employees will be in one group, which will help train them and motivate them. The database is created with age, socio-economic status, and job position of respondents. Identification of different motivational groups of the enterprise's employees enables corporate motivational processes to be tailored to a particular type of employee. Based on this identification, differentiated motivational programs can be created, explicitly targeting individual employee groups with a similar motivational profile.

15.5 CASE STUDIES

The important tasks of HR management strategies are recruitment, performance management, based on which training the employees and risk management in which this section discusses a real scenario with sample data for the better understanding of ML. The important areas are shown in Figure 15.12.

15.5.1 CASE STUDY 1: COMPETENCY-BASED RECRUITMENT PROCESS

Most employers use a pre-employment assessment for separating deserved candidates from the rest in the present competitive world. Since many of the candidates

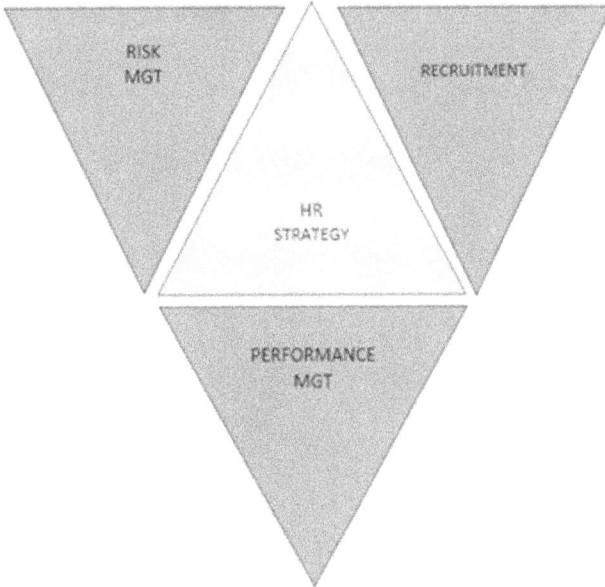

FIGURE 15.12   HR strategy.

have similar qualifications, aptitude tests are a great tool for choosing between the candidates. This case study is to process the candidates' interview performance and prepare the final selection list using ML. It has used three parameters (i) depth of knowledge, (ii) communication skill, and (iii) technical skill. Each parameter is valued as Excellent, Good, Fair, and Poor. The target variable of the recruitment process is the result and its values are **Selected or Not Selected**. The database with parameters and target variables is shown in Table 15.1.

The classification model is built from Table 15.1 to reach out to the result. The two data sets needed for classification are the training data set and test data set for different purposes. The data set used for the training is the one that is made used for the model training, learning and to produce results. This can include both the data and the anticipated output. Training sets have made up the majority of the total data. The data used for the testing purpose are used to evaluate the model for classification that considers the trained data. The sample size is with 100 observations (Table 15.1) and tested with 20 people and the classification result is shown in Table 15.2 with the predicted value.

From the above results of selected candidates, the ranking algorithm is used to generate the rank order.

The confusion matrix (Table 15.3) is used for testing the accuracy of a classification model. This is a summary of the predictive results in a given classification problem. The number of correct as well as the incorrect predictions are then summarized with the count values and are broken down in every class. This is an important key in the confusion matrix. This shows how the model is confused when the predictions are made. It also gives insights not only on the errors made but more apparently the types of errors that are made (Table 15.3).

TABLE 15.1

Applicant Assessment Factors

S. No.	Subject Knowledge	Communications	Class Control	Approachable	Technical Skill	Remarks	Predicted Remarks
1	Average	Average	Average	Average	Average	To be Improved	To be improved
2	Good	Good	Good	Average	Good	Good	Good
3	Good	Average	Average	Average	Average	Good	To be improved
4	Average	Average	Average	Average	Average	Good	To be improved
5	Good	Good	Good	Average	Average	Good	Good
6	Good	Good	Average	Average	Average	Good	To be improved
7	Good	Good	Good	Average	Good	Good	Good
8	Good	Average	Average	Average	Average	Good	To be improved
9	Good	Average	Average	Average	Good	Good	To be improved
10	Good	Average	Good	Excellent	Average	Good	Good
11	Good	Average	Good	Average	Excellent	Good	Good
12	Good	Good	Good	Good	Good	Excellent	Excellent
13	Excellent	Excellent	Excellent	Good	Good	Excellent	Excellent
14	Good	Good	Good	Good	Good	Excellent	Excellent
15	Good	Good	Average	Average	Average	Good	To be improved
16	Good	Good	Good	Good	Good	Excellent	Excellent
17	Excellent	Excellent	Excellent	Excellent	Good	Excellent	Excellent
18	Good	Good	Good	Good	Good	Excellent	Excellent
19	Good	Good	Good	Good	Good	Excellent	Excellent
20	Good	Average	Average	Good	Average	Average	Average
21	Good	Good	Good	Good	Excellent	Excellent	Excellent
22	Excellent	Good	Average	Good	Good	Excellent	Excellent

(Continued)

TABLE 15.1 (Continued)
Applicant Assessment Factors

S. No.	Subject Knowledge	Communications	Class Control	Approachable	Technical Skill	Remarks	Predicted Remarks
23	Good	Good	Good	Good	Average	Good	Good
24	Good	Good	Good	Good	Average	Good	Good
25	Good	Average	Average	Good	Average	To be Improved	To be improved
26	Good	Average	Average	Good	Average	Good	Good
27	Good	Average	Average	Average	Average	To be Improved	To be improved
28	Good	Average	Average	Average	Average	To be Improved	To be improved
29	Good	Average	Good	Excellent	Average	Good	Good
30	Good	Good	Good	Average	Average	Good	Good

TABLE 15.2

Applicant Assessment Factors with Predicted Results

Application Number	Depth of Knowledge	Communication Skills	Technical Skill	Result	Predicted Result
Applicant 1	Fair	Fair	Fair	'Not Selected'	'Not Selected'
Applicant 2	Good	Poor	Fair	'Not Selected'	'Not Selected'
Applicant 3	Excellent	Good	Excellent	Selected	Selected
Applicant 4	Good	Poor	Poor	'Not Selected'	'Not Selected'
Applicant 5	Fair	Good	Good	Selected	'Not Selected'
Applicant 6	Fair	Good	Fair	'Not Selected'	'Not Selected'
Applicant 7	Good	Fair	Poor	Selected	'Not Selected'
Applicant 8	Good	Good	Good	'Not Selected'	'Not Selected'
Applicant 9	Poor	Good	Fair	'Not Selected'	'Not Selected'
Applicant 10	Poor	Excellent	Fair	'Not Selected'	'Not Selected'
Applicant 11	Good	Fair	Fair	'Not Selected'	'Not Selected'
Applicant 12	Fair	Fair	Good	'Not Selected'	'Not Selected'
Applicant 13	Good	Good	Fair	'Not Selected'	'Not Selected'
Applicant 14	Good	Excellent	Good	'Not Selected'	'Not Selected'
Applicant 15	Poor	Good	Fair	'Not Selected'	'Not Selected'
Applicant 16	Poor	Fair	Fair	'Not Selected'	'Not Selected'
Applicant 17	Excellent	Fair	Excellent	'Not Selected'	Selected
Applicant 18	Fair	Good	Fair	'Not Selected'	'Not Selected'
Applicant 19	Excellent	Excellent	Good	Selected	Selected
Applicant 20	Poor	Good	Fair	'Not Selected'	'Not Selected'

TABLE 15.3
Confusion Matrix

	Predicted Class 1	Predicted Class 2
Actual Class 1	TP	FN
Actual Class 2	FP	TN

The definition of the terms are given as
TP - True Positive FN - False Negative FP - False Positive TN - True Negative

15.5.1.1 True Positive

The true positive is when the final condition is marked as matching and correct, indicating the positive condition and denying the null hypothesis [20]. True positive is given with the symbol A. The true positive is given as the following:

$$TP = n_{11} = number\ of\ such\ individuals$$

15.5.1.2 True Negative

The true negative is when the final condition is marked as non-matching and correct, which shows the negative condition and accepts the null hypothesis. True negative is given with the symbol B. The true positive is given as the following:

$$TN = n_{00} = number\ of\ such\ individuals$$

15.5.1.3 False Positive

The false positive is when the final condition is marked as matching and incorrect, which shows the positive condition and denies the null hypothesis. False positive is given with symbol C. The false positive is given as the following:

$$FP = n_{01} = number\ of\ such\ individuals$$

15.5.1.4 False Negative

The false negative is when the final condition is marked as non-matching and incorrect, which shows the negative condition and accepts the null hypothesis. False negative is given with the symbol D. The false negative is given as the following:

$$FN = n_{10} = number\ of\ such\ individuals$$

15.5.1.5 Recall

It is the test based on the probability of accuracy that indicates the model's overall performance in the presence of false negative scenarios. This is calculated as

$$Recall: = \frac{True\ positive}{True\ positive + False\ Negative}$$

15.5.1.6 Precision

It is the test based on the probability for accuracy that indicates the model's overall performance in the presence of positive scenarios. This is calculated as

$$Precision: = \frac{True\ positive}{True\ positive + False\ Negative}$$

15.5.1.7 F1-Measure

It is the cumulative measure to assess the overall impact that the precision and the recall has in a case. The F-Measure is represented between 0 and 1 or 0 to 100 and normally decided on the case and ranges of precision and recall. It is measure by

$$F1 - Measure: = 2 * \frac{(R * p)}{R + P}$$

where R recalls, and p or P is precision.

15.5.1.8 Accuracy

The overall value for the accuracy is obtained by dividing the total number of true cases by all of the cases.

$$Accuracy: = \frac{True\ Positive + True\ Negative}{True\ Positive + True\ Negative + False\ Positive + False\ Negative}$$

15.5.2 CASE STUDY 2: PREDICTION OF EMPLOYEE ATTRITION

In this case study, the sample size is 100 employees with the attributes (i) Employee code, (ii) Department associated with, (iii) Gender as Male/Female, (iv) Age of the Employee, (v) Marital Status as Married or single, (vi) Business Travel as Frequently, Rarely, Not Travel, (vii) Over Time, (viii) Salary as Highly paid, Medium and less paid and the value of the target variable is Resigned and continuing which is shown in Table 15.4. The sample size is with 100 observations and tested with 20 and the classification result is shown in Table 15.5 with the predicted value.

TABLE 15.4

Employee Attributes for Attrition Detection

S. No.	Emp Code	Dept	Gender	Age	Marital Status	Business Travel	Over Time	Salary	Result
1	Emp 1	Production	M	35	M	N	Y	H	Continuing
2	Emp 2	Production	M	32	M	N	Y	M	Continuing
3	Emp 3	Admin	M	30	S	R	N	H	Continuing
4	Emp 4	Admin	F	40	M	R	N	H	Continuing
5	Emp 5	Purchase	M	42	M	R	Y	H	Continuing
6	Emp 6	Purchase	M	40	M	N	Y	H	Continuing
7	Emp 7	Sales	M	32	M	F	Y	M	Resigned
8	Emp 8	Sales	M	31	S	F	Y	M	Continuing
9	Emp 9	Sales	F	27	S	F	Y	L	Resigned
10	Emp 10	Personal	M	35	M	N	N	M	Continuing
11	Emp 11	Personal	F	37	M	N	N	M	Continuing
12	Emp 12	Personal	F	42	M	N	N	H	Continuing
13	Emp 13	IT	M	31	M	R	Y	M	Continuing
14	Emp 14	IT	F	32	M	R	Y	M	Continuing
15	Emp 15	IT	F	29	S	R	Y	L	Resigned
16	Emp 16	Production	M	45	M	N	Y	H	Continuing
17	Emp 17	Production	M	42	M	N	Y	H	Continuing
18	Emp 18	Production	M	41	M	N	Y	H	Continuing
19	Emp 19	Production	M	40	M	N	Y	H	Continuing
20	Emp 20	QC	M	36	M	R	Y	M	Continuing
21	Emp 21	QC	M	32	M	R	Y	M	Continuing
22	Emp 22	QC	F	31	S	R	Y	M	Continuing
23	Emp 23	Design	F	32	S	N	Y	M	Continuing
24	Emp 24	Design	F	37	M	N	Y	M	Continuing
25		Design	M	32	S	N	Y	M	Resigned

(Continued)

TABLE 15.4 (Continued)
Employee Attributes for Attrition Detection

S. No.	Emp Code	Dept	Gender	Age	Marital Status	Business Travel	Over Time	Salary	Result
	Emp 25								
26	Emp 26	Production	M	37	M	N	Y	M	Continuing
27	Emp 27	Production	M	50	M	N	Y	H	Continuing
28	Emp 28	Admin	M	36	M	R	N	H	Continuing
--	--	--	--	--	--	--	--	--	--
--	--	--	--	--	--	--	--	--	--
98	Emp 36	Personal	F	36	M	N	N	M	Continuing
99	Emp 34	Sales	M	37	M	F	Y	M	Continuing
100	Emp 35	Personal	F	38	M	N	N	M	Continuing

To obtain the value of the target variable, the above data set is fed to the classification model. For classification, it considers the above attributes/features and computes whether the employee will be continuing or would resign. The case study envisages whether the employee will continue in the organization or not.

15.5.3 CASE STUDY 3: PERFORMANCE ASSESSMENT FOR EDUCATIONAL INSTITUTION

The sample size consists of 100 employees. The assessment considers Subject knowledge, Class control, and Communication skill, and the values of target variables are excellent, good, and to be improved. The database is shown in Table 15.6 and Table 15.7 shows the factors with predicted remarks.

To obtain the value of the target variable, the above data set is fed to the classification model. For classification it considers the above attributes/features Subject knowledge, Communication skill, Class control, Technical skill, and reach the target as excellent, good, or to be improved which will be helpful for the management to assess the overall performance capabilities of the employees.

15.6 SUMMARY

This chapter brings an insight into the importance of machine learning in human resources management. The impacts and the possible influences of ML in HRM are

TABLE 15.5
Employee Attributes with Predicted Results

S. No.	Emp Code	Dept	Gender	Age	Marital Status	Business Travel	Over Time	Salary	Result	Predicted Result
1	Emp 1	Production	M	35	M	N	Y	H	Continuing	Continuing
2	Emp 2	Production	M	32	M	N	Y	M	Continuing	Continuing
3	Emp 3	Admin	M	30	S	R	N	H	Continuing	Continuing
4	Emp 4	Admin	F	40	M	R	N	H	Resigned	Continuing
5	Emp 5	Purchase	M	42	M	R	Y	H	Continuing	Continuing
6	Emp 6	Purchase	M	40	M	N	Y	H	Continuing	Continuing
7	Emp 7	Sales	M	32	M	F	Y	M	Resigned	Resigned
8	Emp 8	Sales	M	31	S	F	Y	M	Continuing	Continuing
9	Emp 9	Sales	F	27	S	F	Y	L	Resigned	Resigned
10	Emp 10	Personal	M	35	M	N	N	M	Continuing	Continuing
11	Emp 11	Personal	F	37	M	N	N	M	Continuing	Continuing
12	Emp 12	Personal	F	42	M	N	N	H	Resigned	Continuing
13	Emp 13	IT	M	31	M	R	Y	M	Continuing	Continuing
14	Emp 14	IT	F	32	M	R	Y	M	Resigned	Continuing
15	Emp 15	IT	F	29	S	R	Y	L	Resigned	Resigned
16	Emp 16	Production	M	45	M	N	Y	H	Continuing	Continuing
17	Emp 17	Production	M	42	M	N	Y	H	Resigned	Continuing
18	Emp 18	Production	M	41	M	N	Y	H	Continuing	Continuing
19	Emp 19	Production	M	40	M	N	Y	H	Continuing	Continuing
20	Emp 20	QC	M	36	M	R	Y	M	Continuing	Continuing

TABLE 15.6
Performance Assessment Factors

S. No.	Emp No.	Subject Knowledge	Communications	Class Control	Approachable	Technical Skill	Remarks
1	Employee 1	Average	Average	Average	Average	Average	To be improved
2	Employee 2	Good	Good	Good	Average	Good	Good
3	Employee 3	Good	Average	Average	Average	Average	To be improved
4	Employee 4	Average	Average	Average	Average	Average	To be improved
5	Employee 5	Good	Good	Good	Average	Average	Good
6	Employee 6	Good	Good	Average	Average	Average	To be improved
7	Employee 7	Good	Good	Good	Average	Good	Good
8	Employee 8	Good	Average	Average	Average	Average	To be improved
9	Employee 9	Good	Average	Average	Average	Good	To be improved
10	Employee 10	Good	Average	Good	Excellent	Average	Good
11	Employee 11	Good	Average	Good	Average	Excellent	Good
12	Employee 12	Good	Good	Good	Good	Good	Excellent
13	Employee 13	Excellent	Excellent	Excellent	Good	Good	Excellent
14	Employee 14	Good	Good	Good	Good	Good	Excellent
15	Employee 15	Good	Good	Average	Average	Average	To be improved
16	Employee 16	Good	Good	Good	Good	Good	Excellent
17	Employee 17	Excellent	Excellent	Excellent	Excellent	Good	Excellent
18	Employee 18	Good	Good	Good	Good	Good	Excellent
19	Employee 19	Good	Good	Good	Good	Good	Excellent
20	Employee 20	Good	Average	Average	Good	Average	Average
21	Employee 21	Good	Good	Good	Good	Excellent	Excellent
22	Employee 22	Excellent	Good	Average	Good	Good	Excellent

(Continued)

TABLE 15.6 (Continued)
Performance Assessment Factors

S. No.	Emp No.	Subject Knowledge	Communications	Class Control	Approachable	Technical Skill	Remarks
23	Employee 23	Good	Good	Good	Good	Average	Good
24	Employee 24	Good	Good	Good	Good	Average	Good
25	Employee 25	Good	Average	Average	Good	Average	To be improved
26	Employee 26	Good	Average	Average	Good	Average	Good
27	Employee 27	Good	Average	Average	Average	Average	To be improved
28	Employee 28	Good	Average	Average	Average	Average	To be improved
⁞	⁞	⁞	⁞	⁞	⁞	⁞	⁞
⁞	⁞	⁞	⁞	⁞	⁞	⁞	⁞
⁞	⁞	⁞	⁞	⁞	⁞	⁞	⁞
98	Employee 32	Excellent	Excellent	Excellent	Good	Good	Excellent
99	Employee 33	Good	Good	Good	Good	Average	Good
100	Employee 34	Average	Average	Average	Average	Average	Average

TABLE 15.7
Performance Factors with Predicted Remarks

S. No.	Subject Knowledge	Communications	Class Control	Approachable	Technical Skill	Remarks	Predicted Remarks
1	Average	Average	Average	Average	Average	To be Improved	To be improved
2	Good	Good	Good	Average	Good	Good	Good
3	Good	Average	Average	Average	Average	Good	To be improved
4	Average	Average	Average	Average	Average	Good	To be improved
5	Good	Good	Good	Average	Average	Good	Good
6	Good	Good	Average	Average	Average	Good	To be improved
7	Good	Good	Good	Average	Good	Good	Good
8	Good	Average	Average	Average	Average	Good	To be improved
9	Good	Average	Average	Average	Good	Good	To be improved
10	Good	Average	Good	Excellent	Average	Good	Good
11	Good	Average	Good	Average	Excellent	Good	Good
12	Good	Good	Good	Good	Good	Excellent	Excellent
13	Excellent	Excellent	Excellent	Good	Good	Excellent	Excellent
14	Good	Good	Good	Good	Good	Excellent	Excellent
15	Good	Good	Average	Average	Average	Good	To be improved
16	Good	Good	Good	Good	Good	Excellent	Excellent
17	Excellent	Excellent	Excellent	Excellent	Good	Excellent	Excellent
18	Good	Good	Good	Good	Good	Excellent	Excellent
19	Good	Good	Good	Good	Good	Excellent	Excellent
20	Good	Average	Average	Good	Average	Average	Average
21	Good	Good	Good	Good	Excellent	Excellent	Excellent
22	Excellent	Good	Average	Good	Good	Excellent	Excellent

(Continued)

TABLE 15.7 (Continued)
Performance Factors with Predicted Remarks

S. No.	Subject Knowledge	Communications	Class Control	Approachable	Technical Skill	Remarks	Predicted Remarks
23	Good	Good	Good	Good	Average	Good	Good
24	Good	Good	Good	Good	Average	Good	Good
25	Good	Average	Average	Good	Average	To be Improved	To be improved
26	Good	Average	Average	Good	Average	Good	Good
27	Good	Average	Average	Average	Average	To be Improved	To be improved
28	Good	Average	Average	Average	Average	To be Improved	To be improved
29	Good	Average	Good	Excellent	Average	Good	Good
30	Good	Good	Good	Average	Average	Good	Good

emphasized. The intelligent way in which the human resources are handled using machine learning methods is also discussed with relevant examples. The ML methods can thus contribute a lot to efficient human resource management.

REFERENCES

Faggella, D. 2019. Machine Learning in Human Resources – Application and Trends. Business Intelligence Analytics.

Hitka, M., Lorincová, S., Ližbetinová, L., Bartáková, G.P., and Merková, M.A. 2017. Cluster analysis used as the strategic advantage of human resource management in small and medium-sized enterprises in the wood-processing industry. *BioRes*. 12(4), 7884–7897.

Karabey, Ö.F. 2019. HR based ML Project, Employee Resignation. Data-Driven Investor.

Latheef, N.A. 2017. Machine Learning in Human Resources - Applications and Trends. Towards Data Science.

Matyunina, J. 2019. How Machine Learning is changing in the HR Industry. Codetiduron.

Tomassen, M. 2016. Exploring the Black Box of Machine Learning in Human Resource Management. Master of Science Thesis, University of Twente, The Netherlands.

Varghese, D. 2018. Comparative Study on Classic Machine learning Algorithms quick summary of various ML algorithms. Towards Data Science.

16 Machine Learning Models in Product Development and Its Statistical Evaluation

V. Kaviyarasu

Assistant Professor, Department of Statistics, Bharathiar University, Coimbatore, India

CONTENTS

16.1 INTRODUCTION

Manufacturing is playing a vital role in our country's economic development, and it is also considered one of the backbones of our nation. The industrial ministry has claimed that India's manufacturing sector's contribution towards the country's Gross Domestic Product (GDP) is a key feature in economic growth, which is 20.5% is higher than the global average GDP contribution in India. Hence, our honorable prime minster initiated **MAKE IN INDIA** scheme, which was a very popularized scheme suggested by the central government and encouraged many young minds to start their concerns. The Indian government has decided to uplift the manufacturing sector's share value from 20% to 24% in the vision of 2022, which shows that the Indian manufacturing sector continues to grow in a positive direction. The industrial manufacturing sector plays a vital role in the Indian economy with diverse fields such as manufacturing machinery and equipment, electrical products, electronic products, metal products, cement, building and construction materials, and rubber and plastic products in automation technology products. Manufacturing is a blend of art, economics, science, and technology, which was very popular in south India, which broadens social sense, engineering sense, and economic sense. Manufacturing started 6,000 years ago when human beings used sharp and sturdy materials as cutting tools and their bodies as machine tools.

The growth of smart manufacturing is increasing day by day towards the modern development and technological advancements. To meet global challenges and competition, smart manufacturing came into existence. It is moving towards production efficiency, labor shortage, and quality products to meet international markets' standards. The global competition increases the producers to think smart manufacturing is technology-driven so that the manufacturer is ready to meet the requirements of the modern industries. It brings the development in industries to enhance, capture, to build, and understand data. The implementation of smart manufacturing becomes essential in optimizing the production operations; improve the performance and quality. In the United States, two major companies highlighted the importance of the Smart Manufacturing Leadership Coalition (SMLC) and Digital Manufacturing and Design Institute (DMDI). These organizations highlighted that potential productivity towards efficiency might increase smart manufacturing ranging from 5% to 30% in the near future.

Machine learning gives vital information in improving the standards of the smart manufacturing sector. Manufacturing products may or may not be very expensive but involve complex processes for those involved and need the right tools to integrate data resources to develop quality standard products. In such cases, artificial intelligence and machine learning have become more prevalent in production and assembling items, which reduces the cost of the item and saves the time of production. Forty percent of the potential values gained by analytics come from artificial intelligence (AI) and machine learning (ML). In the last five years, it is observed that exponential growth in technologies may help engineers to build models that drive functional improvements. Machine learning techniques support the applications of artificial intelligence that can enhance automatic production, which learns and improves from experience without being explicitly programmed.

16.2 METHODOLOGY FOR MODEL BUILDINGS

Model building is not an easy way of representing real-world problems towards processes. The significant characteristics are smart manufacturing and its screening methodology, which has multiple complex issues involved. This methodology's primary objective is to develop a suitable model to study and execute a proper analysis process. Hence, using machine learning models, a product can be produced better by supporting its real-time data. There are several models available for the development of a product in an industry. For instance, the mathematical model describes a mathematical problem or concept towards achieving its goals. Developing a model in terms of production and control strategies employed in the manufacturing unit before going to marketing forms mathematical modeling helps to understand the system to study the need for control strategies employed in manufacturing units through various components involved in production strategies.

A model that has the possibility of measuring observations may be called a quantitative model. A product, a device, or any tangible thing used for experimentation may represent a physical model. An excellent mathematical model can develop a new problem, further considering a new formulation of the situation without affecting significant changes in framing the objectives and their assumptions, making the model more suitable. Models can be framed by the degree of abstraction or based on the data's past performance with information supported by the technology under consideration. They can be categorized into a language model and a case studies model. Models by functions are coined and classified as Descriptive model, Predictive model, and normative model. By their structure, models are coined as iconic models, analog models, and symbolic models, and by nature, they are classified into a deterministic model and a probabilistic model. Models by the extent of generality are categorized as general models. General models are termed as simulation and heuristic models. Model development becomes one of the critical factors for any sort of product development.

16.2.1 PREPARE THE DATA

Data preparation and handing is an essential requirement in smart manufacturing technologies. A data warehouse is necessary, containing consolidated data from various sources, augmented with summary information, and covering historical information. It can be viewed in two aspects: a business perspective and another from a technological standpoint. In the data preparation, one must know the type of data to be studied and analyzed, whether the data supports it is numeric or not, data volume, and nature of data to be stored and analyzed.

The data and information technology are associated with technological support, making smart manufacturing a reality with the information technology solution providers. When you prepare the data for storage, one should understand the importance of various attributes involved in the process. In reality, the number of variables under study is essential in which multiple numbers of observations are involved. The data collected and stored is quite long, and it can be handled by numerous software. For data cleaning and enrichment, the software is used. Further software helps us study reality through pattern recognition and its associated techniques to measure the solution provider's quality standards.

16.2.2 Perform Data Analysis

Data analysis is a crucial method to appropriately processing the data. It involves selecting the data, modeling the data, cleaning the data, updating the data, and transforming the data. Here, one should assess the importance of data and its purpose and study the relationship between variables considered. In a smart manufacturing inspection process, one should understand the critical importance of the data and preprocessing techniques. It investigates the production unit so that it meets the standards prescribed by the engineers. It also incorporated some graphical representation of data and became a guiding star to carry out the statistical analysis.

The primary purpose of data analysis is to study the patterns involved in the process. In our day-to-day life, whenever a decision is to be taken in some circumstances, we need the data's past performance. From this, one can understand the customer's important behavior and their need so that the organization can be planned accordingly and meet the customer's expectations. Both the producer and consumer will be benefited from the business point of view.

16.3 PRODUCT DEVELOPMENT

Many manufacturing companies understand their customer needs and their business to run appropriately. They execute their business to meet their customer needs in day-to-day activities and involve themselves in product development. When a new product is to be launched, the management may study the past performance and proper understanding of data may reveal how their product meets the essential to satisfy the market's customer demands. Valuable data is essential for the product developer to involve himself in manufacturing their products by minimizing their risk involved in the process, and a new product can be developed. Here, a set of ideas is collected together and put into action to make a new product with proper planning and modeling. The product concept may help in better strengthening the idea of new product development. Nowadays, product development moves to the next stage of automatic production due to technological advancements. The various stages involved in the new product development are given in Figure 16.1.

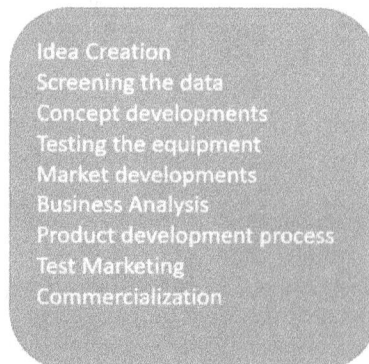

Idea Creation
Screening the data
Concept developments
Testing the equipment
Market developments
Business Analysis
Product development process
Test Marketing
Commercialization

FIGURE 16.1   New product developments criteria.

During the development of new products, the product manager is responsible for assessing its need and purpose. The necessity arises for the investments related to product development, their technical challenges, and product cost. The decision-making process can be controlled to guarantee the additional costs of the product and critical conditions for the "time-to-market." The main reasons for technical changes are as follows:

1. Product content improvement, towards the consequence faced by the marketing people and requests from the marketing section
2. Quality-level development towards the assembly of the product for market alignment (style, functionality, reliability), considering the product's contents
3. Direct material cost reduction
4. Transformation of cost reduction towards "making" the product parts
5. Production of non-quality item towards cost reduction
6. Product returns after sales because of non-quality or repair

16.4 SMART MANUFACTURING

The word SMART stands for Supplier, Model, Approved, Replaceable, and Total. The smart machine concept has many advantages over traditional manufacturing systems. The modern manufacturing systems will lead to safe, secure, self-aware, flexible machines and can meet both the producer and consumers' demands. With the help of technological support, a uniform production process is possible, and the product can change its shape and size as per the consumer's requirements (Radu Godina and Joas Matias, 2019). A manufacturing system is said to be fully automated if it can develop the process and solve the problem without any interactions (Figure 16.2).

According to the National Institute of Standards and Technology (NIST), smart manufacturing systems are "fully integrated, collaborative manufacturing system that responds in real-time to meet changing demands and conditions in the factory,

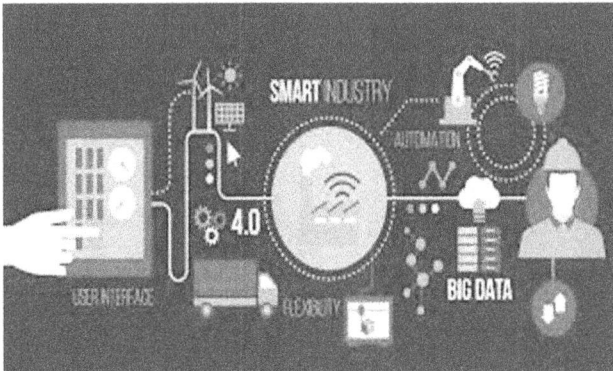

FIGURE 16.2 Smart manufacturing systems.

in the supply networks and customer needs." The key characteristics of smart machines include the following:

Self-awareness – This industrial revolution creates more self-awareness during the manufacturing process. It is more effective in using data generated through the process and interconnected one with the other by the smarter machines that communicate with the operator. Here the machine is enabled with sensors that communicate with each other and produce automated decision-making in the factory.

Safety and Security – It can be built with fundamental design. Smarter machines will improve the safety of the products and minimize the security risk of increasing the operators' security. It is exclusively focused on more intelligent products.

Connectivity – Smart machines may connect one among the other through network technology. This enables the manufacturer to share data and plan, helps the developer with traditional stand-alone machinery and automation. Smart machines will bridge the IT/OT gap, and the production data can be used in many ways to help the management make appropriate decisions.

The smart manufacturing leadership coalition (SMLC) defines smart manufacturing as "the ability to solve existing and future problems via an open infrastructure that allows solutions to be implemented at the speed of business while creating advantaged value." In recent days due to technology advancements and connectivity improvements there is unprecedented access to contextualization. This enables the smart manufacturing sector to create an open atmosphere for the manufacturing industries where fact-based decisions can be decided, and decision-makers can take the appropriate decisions. The companies are confronted to manage manufacturing and execute the relevant task to be achieved. Manufacturers always will have the ability to handle the applications of their products through their market (Figure 16.3).

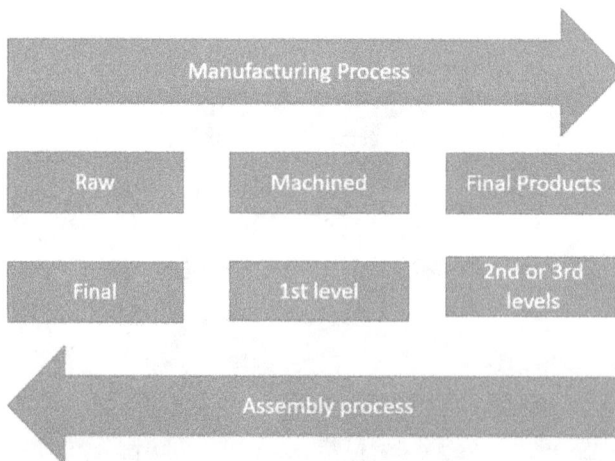

FIGURE 16.3 Production flow.

Smarter manufacturers not only develop and capture the data, and also they can understand the utility of data. As a result, the identity captures the data preprocesses in the smart manufacturing sector. It depicts the complexity involved in the inherent development of the process within the system. Three smart manufacturing levels are identified towards the enterprise management system, the operating system, and the product creation system.

Machine learning supports the smart manufacturer to do better production where the robots can help with their tools. In some aspects, together with detailed precision, this analytics method can identify the important situations involved in it, the automated process technique can develop outputs that are free from errors. The amount of data is increasing daily, so the manufacturing people's businesses need to leverage smarter solutions to take their entire methods efficiently and scalably. Such data helps a lot in identifying the terms in automating the processes for even predicting and monitoring.

16.5 QUALITY CONTROL ASPECTS

Quality control is an essential step in every production system. A lot of business investments aim to reinforce this process to grant a higher performance product. Quality can be defined in a few ways towards satisfying customer needs, fitness for use, and conformance to standards (Jaya Chandra, 2001). Business people always need higher quality in their manufactured products to achieve their goals. Quality is very important because the manufacturer focuses on the design, development, and manufacturing of products to properly understand their concepts and methods to improve the product quality. The quality control technique provides the new techniques necessary to assure the quality of the manufacturing products towards enhancing their product standards (Figure 16.4).

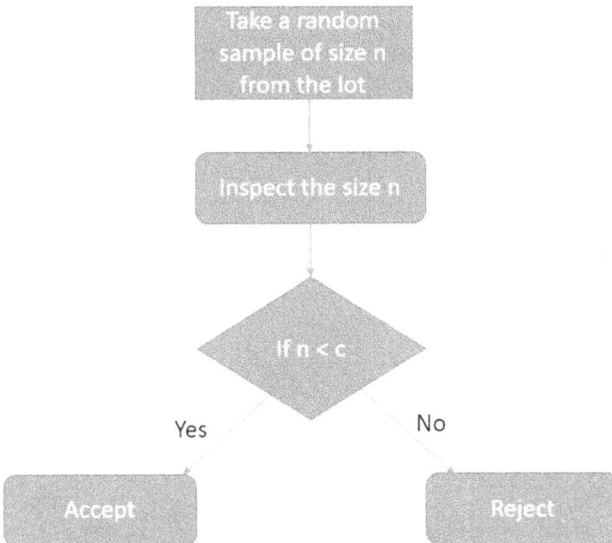

FIGURE 16.4 Quality checking processes.

Quality control involves a collection of procedures that are implemented to ensure the quality of the manufactured product or performed service adheres to a defined set of quality criteria to meet the customer's requirements. This method is based on the statistical techniques to determine and control the quality through sampling. Random sampling, probability, and statistical inferences are used to develop the process, using this method to control the product's quality. There are two types of quality control tools, which include process control techniques and product control techniques. Process control techniques control the product development process through every stage of production. In contrast, the product control technique involves checking their units and determining their lot if they are within their specifications towards the final product before going to market. Here both the producer and consumer can determine their quality checking.

The main aim of statistical testing is to develop corrective measures in the inspection process. Statistical control helps manufacturers to meet the needs of consumer demands for their best products. The opportunity available in smart technologies and data processes is much applicable and becomes a need for these industries. It becomes necessary to study the focus on industries and their processes with the most significant background. Nowadays, it is easy to determine whether a device is properly functioning or not quickly. Classifying the defective units, misaligned machine, or wrong behavior of a process is very critical to the end line. There are thousands of TVs, cell phones, tablets, iPad, Android systems, computers, and other electronic devices produced every year. The development point is to be increased every year and for the next few years to come. There are two types of probability distribution: discrete probability distribution and continuous probability distribution. These probability distributions are applied in inspection of various productions as shown in Table 16.1.

Leading manufacturers may take a proactive approach to streamline their operations. Companies that may take the extensive usage of artificial intelligence, which are the benefits of improved efficiency, decrease their time simultaneously increasing customer satisfaction. Deep learning and neural networks can help develop the performance, availability, and quality of products to be assembled and strengthen the machine towards quality products.

TABLE 16.1
Types of Productions

Discrete Parts and Assembly	Batch and Continuous Process
Motor vehicles and their units	Food
Aerospace products and their units	Chemicals
Constructive metals	Oil, gas
Plastic and rubber items	Electricity
Furniture and alloyed products	Paper
Electrical equipment and appliances	Primary metals

16.6   MACHINE LEARNING METHODS

Machine learning techniques play an essential role in research and the industrial revolution. It plays a predominant role in developing the tools and techniques that can be used in the new modernized data-driven world. A machine learning algorithm is also called model building, a mathematical expression representing a real-time problem. The aim is to select the proper data which go insight and develops modern techniques. For instance, a windmill manufacturer wants to monitor his wind reading calculation. It is an important piece of equipment to capture the video data through algorithm trained and to identify the dangerous cracks in their processes. The important methods using which one can build machine learning knowledge and their skills (Jared Dean, 2014) are:

- Regression Analysis
- Classification
- Clustering

16.6.1   REGRESSION ANALYSIS

The regression method comes under the heading of supervised machine learning. This method helps us to predict/explain a particular value based on a set of data. In some situations, one may need to know how far one variable depends on another variable. For example, when you want to predict the property price based on previous price and nearby property price, data are used to check similar properties. In such a situation, one can use the simplest linear regression method. Here, one can use the simple regression equation to obtain the simple line $Y = mx + c$ for the data set (Figure 16.5).

Once the linear regression model is composed with any data set in terms of pairs (X, Y), the position and slope of a line can be calculated. In other words, calculate the slope of the equation and obtain the Y-intercept for testing the line. The linear regression is studied well in machine learning to understand the statistical concepts more deeply. It helps us to create a linear regression model between the dependent variable and independent variable. It can be studied through predictive modeling for the given data concerned with reducing the error in the problem. It provides a clear idea between the input and out variable under the study, which was widely used in machine learning algorithms. There are many names used for linear regression. They are linear models, simple linear regression, multiple linear regression, ordinary least square method, etc. These are popular because of their simplicity to apply to real-world problems.

16.6.2   CLASSIFICATION

The classification method is the supervised machine learning technique, and here classification is used to estimate the association between classifying the objects in classes. If classes are created with data, then it is called a priori classification; however, if the classes are created empirically then it is called empirical classification. For example, one can predict whether an online customer will buy a product or not.

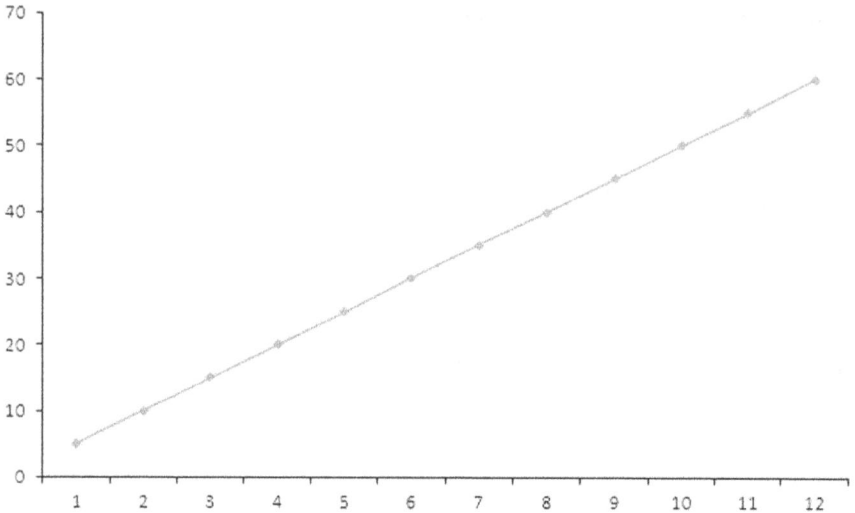

FIGURE 16.5 Linear regression.

The output can be very simple such as yes or no that is buyer or not buyer. In classification methods, it can be restricted only to two-way classes. A classification method, in which few classes have been pre-defined towards this method's needs, may train the machine system to allocate various objects into their classes. It is developed based on a sample taken from here, so each object is known, and the class attribute is unknown, which can be developed by the classification method.

The regression problem and classification problem have many similarities. Each is related to the other, and sometimes one method may transform into another form if it merely requires changing the variables from either side of these methods. Classification techniques have several applications they can predict based on the customer behavior, prediction towards direct responses received through the mail or identifying the customers who switch their company, debit and credit card applications, and students' categorization in the entrance test.

16.6.3 CLUSTERING

Clustering is a statistical technique for organizing the groups into similar objects that can be made by divided into subgroups with several various statistical algorithms and techniques. Clustering methods can be classified into three main divisions such as supervised, unsupervised, and semi-supervised clustering.

16.6.3.1 Supervised Clustering

In this supervised clustering method, one has to find clusters with high probability density values concerning individual classes that can be categorized into groups. Moreover, in supervised clustering, a target variable is identified. The data set of that variable becomes a new small cluster. One can keep the number of clusters as small as possible and similar objects are assigned to these clusters through similarity of the cluster for a given distance form.

16.6.3.2   Unsupervised Clustering

In the concept of unsupervised clustering, when the label is absent, one can find similar objects within the same cluster and which have dissimilarity with other objects. It is also used to maximize the intracluster similarity and to minimize the inter-cluster similarity, based on similarity or dissimilarity measurements. It can be used to the specific objective of the function. K-Means and hierarchal clustering techniques are the most important and widely used unsupervised clustering techniques in unsupervised methods.

16.6.3.3   Semi-Supervised Clustering

This method is a similarity measure between supervised and unsupervised clustering. Here the label is not known, only a part is given, and the remaining is a small amount of labeled data, and a large amount of unlabeled data is present. The domain information can be obtained in a pair of items in the observations. When the training data set does not contain all ground truth, classes are masked entirely to understand the semi-supervised clustering. Generally, cluster analysis is used in many applications, such as data analysis, image processing, market-research, and pattern recognition methods.

16.7   STATISTICAL MEASURES

In statistical measures, there are many types of literature among them, two main popularly used methods are descriptive statistics and inferential statistics. In descriptive statistics, one can describe your sample size, define the center of your data, and describe your data's spread and its relative distribution. Further, these data can be used to compare one group to another group to draw a suitable conclusion. The statistics have a four-step process, which consists of the following:

- Collecting data
- Classifying data
- Analyzing data
- Interpretation of findings includes graphics
- Drawing suitable conclusions

The above step-by-step process is used to examine the data science and assess whether the given data describing its domain in statistics or extensions of statistics.

The two important statistical measures are descriptive statistics and inferential statistics. In descriptive statistics, one can study the importance of measures of central tendency and measures of dispersion. The measure of central tendency deals with the various statistical measures such as arithmetic mean, median, mode, and weighted mean (Bruce Ratne, 2017). One can study the different types of dispersion in dispersion measures such as range, interquartile range, and standard deviation.

In inferential statistics, mostly a sample is taken from the population, and inferences are usually drawn for the people. Many research studies involve a larger population. One can't go for complete enumeration, so a sample is usually drawn and tested for inspection. Based on the sample, one can infer that the population either accepts or refuses to accept. In such situations, lots are formed based on the production; further, it can be estimated and enumerated under the circumstances involved in it, such as inferential statistics.

16.8   ALGORITHM FOR DATA ANALYTICS

Machine learning algorithms are very much important for supporting data analytics to refine the data. There are many such algorithms are available in the literature for the selection of methods in data-based analytics. One should understand the real-time problem and choose the relevant data to further study by supporting their methodology, which gives an accurate and efficient data classification method. Many such methods are available: k-means algorithm, neural networks, decision trees, k-nearest neighbor, and genetic algorithm, etc. Before applying these algorithms, one should have clarity about their data to be processed and their attributes. Further, one may find the relevant techniques to analyze and predict their findings based on the methods under the machine learning algorithm like clustering, classification, or regression methods, which are more appropriate methods for the given problems.

16.9   REAL-TIME APPLICATIONS

Suppose a cell phone manufacturing company decided to introduce a new model to the market. Thus the company knows about their features of their product and their feedback of their product. In the digital era, a vast amount of data is automatically or semi-automatically collected, recorded, and gathered for the existing products based on the product's feedback. Based on the input, the company should go for a new product. The company's diagnosis of their current product, faults, serviceability, and product requirements show that the new product should come without any drawbacks given by the customers from existing products. Decision-makers should think about whether the information obtained from the database is true or not, which is to be verified before concluding. Later, they should develop a new solution based on raw data that may help their decision-makers identify their unique patterns in the data.

Here, one should remember the relationship between the data models and processes verified and investigated by the quality engineers via screening methods. Various statistical measures are developed to identify the data patterns and make a new product through the scientific way. Decision tree models will identify the root cause of the problem and make a new solution for the manufacturers. Time-series methods with the similarity matrix may investigate the problem, and forecasting can be done. After proper execution of the model, one can find the company's manufacturing sector's successful need. Various techniques will address the problem related to their study of whether the company's products may take advantage of big data architecture. Few other illustrations for the study are given below:

- Pattern analysis can be done for data with manufactured electronic devices
- Big data analysis can be used to set up their new business
- Social media analysis
- Brand reputation
- Monitoring new trends in technology
- Call center performance
- Retail market quality and claim risk monitoring

16.10 RESULTS

The technology infrastructure is increasing year by year with the support of industry towards the manufacturing process. Nowadays, smart manufacturing has become a pioneering method in the global market with technology adaption. Artificial intelligence and machine learning methods enable a machine to think and to act accordingly. Humans have been observed with automation since the beginning of technology adaption. Artificial intelligence enables machines to think without any human intervention, a broad area of computer science. Machine learning is a subset of artificial intelligence that uses a statistical learning algorithm to build smart systems. The machine learning systems can automatically learn and improve without explicitly being programmed. The machine learning algorithms can be categorized into three classifications such as supervised learning, unsupervised learning, and reinforcement learning.

Nowadays, the manufacturing process may reduce capital, human effort, raw material, and other energy costs that impact productivity. The software will be continued to develop in two separate tracks. One route is the software to be created by commercial users, and the other route is for the community where the vendor work is done mostly to buy volunteers and few staffs were paid with salary. As a science of predicting, these algorithms will always continue to increase with better prediction. Machines will find a better and better result to find meaningful patterns in data with skilled software engineers may develop more efficient software for their utility. Many organizations are spending crores of money in the manufacturing sector to establish their products and meet competitiveness in the global market with two important challenges: minimizing the wastage and maximizing product acceptance.

In the automobile industry, products are assembled which are made with robots used heavily towards the achievement of the process. In such a situation, humans have to manage the equipment and inspect these items to be free from faults. No matter how technology increases, such advanced computer technology will not replace human efforts for their problem-solving. Human imagination is the ultimate to make a new innovative product.

16.11 CONCLUSION

Today, people talk about industrialization, which is called Industry 4.0, that is marching towards digitalization in manufacturing. Cloud technologies, the Internet of Things, and cyber-physical systems are technological supports that help make manufacturing more accurate. The first application was seen in Germany, and some studies indicate the manufacturing firms from developing countries have started to use these technologies.

The industry can use advanced technologies and some proposed ideas to upgrade and transform from traditional manufacturing mode into a more modernized or advanced manufacturing mode. In India, the fastest-growing economy is because of the manufacturing sector GDP growth rate, given by outlook for 2020, they said the GDP would rise from 6.1% to 7.4% in 2024. The manufacturing sector may provide many jobs in all fields, and it indirectly supports increasing all other sectors.

Here, a systematic framework has to frame towards the need for smart industrial manufacturing in today's world; it is proposed to have a suitable design, managing, monitoring, control, and scheduling have to be adopted. Secondly, a systematic framework towards the model building's methodology has to be made, and the need for model building and its importance is to be understood. Thirdly, product development and its importance in the competitive global market has to be kept in mind.

This framework provides an idea towards the mathematical model building or statistical model to be constructed and their importance are addressed. It continued to support the various statistical measures involved in understanding the data collection, visualization, analysis, and interpretation of machine learning model buildings' statistical measures, and their associated methodology is explained. Today, supply chain management plays a crucial role in the manufacturing sector, making us availability of goods towards the standards everywhere. One successful application is elaborated for modern smart manufacturing systems, and it paves the way for Industry 4.0 to enable smart manufacturing systems to come into existence.

ACKNOWLEDGMENTS

I acknowledge Our Honorable Vice-Chancellor Prof. Dr. P. Kaliraj, Vice-Chancellor, Bharathiar University, for his initiative and opportunity to write this chapter. Further, I acknowledge Prof. Dr. T. Devi, Professor and Head, Department of Computer Applications for her service and unknown referees for their valuable suggestions and guidance for bringing this chapter successfully.

REFERENCES

Bruce Ratner (2017). Statistical and Machine learning Data Mining: Techniques for Better Predictive Modeling and Analysis of Big Data, CRC Press, Florida.

Jared Dean (2014). Big Data, Data Mining, and Machine Learning, John Wiley and Sons, New Jersey.

Jaya Chandra (2001). Statistical Quality Control, CRC Press, UK.

Radu Godina and Joas Matias (2019). Quality Control in the Context of Industry 4.0, International Joint Conference on Industrial Engineering and Operations Management and Industrial Engineering and Operations Management, Lisbon, Portugal, volume 281. pp 177–187.

17 Influence of Artificial Intelligence in Clinical and Genomic Diagnostics

E. Kiruba Nesamalar[1], J. Satheeshkumar[2], and T. Amudha[2]

[1]Assistant Professor, Department of Information Technology, Women's Christian College, Chennai, India

[2]Associate Professor, Department of Computer Applications, Bharathiar University, Coimbatore, India

CONTENTS

DOI: 10.1201/9781003175865-17

17.1   ARTIFICIAL INTELLIGENCE

Artificial intelligence (AI) is an indispensable domain in today's technological arena, which involves planning, learning, and processing tasks to robots in such a way that it can be programmed to execute actions like humans. It can be used for problem-solving and learning that manipulate objects to achieve certain goals. AI works on the principle of human intelligence that can be used to solve complex tasks.

AI is defined as "The branch of computer science that is concerned with the automation of intelligent behavior" – **by Luger and Stubblefield** in 1993. AI is designed in such a way to solve challenging problems in computer science, software engineering, and operation that include advances in computer power and amounts of data. It can be used in various fields like information technology, mathematics, linguistics, and philosophy. AI can be used in multiple branches of computer science, which include logical, search, pattern recognition, representation, and inference, reasoning, learning, planning, epistemology, and ontology.

17.1.1   BRANCHES OF COMPUTER SCIENCE

Various dimensions of problems and solving methods are categorized as follows:

  i. **Logical AI** – It refers to the goals and the appropriate actions for achieving the specific objectives, represented through mathematical logic.
 ii. **Search AI** – It examines a substantial number of potential solutions that are found to be highly promising and proven to be successful in diverse domains.
iii. **Pattern Recognition AI** – It interprets various patterns and is applicable in real-world image analysis that involves complex and similar patterns.
 iv. **Representation** – It makes mathematical logic that is used to represent the facts about the world.
  v. **Inference** – They are used to infer some facts, utilizing mathematical logical deduction.
 vi. **Reasoning** – It is far from the human mind that includes active research progress in developing intelligent systems.
vii. **Learning** – They are used to learn mathematical logic from previous facts, knowledge, and behavior.
viii. **Planning** – It starts with general facts about a particular matter and situation to achieve a goal. They can be performed by a series of action strategies.

ix. **Epistemology** – This refers to the theory of knowledge for solving real-world problems, with special reference to the scope and validity of knowledge.

x. **Ontology** – This is a representation of different kinds of objects associated with properties and behavior through some conceptual relationships.

xi. **Heuristics** – It is a method of finding a problem-solving strategy that is associated with AI. A heuristic is the rule of thumb that can be effectively used on a trial and error basis on most of the problem domains.

xii. **Genetic Programming** – It is a method of creating a computer program from a high-level statement in a problem. Also, automatically used to solve the problem.

AI has broader applications in domains such as cybernetics and brain stimulation, the symbolic approach, cognitive simulation, logic-based, anti-logic, knowledge-based, statistical, and soft-computing approaches. Various algorithms often play an important part in the structure of AI to solve processing tasks quickly. AI is classified into two types, such as weak and strong. *Weak AI* occurs in a system that is designed to carry only a particular job. Examples include personal digital assistants such as Alexa from Amazon and Siri from Apple. *Strong AI* is a more complex system that carries on tasks like humans. Examples include self-driving cars, unmanned vehicles, and hospital operating rooms.

AI has both positive and negative sides. The advantages of AI include solving problems, handling information, realizes overloaded information, provides improved interfaces and powerful computers. Disadvantages of AI include increasing cost, slow in software development, and less experienced programmers available.

17.1.2 APPLICATIONS OF ARTIFICIAL INTELLIGENCE

AI expert systems are embedded in products, shipping and trading, marketing, warehouse optimization, healthcare, industry, music, and self-driving cars. Other applications in AI include streamline of trading, workstation maintenance in space, and satellite controls.

Medical AI applies computer-based procedures in clinical diagnosis and recommends personalized treatments. It can identify the significant associations among data, which helps in the accurate diagnosis and treatment plans. There are various medical procedures and systematic health informatics such as AI and machine learning in medical diagnostics, medical data mining and knowledge discovery, medicinal and therapeutic expert systems, automated patient monitoring, and AI in drug discovery. AI is good in the detection of meaningful association in data sets such as DNA or drug information.

DNA-based applications use analysis software for identifying a sequence in DNA to provide biosecurity, bio-intelligence, and IP protection. Genetic engineering plays a predominant role in AI by providing techniques of design and synthesis of DNA sequences easier. It may not be easier to implement techniques using biological weapons, so it is better to handle software tools that facilitate synthetic DNA sequences analysis. The technology uses history and culture that have similarities of sequence in DNA to identify signatures and origin of DNA. The most common technique in AI is BLAST, a comparison technique for short sequences of DNA sets.

17.2 MACHINE LEARNING

Machine learning (ML) is a subset of AI that provides computers with the capability to learn and understand concepts without being explicitly programmed. It provides algorithms to construct a model by using the relevant domain-oriented data, further classified into training data and test data in order to predict the results based on historical data and experiences. ML techniques are applicable in diverse real-life applications such as weather forecasting, fingerprint matching, and disease prediction.

"ML is based on algorithms that learn from data without relying on rule-based programming" – McKinsey & Co. It is defined as the study of computer programs that learn algorithms and build statistical models to infer and provide patterns without being explicitly programmed. Approaches in ML include supervised learning, unsupervised learning, and reinforcement learning, which are further categorized based on the signaling and feedback strategies utilized by the ML models.

17.2.1 Approaches of Machine Learning

The major categories of machine learning approaches are as follows:

  i. **Supervised Learning** – It is a type of classification model in which a machine is trained, and the class variables are to be presented for mapping inputs to the outputs.
  ii. **Unsupervised Learning** – It is a process of learning when training with data, class, or target variables is not present but discovered by hidden patterns of data.
  iii. **Semi-supervised Learning** – This is a combination approach of supervised and unsupervised learning. A set of data is fed to the system with a small amount of data along with a class variable and a large amount of data without a class variable.
  iv. **Active Learning** – The User plays an active role with machines. It will ask questions to the user and responds back to the user based on the data and segregates the data based on the class, and predicts the result.
  v. **Reinforcement Learning** – A computer learns to interact with an environment, and must perform a certain goal, by a trial-error method.
  vi. **Deep Learning** – This method is one of the recent development where intelligence is used to process data to detect objects, recognize speech, translate language, and make decisions by drawing data that is both structured and unlabeled.

ML can be used in various branches of computer science, which include computational learning theory, grammar induction, and meta-learning. Also, various cross-disciplinary fields include adversarial ML, predictive analysis, quantum ML, and robot learning.

There are various challenges in ML. The advantages of ML include continuous improvement, quick identification of patterns, minimum or otherwise nil support needed from humans, efficient management of data with various varieties, and dimensions over a wide range of applications. ML has few weaknesses like data acquisition, time and resources, interpretation of results, and high-error susceptibility.

ML needs to learn from past data, builds solution models based on a prediction from past data, and effectively predicts the output/outcome whenever it receives new data. It generally divides 60%/70% of data for training purposes and 40%/30% of data for testing purposes, respectively. The accuracy of output depends upon the quantity of data employed in building the ML model. ML techniques have various noble features, including continuous data-driven learning behavior leading to automatic improvement in the predictions.

Significant applications of ML include image recognition, speech recognition, traffic prediction, product recommendations, self-driving cars, email spam, malware filtering, virtual personal assistant, online fraud detection, stock market trading, and medical diagnosis.

17.3　INFLUENCE OF ARTIFICIAL INTELLIGENCE IN MACHINE LEARNING

The fundamental concept of machine learning is the ability of machines to learn from experiences and adapt as per the environment. Artificial intelligence is the ability of machines to make decisions and dynamically perform smart tasks by applying the gained knowledge. AI and ML will always go hand in hand and the conglomeration of these two technologies can bring newer insights in giving solutions to various real-world problems. The goal of AI is to understand human intelligence and imitate their behavior which requires knowledge. It also initiates problem-solving and analytical reasoning power to machines, which makes them perform complex tasks.

17.3.1　CLASSIFICATION OF AI

AI approaches are classified into two major types such as vertical and horizontal AI methods. Vertical AI is one that focuses on a single job, similar to scheduling a meeting, and performs the task well. Horizontal AI is one that handles multiple tasks. Examples include Cortana, Siri, and Alexa. AI is achieved by analyzing data and solves an issue using analytical problem-solving techniques to allow complex algorithms that perform similar tasks. It is an automated decision-making system where it can learn, adapt, suggest, and take actions automatically and therefore machine learning can learn from their experience. ML is a subset of AI that applies algorithms to solve issues that are complex in nature and also uses computer science and statistics to predict rational outputs.

AI also uses applications such as self-driving cars, natural language processing, and deep learning with machine learning. It is used to complete specialized tasks through the efficient processing of enormous data and information. It is used in various sectors like retail, healthcare, manufacturing, and banking. AI can also be incorporated with machine learning to obtain developments in other areas of science such as biometrics, automatic speech recognition, and even other human-related issues.

17.3.2 UTILIZATION OF AI

i. **Anti-Captcha** – It is used by humans to break CAPTCHA either directly or by solving photographic images.
ii. **Content Development** – It is used as a check-cashing system that relies on humans to compare and perform a financial transaction enrolled with the system. Thus, results with accuracy by biometric techniques.
iii. **Data-tagging** – It provides users with the metadata for unstructured data like images, audio, or video files.
iv. **Distributed Proofreaders** – It eliminates the need for error in the book created by human intervention, done by creating the optical character recognition process.
v. **Spam Prevention** – It is done by accomplishing humans to vote on emails which they receive as spam or not. If a certain threshold is reached, then a particular piece of email is said to have a high degree of accuracy that is predicted to be considered spam.

Therefore, artificial intelligence incorporated with machine learning makes complex tasks for humans to be solved easily. Such a problem can be easily integrated with the advancement of technologies to make it much easier and also less time-consuming, which is said to process tasks in a faster manner.

17.4 MEDICAL MACHINE LEARNING

17.4.1 COMPUTER TECHNIQUES USED IN MEDICAL ML

Medical ML takes the help of computer algorithms in clinical diagnosis, treatment planning, and prescriptions. It is highly capable in the detection of notable relationships among data, which helps in the diagnosis and customized treatment plans. It helps to build 3D models that predict results for brain tumors and other related problems. The difficulties faced by data mining techniques in processing the non-numerical features of biological sequences can be handled well by using ML techniques. Sequence classification predicts the category of DNA sequence from its structural similarity. It also predicts its functionality by analyzing the relationship among various attributes and identifies the genetic functions in DNA fragments.

17.4.2 METHODS FOR CALCULATING BIOLOGICAL SEQUENCE PATTERNS

Two methods are generally used to calculate biological sequence patterns, such as heuristic and exhaustive search methods. The heuristic approach is an iterative

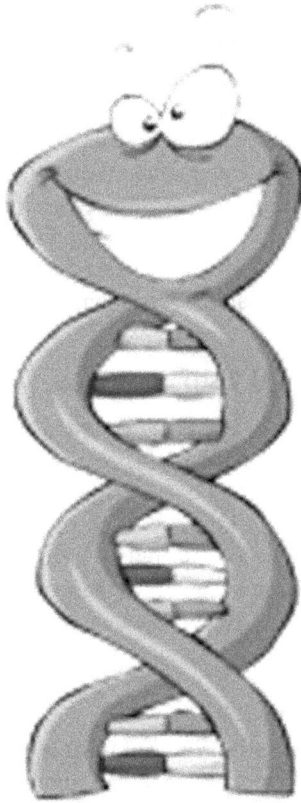

FIGURE 17.1   DNA molecule.

process. The advantage of this method is reduced complexity, and it is mainly suitable for DNA sequences. The disadvantage of this approach is the consideration of local optimum. Exhaustive search techniques are widely used in finding feasible solutions and arriving at the best solution as well. DNA molecule prediction requires a description of the biological significance of DNA sequences, that they may require sensitive and specific data. A DNA molecule is shown in Figure 17.1.

The four major research areas with DNA sequences are sequence alignment, pattern matching and analysis, data clustering, and classification. It has become quite necessary to identify a suitable ML technique to study and analyze the DNA sequence that shows performance improvement as well as the reduction in training time of data.

17.5   INFLUENCE OF AI AND ML IN CLINICAL AND GENOMIC DIAGNOSTICS

Artificial intelligence and machine learning help develop a variety of simulations through automated and computerized models that otherwise require human intelligence. In recent advances, various branches of AI algorithms have been implemented in medical applications. AI techniques in medical diagnosis are used to make a study and interpret based on the health data available. They are mainly used to analyze data sets that are huge in size and complex to process. Intelligent machines train themselves through the data that humans already interpret for learning purposes and apply the knowledge to interpret similar data, leading to better identification and forecasting of diseases. The AI interpretation can be classified based on various techniques applied such as image analysis, time series prediction, speech processing, and natural language recognition, which are suitable for clinical diagnostics. Thus, AI systems are used to integrate a variety of complex features and multiple concepts and arrive at decisions similar to human interpretation.

17.5.1 CLASSIFICATION OF AI USED IN MEDICAL DATA

Computer scientists, medical researchers, doctors, and clinical specialists work together in the development of AI and ML research in the field of medical data analysis. An enormous quantity of data in the areas of medical diagnosis and treatment is matched with social information to offer reliable and safe healthcare systems. Intelligent algorithms are machines used to perform various types of medical diagnostics and treatment recommendations with high accuracy and re-duced medical costs over time. AI will augment and assist human experts in un-dertaking repetitive tasks that require much precision and high levels of dexterity.

17.5.1.1 Computer Vision

Computer vision is a multidisciplinary domain that acquires and analyzes images to gain better and accurate interpretation for the automation of tasks. This process provides a way to understand the meaning of images. The process flow of computer vision includes image acquisition, preliminary processing, extraction of desired features, pattern recognition, labeling, and categorization. Convolutional neural network (CNN) is a type of deep learning methodology used in performing computer vision-related tasks. Using CNN, input images are known as filters that are used to detect the image [1].

The detected features are said to be patterns that include the presence of complex images. Applications of computer vision include Surveillance, image recognition, and autonomous vehicles. Medical imaging applications include cardiac MRI, echocardiograms, radiographs, stoke detection, and mammography. Vision technology is well suited in genomic testing procedures, which extract phenotypic features to provide recommendations of molecular testing performed by a pathologist [2].

17.5.1.2 Time Series Analysis

Time series analysis methods are widely applicable to analyze continuous and streaming data in the healthcare domain such as echocardiogram data, temporal data processing, forecasting the future scenario, and detecting a sequence of observa-tions applied on an ordered data. The advantage of time series analysis is its cap-ability in the efficient detection of data associations, learn the sequential data statistics, and make predictions by using conventional approaches such as Markov stochastic modeling techniques. Deep learning models, such as recurrent neural networks, are used in sequential analysis tasks. Applications of time series analysis include share market predictions, weather forecasting, and projection of environmental occurrences. AI and ML techniques are applied to automate medical appliances such as electrocardiograms for improved monitoring and analysis. In genomic sequence data, they appear as detection of functional DNA sequences for gene splicing and functions.

17.5.1.3 Automatic Speech Recognition

Speech recognition is useful for detecting neurological disorders, which comprise a collection of language interpretation procedures. Speech recognition algorithms allow the processing of basic elements such as tempo, pitch, and volume. Advanced algorithms identify specific features in audio data such as temperaments and emotions. These techniques are used to address medical and health information barriers. Applications of speech include voice control and assistance, online banking using voice, voice biometry, transcriptions, and so on. Speech recognition is applied to detect diseases such as Alzheimer's disease, Parkinson's disease, and coronary artery disease.

17.5.1.4 Natural Language Processing

NLP is widely applicable in data collection and information extraction in the patient's electronic health records. These algorithms take the document as input and produce a useful transformation of the document as output. The transformation performed is language interpretation, classification of documents, and preparation of summary. NLP algorithms involve syntactic analysis followed by semantic analysis of the text. Challenges of NLP include the extensive vocabulary, range of available synonyms, expressions, jargon, and similar terminologies that convey the same meaning.

NLP is effectively used in the medical field to synthesize and make predictions on current and future diagnosis. NLP is also used with AI-based chatbots for interaction purposes and includes approaches of EHR data in terms of high dimensionality and incompleteness. When combined with genomic data it is used to predict rare disease diagnosis resulting in automated genetic diagnosis accuracy.

17.5.2 AI in Clinical Genomics

AI applications efficiently perform complex works, which are difficult and repetitive for humans to carry out and address errors with standardized methods. Annotation of genomes, genotype-to-phenotype, and phenotype-to-genotype predictions, and variant classification are certain approaches in clinical genomics. Genome analysis and its flow diagram are shown in Figure 17.2.

Genomics is a multidisciplinary scientific domain that centers around the study of genome structure, function, mapping, modification, etc. A genome is a collection of DNA in an organism that includes all genes. It divides into several subsets such as regulatory and structural genomic. Regulatory genomics is a study of genomic features and ways of implementing an expression, whereas structural genomics is a

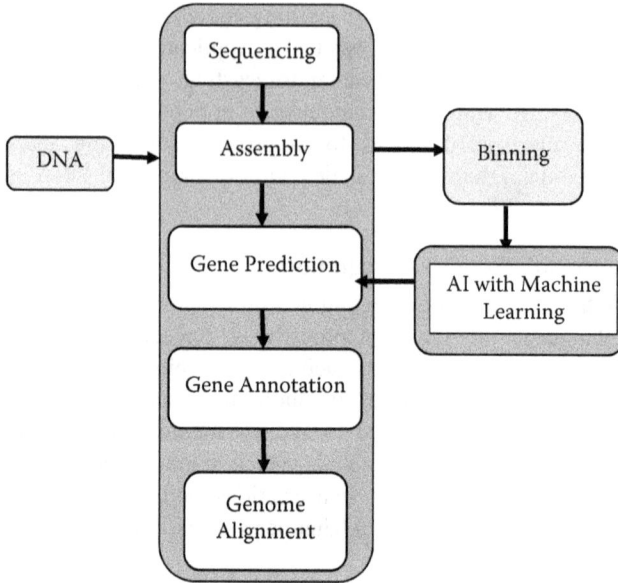

FIGURE 17.2   Flow diagram of genome analysis.

study in exploring the characteristics of genome structures. Functional genomics is a study describing gene functions and interactions and a genome analysis involves a set of phases such as sequencing, assembly, gene prediction, gene annotation, and genome alignment. Three main phases provide a better understanding of genetic analysis, such as DNA sequencing and assembly of DNA that represent original chromosomes, and analysis must be done to represent data.

Once the DNA set has been collected, pre-processing is said to be performed for further analysis. First, DNA sequencing is defined as the process to determine nucleotide order in a specific DNA molecule that performs in order to understand its functions and its effects on an organism. It also involves alignment and merging of fragments to reconstruct the DNA into smaller pieces, so that genome can be analyzed easily. Second, the process of genome assembly takes a considerable quantity of small DNA strand sequences from DNA sequencing and puts them together to create the actual chromosomes from where the DNA originated. Next, binning is an unsupervised approach of clustering DNA which reads sequences into an individual genome by appropriate ML methods to identify feature patterns of DNA sequences. AI can be implemented in various subsets to have an incredible value to the genomic industry. Regulatory genomics predicts the enhancement of gene expression, functional genomics helps in classification of mutants in functional and classification of activity, and structural genomics helps to classify structures of protein structures and make connection establishment with it. The analysis of the DNA phase brings discoveries and knowledge of genomes that can be applied in relevant situations. Gene prediction refers to the process of identifying regions of DNA genomes that are used for encoding and also includes protein sequences such as RNA genes which is useful for the predictions of functional DNA elements. Gene annotation is the process of identifying the location of genes and their relevant code in a specific genome that may process the possible function of genes. Finally, gene alignment is a way of arranging the DNA or protein sequences that is useful for identifying regions based on the types of genomic analysis and alignment based on the structure. It is considered to be the final step of DNA analysis that makes discoveries of genomic data [3].

17.5.2.1   Variant Calling

Genome interpretation is a high-precision task, and a variety of benchmark tools are available for variant calling, based on preparation and technology, which are also unpredictable in nature. Statistical techniques help to reduce biased errors with high accuracy. A deep variant, a CNN-based technique that brings out certain standard variant-calling tasks, provides improved accuracy due to the identification of complex dependencies in sequencing data.

17.5.2.2   Genome Annotation and Variant Classification

Genome annotation identifies the elements in the genome sequence by adding meaning to the sequence. Genes rely on the documentation of the genetic variants through proper information and genomic element functionality. AI techniques help improve knowledge by mapping phenotype-to-genotype predictions based on the influence of genetic variations found in the functional elements [4].

17.5.2.3   Coding Variants Classification

Various techniques are reported in the literature towards the implementation of classification, but they are integrated with deep learning techniques that outperform certain machine learning approaches. Deep learning technique, also called Deep Neural Networks (DNN), is later named Deep Artificial Neural Networks (DANN) based on the improved performance. It can be helpful in clinical genomic data analysis. AI techniques are proven to be promising in predictive analytics of DNA and sequence data with a minimum set of attributes. Primate AI is an approach used by CNN known as pathogenicity for cross-species information. It is an important classification tool for clinical diagnosis. Deep generative models are used to predict effective genetic variants and the absence of pathogenic prediction tools. It is the variant of a neural network used to study the replication of the distributed data, analyze, find, and deliver unobserved data [5].

17.5.2.4   Non-Coding Variants Classification

In the field of genomics, finding and predicting the pathogenic variants quite often poses a challenge to the researchers. AI algorithms improve the understanding and interpretation of non-coding variants in genes. Gene splicing plays a key role of up to 10% of pathogenic genetic variation, but on the other hand, it is hard for in-teractions of DNA gene splicing. Splice AI, a 32-layer deep neural network predicts both forms of splicing from sequence data, the canonical and non-canonical, which are used for long-range information. Deep learning approaches improve the ability of regulatory issues and predict genetic variation. Deep SA is a structured neural network model, trained on extensive functional genomics data, and simultaneously produces predictions which influence genetic variants.

17.5.2.5 Phenotype–Genotype Mapping

Human genomes consist of abundant genetic variants, labeled or predicted to be pathogenic based on individual health status. The process of molecular diagnosis of diseases requires the discovery and determination between the phenotype of the individual and the estimated result as a pathogenic variant. AI algorithms are extremely good in phenotype–genotype mapping, abstraction and interpretation of medical images and electronic health records, and high precision diagnostics.

17.5.2.6 Genetic Diagnosis

Clinical diagnosis is treated in the form of gene sequencing or phenotype analysis of genetic information. Deep-Gestalt, a neural network-based facial recognition and analysis technique performs well in a precise form and molecular gene diagnosis is mapped to a similar diagnosis, which combines with genomic data that extracts phenotype features from pictures of faces. Genetic patterns and disorders are recognized by analyzing facial features and make confirmations for DNA testing. AI-based systems can predict genomic representation present on distinct genomes through the embedded phenotypes present in clinical images [6].

17.5.2.7 Electronic Health Record (EHR) to Genetic Diagnosis

Phenotypes of diseases may be complex at times, captured through medical imaging and biochemical testing done at different stages during diagnosis. The findings are recorded in detail in an EHR where doctors analyze the documentation to perform diagnosis and provide prescriptions. AI-based algorithms are generally good at pattern recognition and in extracting significant information from the EHR. This system has been trained on a statistical model based on the divisions to generate a diagnostic system. Along with genomic data, AI algorithms and genome interpretation could easily provide accurate genetic diagnostics. Literature suggests that AI-based phenotype-to-genotype mapping results in highly improved diagnosis in genetic testing and also in genetic disorder identification [7,8].

17.5.2.8 Genotype–Phenotype Predictions

The primary goal of genetics is to forecast future disease at risk during diagnosis. Many statistical approaches are available for risk prediction in complex diseases. An application of ML is the genomic prediction of height that accurately predicts the height within the permissible limits to improve statistical techniques. Genotype-to-phenotype prediction integrates a range of health-related information and associated risk dynamics for identifying the possibility of disease prevalence. AI techniques can always handle an enormous volume of data with immense complexity.

Various challenges and limitations are embedded with AI like the ability to interpret complex medical data. Regulatory issues are quite often faced with AI, in which the AI algorithms lead to quite a few ethical and regulatory issues on data privacy, comprehensibility, and generalizations. Such challenges in the applicability of AI can be handled through the development of better practices towards data protection, fairness standards to minimize data, and allow continuous improvement of algorithms. AI interpretability is based on the volume, accuracy, and reliability of data, which work well for medical diagnosis with massive data. When dealing with complex data, AI task outputs are challenging in nature. AI can improve health-related communications among diagnostic users, clinical experts, and individuals. Data and machine bias must be pointed out when analyzing the interpretability of different data types and segregating them based on training and testing data for further analysis [9,10].

17.6   CONCLUSION

AI systems are proven to be extremely good at clinical diagnostics, mainly image-based diagnosis for analysis. AI finds a wider application in the extraction of phenotype information, EHRs, and other genetic analysis. Deep learning techniques improve variant calling, genomic annotation, variant classification, genetic diagnosis, and prediction. Various genomic tools are available in interpreting complex data, and performing recurring tasks, which is well suitable for genomic data by the advanced usage of CNNs and RNNs. Current DNA sequencing technologies allow generations of genomic data that require numerous data which tend to be time-consuming, high-priced, and unpredictable across collection spots. AI technology has profound applications in diverse forms of clinical and genomic diagnosis, which could substantially help healthcare professionals.

REFERENCES

1. Fragkiadaki, K., Levine, S., Felsen, P., and Malik, J., "Recurrent network models for human dynamics," in Computer Vision (ICCV), 2015 IEEE International Conference on. IEEE, Santiago, Chile, 7-13 Dec. 2015, pp. 4346–4354.
2. Milford, M., Shen, C., Lowry, S., Suenderhauf, N., Shirazi, S., Lin, G., Liu, F., Pepperell, E., Lerma, C., Upcroft, B., et al., "Sequence searching with deep-learnt depth for condition-and viewpoint invariant route-based place recognition," in Proceedings of the IEEE Conference on Computer Vision and Pattern Recognition Workshops, 2015, pp. 18–25.
3. David, O.E., Netanyahu, N.S., and Wolf, L., "Deepchess: End-to-end deep neural network for automatic learning in chess," in International Conference on Artificial Neural Networks, Springer, 2016, pp. 88–96.
4. He, K., Zhang, X., Ren, S., and Sun, J., "Delving deep into rectifiers: Surpassing human-level performance on ImageNet classification," in Proceedings of the IEEE International Conference on Computer Vision, 2015, pp. 1026–1034.
5. Devin, C., Gupta, A., Darrell, T., Abbeel, P., and Levine, S., "Learning modular neural network policies for multi-task and multirobot transfer," in Robotics and Automation (ICRA), 2017 IEEE International Conference on. IEEE, 2017, pp. 2169–2176.
6. Mohamed, S. and Rezende, D.J., "Variational information maximisation for intrinsically motivated reinforcement learning," in Advances in Neural Information Processing Systems, 2015, pp. 2125–2133.

7. Ryu, J. and Cho, S.B., "Towards optimal feature and classifier for gene expression classification of cancer," Lecture Note in Artificial Intelligence, 2012, 2275, pp. 310–317.

8. Quinlan, J.R., "The effect of noise on concept learning," in Michalski, R.S., Carbonell, J.G., and Mitchell, T.M. (eds) Machine Learning: An Artificial Intelligence Approach. San Mateo, CA: Morgan Kauffmann, 2016, 2, pp. 149–166.

9. Zhu, Y., Mottaghi, R., Kolve, E., Lim, J.J., Gupta, A., Fei-Fei, L., and Farhadi, A., "Target-driven visual navigation in indoor scenes using deep reinforcement learning," in Robotics and Automation (ICRA), 2017 IEEE International Conference on. IEEE, 2017, pp. 3357–3364.

10. Xu, Y., Selaru, M., Yin, J., Zou, T.T., Shustova, V., Mori, Y., Sato, F., Liu, T.C., Olaru, A., Wang, S., Kimos, M.C., Perry, K., Desai, K., Greenwood, B.D., Krasna, M.J., Shibata, D., Abraham, J.M., and Meltzer, S.J., "Artificial neural networks and gene filtering distinguish between global gene expression profiles of Barrett's esophagus and esophageal cancer," *Cancer Research*, 2012, 62:3493–3497.

18 Applications of Machine Learning in Economic Data Analysis and Policy Management

Brijesh Kumar Gupta
Product Manager - Data Analytics, IBS Software, Bengaluru, India

CONTENTS

Governments, policymakers, and regulators are increasingly adopting digital tools to enhance their capability to achieve better governance and control of the economy. This chapter delves deep into the details of machine learning in the context of economic policies and how economists are leveraging technology advancements to make robust and effective economic policy decisions. We will cover the following pointers by taking the references to real-world examples and economic situations.

- Goals of economic policies and broad areas under consideration for policy creation

DOI: 10.1201/9781003175865-18

- Current methods and thought process to analyze, measure, and modify policies
- Overview of common machine learning techniques and algorithms
- Applicability of advanced machine learning methods in economic data analysis
- Case studies undertaken by economists and regulators across the world

18.1 GOALS OF ECONOMIC POLICIES

We might not use the term "economics" "on a daily basis but we practice many of the economic principles in our day to day life; e.g., different household members taking care of various household activities, buying groceries and other essential items, trading off between luxury services and future savings, etc. All these activities and particularly the decision making involved in these activities are driven by a set of objectives. Those may be either short term objectives or medium to long term. This is what we refer to as household economics. Magnifying the scope and the activities of a household to society, jurisdiction, county, states, and finally to the national level makes it the branch of social study that is called Economics. Government as the head of an economy weighs its options pertaining to production, distribution, consumption of goods and services and its impact on revenue, spending, growth, and well-being of its citizens to formulate the objectives and underlying policies.

Over a period of time, since the concepts of currency, bank, debt, and tax were first introduced by different tribes in small societies or, at a scale, by countries and governments, the fundamental principles and objectives have been routinely altered by Intellectuals and economists. These experts either saw the flaws in existing economic principles or felt the need for upgrade due to changing ecosystem and preferences. Evolution of various entities such as corporations, jobs, demand from societies, and role of money further gave a boost to the need for new principles and frameworks that can be applied to streamline the functioning of an economy.

In an economic framework, a citizen is well placed if he has income-generating employment, access to essential goods and services and aspirations to grow with his hard work and skills to achieve a better lifestyle and means to live a comfortable life. These factors, as explained in Figure 18.1, can be termed stable prices, maximum employment, and economic growth which in combination makes the overall objective of a well-functioning economy. Though, there are different schools of thoughts on how to achieve a well-functioning economy which would serve its citizens better. For example the ideas of classical economics vs Behavioral economics. A fundamental assumption in classical economics is that players are rational and, given the desired information they will make decide and act rationally. While followers of behavioral economics, on the other hand, assumes people to be irrational actors who are biased in several ways. Under this assumption, all possible information does not guarantee consistency in decision making. "Understanding the difference between decision making behaviors of rational actors and largely irrational ones" is at the core of behavioral economics. At times, the difference in opinions is so intense that the approach to handle the economy can divide the whole

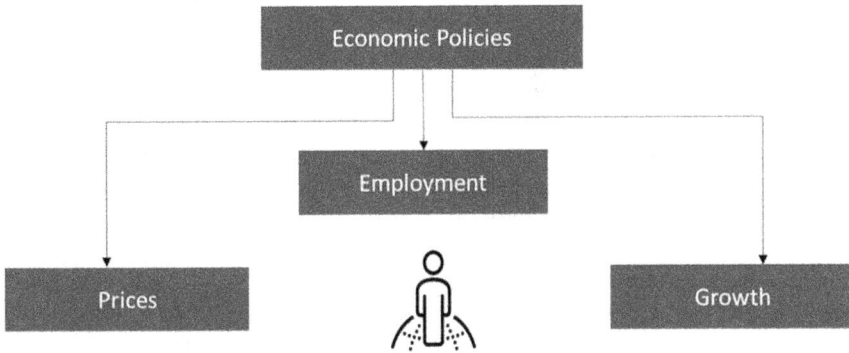

FIGURE 18.1   Goals of economic policies.

world into different blocks. For example, capitalist vs communist approach of the role of government in driving the economy or Keynesian economics vs classical economics which differs in the role of fiscal policy during slowdown or recession.

While distinct groups posit different viewpoints on various economic factors, economic policies are triggered by the economic situation in the economy but often shaped by prevailing ideologies in governments, institutions, and intellectual debates in that country. This is where policymakers take the driving seat in formulating the economic policies for the country. Before diving deep into the policymaking process and analytical techniques, it will be worthwhile to understand the broad horizon of policymaking and touchpoints to impact the flow of resources in a country.

18.1.1   AREAS UNDER CONSIDERATION FOR ECONOMIC POLICY CREATION

There are multiple ways governments and regulators can intervene in the functioning of an economy. At a macro level, as highlighted in Figure 18.2, two major policy touchpoints are fiscal and monetary policies. While fiscal policies deal with government spending and taxation, monetary policies deal with money supply. Together, these policies are assumed to achieve goods market equilibrium, money market equilibrium, and balance of payments as explained below.

Fiscal Policies	Monetary Policies
Taxation	Interest Rates
Gov Expenditure	Availability of Money
Fiscal Borrowing	Reserve Requirements

FIGURE 18.2   Macroeconomic (fiscal, monetary) policy space.

- Goods market equilibrium: The quantity of goods and services supplied is equal to the quantity demanded.
- Money market equilibrium: The quantity of money supplied is equal to the quantity demanded.
- Balance of payments equilibrium: The current account deficit is equal to the capital account surplus so that the official settlement's definition of the balance of payments equals zero.

Macroeconomic policies alone cannot achieve the intended goals of a well-functioning economy. In order to understand the further scope of economic policies and how they help in desired outcomes, we need to bring in the two factors of production, capital and labor, in the discussion. In recent times, technology has also been deemed as an important factor for production as it has the potential to transform the way economies operate. However, for the time being, we will focus on two traditional factors of production. The domestic and international flow of capital and labor further augments the horizon of economic policies that policymakers deal with. Conventionally, there are five major areas and associated subareas (refer Table 18.1) that play a major role in controlling the chunk of economic activities in a country.

18.2   CURRENT METHODS AND THOUGHT PROCESS TO ANALYZE, MEASURE, AND MODIFY POLICIES

Economic analysis is a continuous journey in policy recommendations and new policy formation. This process is, often, exhaustive and requires skills from a wide

TABLE 18.1

Critical Areas for Economic Policy Management

Policy Areas	Policy Elements
Sectorial Policies	• Agriculture Reforms
	• Manufacturing Controls
	• Services Sector Policies
Trade and Flows	• Export promotion
	• Competition
	• Exchange Rate Policies
Labor and Land	• Labor Utilization and Productivity
	• Employment Policies
	• Land Acquisitions
Financial Markets	• Capital Market Controls
	• Banking Regulations
	• NBFC and other FIs Regulations
Other Services	• Environment
	• Health and Education
	• Data Privacy

range of experts, e.g., data, psychology, economics, analytics, machine learning, and specialists from particular fields such as finance, manufacturing, and trade about which the analysis is being performed. Economic analysis finally connects the dots between various areas and subareas such as fiscal, monetary, industrial, trade, and taxations, etc. and helps understand the cross effects of various government initiatives and programs. Strategically, the economic analysis contains the following steps and varies based on the scope and possible impact.

- Solidify Problem Area and Objective of Analysis
- Factor Identification
- Economic Data Collection
- Building Analytical Models and Forecasts
- Interpretation of Data and Outputs
- Identify the Associated Economic Conditions and Policies
- Build Connected Graph Structure
- Define Scenarios, Validate, and Recommend

Experts have followed a combination of qualitative and quantitative techniques depending on the scope of analysis and its effects on the economy. A complete quantitative method is not good for many reasons. Mathematical equations derived from the fundamental economic principles and collected data at hand can provide the concrete value judgements of individuals only to the extent we can collect the data and process it. Given the time and resource constraints, a combinatory approach has proven to be more efficient and effective; e.g., a decision about Interest rates is taken based on trailing data analysis of Inflation, GDP growth, and the output gap. But factoring in the exogenous factors such as monsoon, change in demographics, business cycle, and investor sentiments are to be included qualitatively and handled with scenario creation and validation exercise to reach to final policy decision. Understanding the details of each of these steps is important to figure out the gaps and how modern technologies such as AI, machine learning, and deep learning can play an important role to bridge these gaps.

- **Solidify Problem Area and Objective of Analysis:** Defining the analysis objective is where the foundation of anatomy is laid. Taking a cautious approach, in this stage, ensures that the results of the analysis can be utilized for economic policy formation in a tangible manner; e.g., a group of analysts or policy committee working on the objective of growing employment in the country would have multiple directions to improve upon. The analysis can focus on specific sectors such as manufacturing, mining, or textile. A further drill down will bring the focus to the employment of either skilled labor vs unskilled labor. Another dissection will involve the elements, which drives the demand for skilled labor, such as technology, ownership, or innovation. A single broad-based study may not reveal the real picture and can potentially distort the influence of various accounted factors by distributing the impact of largely varying latent factors. In summary, there is no shortcut to this process.

- **Factors and Variables Identification:** In traditional economic analysis exercises, factor identification is largely driven by knowledge of economists and sectoral experts. It involves gathering the list of variables which can have the potential impact on the intended outcome, either in a positive or negative manner. These factors are shortlisted based on either the previous studies performed by economists in other parts of the world or theoretical hypothesis mentioned in literature.

In order to analyze the exchange rate volatility in a country, analysts compile the group of factors such as international trade, tourism, capital flows, etc. which have a direct or indirect association with the exchange rate movements. They further list down the specifics of each factor to maximum knocked-down levels where a group of "n" variables are good enough to capture the variability of that factor. While the trend is evolving, a bunch of studies are still performed without the involvement of industrial experts and lacks the changing nature of businesses and the economic environment. The outcome of this phase provides the reference for data collection and source identification. The two steps mark the first milestone and provide the contour and design of overall analysis. Together, it help analysts focus on the details of execution.

- **Economic Data Collection:** Data collection is assumed to be the important gateway where attention inclines towards execution rather than exploration. But an outright statement that "Rest of the steps do not involve any exploration" is wrong. Various governments, agencies, public institutions, and multilateral establishments collect a vast amount of data at different levels. This phase is performed in two steps.
  - Identifying the Data Sources
  - Collection and Mapping of Desired Variables

Given the list of factors and variables from the previous steps, analysts do a thorough search of data sources which have partial or full overlap with the variables in question. This is where analysts end up finalizing more than one data source to perform the analysis. These data sources are validated against the credibility of the collection agency, the timeframe of data available, and feasibility of downloading or exporting data.

At times, even if the variables are capture in a data source, they are not in the right format or to a level where it can be leveraged in the study. Sometimes with certain transformations and aggregations, those variables can be included in the study. The variables, which are not found in any of the available data sources, are treated in one of the following two ways. 1. Define the proxy variables. 2. Buying the data from professional data collection agencies. Proxy identification is a highly sought-after mechanism to address the need for missing variables. At the end of this phase, analysts ensure that they have sufficient data to start the data processing and analysis.

- **Building Analytical Models and Forecasts:** This is the mid-point and backbone of economic data analysis process. Given the variety of possibilities, methods, and tools, approach in this phase differs from analyst to analyst and study to study. We will not be delving deep into all varieties of methods and tools in this section but will focus on the key activities which are expected and performed in the phase.
  1. Data Processing and Structuring
  2. Exploratory Data Analysis
  3. Transformations, Aggregations, Derivations, and Statistical Checks
  4. Identify the Sample Data
  5. Selection of Right Analytical Methods
  6. Leveraging the Appropriate Tool
  7. Collection of Analysis Results
  8. Multiple Iterations to Fine-tune the Accuracy and Clarity of the Results

  The first three activities are analogous to preparing the raw material which is data in this case. Analysts find a hard time juggling with disparate data sets, containing information at different levels. Data in economic analysis are constructed in any of the four ways: Time Series, Cross-Section, Pooled, and, Panel data. The majority of the ad-hoc data processing tasks are performed in excel files. For more systematic analysis, analysts also use SAS, MATLAB®, and SPSS kind of tools. These tools provide basic to advanced level of data processing and visualization mechanism.

  Once the final data set is created with the right format of dependent and independent variables, a sample or full data set is used for a further level of modeling and forecasting. Stata, EViews, MATLAB, Gauss, and Mathematica are few popular tools used by the community of economists around the world. These tools differ in their ease of usage and number of supported models. Majority of economic analysis resolves around regression techniques due to its solid foundation, complete transparency, and control. In order to adjust the various complexities in data arising due to endogeneity, asymmetricity, nonlinearity, etc. various tests are performed and regression techniques are customized to neutralize the impact of these complications. In the last leg of this phase, the outcome of these models is collected and different data samples are used to validate the consistency in the results.

- **Interpretation of Data and Outputs:** As a consequence of this analysis, economists receive various outcome matrices. These matrices are analyzed to conclude the sanctity of the modeling exercise and its qualitative and quantitative results. Following are a few outcomes of results interpretation exercise.
  - The explanatory power of the aggregated data and model used
  - Impacts of various factors on the dependent variable
  - Quantification of the absolute and relative impact

- Importance of features
- The combined effect of two or more variables
- Seasonality, cyclicity in time series data such as consumption, demand, etc.

Activities so far mark the second milestone where quantitative results of various factors and their impacts are available to be utilized in decision making and policy creation.

- **Identify the Associated Economic Conditions and Policies:** This step is another important gateway wherein economists start connecting the results of the analysis with the overall objective of the whole exercise, i.e., policy creation or recommendation. There are certain evidence and economic situations, and risks which are difficult to quantify or get the concrete data points. Apart from this, there are certain policies which are already into effect and needs to be taken into consideration before recommending the new ones; e.g., a decision by the government to augment the existing borrowing programs is not only impacted by the government revenues, projected expenditures, but also existing borrowings in current fiscal, type of investors in government borrowing programs, goals of central banks in terms of liquidity and interest rate, prevailing inflation environment, and some geopolitical risks such as import of key goods and services. These are uncertain risks and are qualitatively accounted for in finalizing the policy recommendations.
- **Build Dependency Graph or Structure:** Various unpredictable risks and geopolitical scenarios are intertwined with each in a complex manner. These factors are connected as either cause-effect pairs or produce circular dependency. In this step, clear visibility of all the associated risks and their dependencies are established to avoid any gaps in decision making. In reality, a large set of economic policies do not achieve its intended effects. This is not surprising as economic situations, human behaviors, black swan events, and geopolitical scenarios are not always predictable. Comprehensiveness and caution in economic analysis can only mitigate these risks and help improve the odds of achieving the intended policy outcomes.
- **Define Scenario, Validate, and Recommend:** This step is the culmination of various qualitative and quantitative exercises which are conducted so far. Based on the final results and dependency structures, few most probable scenarios are built. Economists run through these scenarios with various experts, consulting groups, and advisors to come up with final recommendations. Different economic policies are formed in different government structures and regulatory committees who have the legal authority and legislative power to approve and finalize the policy recommendations; e.g., in India, monetary policies are finalized by a collective voting procedure among monetary policy committee members on a periodic basis. On the other hand, decisions about tax, government spending, and other fiscal measures are taken by designated ministries in the government. Similarly, other institutions such as Market Regulator (SEBI), Competition Commission of India (CCI),

and Reserve Bank of India (RBI) are tasked to finalize and implement capital markets policies, anti-trust regulations, and banking and financial sector policies, respectively. These institutions rely on emerging trends and insights from the economic analysis conducted by analysts, economists, and industrial experts.

18.3   OVERVIEW OF COMMON MACHINE LEARNING ALGORITHMS, TOOLS, AND FRAMEWORKS

Machine learning (ML) is a combination of advanced data analytics and data processing workload automation technique which turns out to predictive if the number of futuristic knowns fairly outnumber the unknowns about the future. Given the industrial adoption of ML in various fields such as banking, healthcare, and insurance, etc., the interest and development in machine learning has grown manifold. A large open-source community has taken the machine learning techniques from research organization to business domains who are reaping exponential benefits from these techniques and algorithms.

As explained in Figure 18.3, at the core of these algorithms is data which feeds into ML algorithm and generate insights. Industrial Revolution 4.0, which is all about digital technologies, has created a parallel world that characterizes the environments and behavior of entities/actors in the real world. The pace of formation of this digital world can be measured with the speed at which physical information is getting converted into digital information. Industries and players who are capable of capturing and simulating the vast amount of information from hysical entities (customers, assets, actions, nature, documents, etc.) to digital storage are the ones who are riding the digital wave of the current era.

Analytics is the traditional way using which the majority of data-driven decision making was performed until a few years back. Economic policy analysis also hinged on advanced statistical techniques and few mathematical equations (e.g., regression, decision trees, etc.) which are considered basic machine learning techniques) for a long period. Based on training behavior and data requirements for training, machine learning algorithms can be divided into the following four types.

- **Supervised (Inductive) Learning:** Learns from a combined set of features and output in training data, e.g., tree-based algorithms, regression, and boosting algorithms, etc.
- **Unsupervised Learning:** Training data does not include labels/output. Algorithms understand the pattern using distance/matrix-based techniques, e.g., clustering, principal component analysis (PCA), autoencoders.
- **Semi-supervised Learning:** Learns from partially labeled data and uses an iterative approach to learn the patterns.
- **Reinforcement Learning:** An exploration-exploitation based technique which uses agent, environment, and reward functions to learn the pattern and achieve the pre-defined objective function.

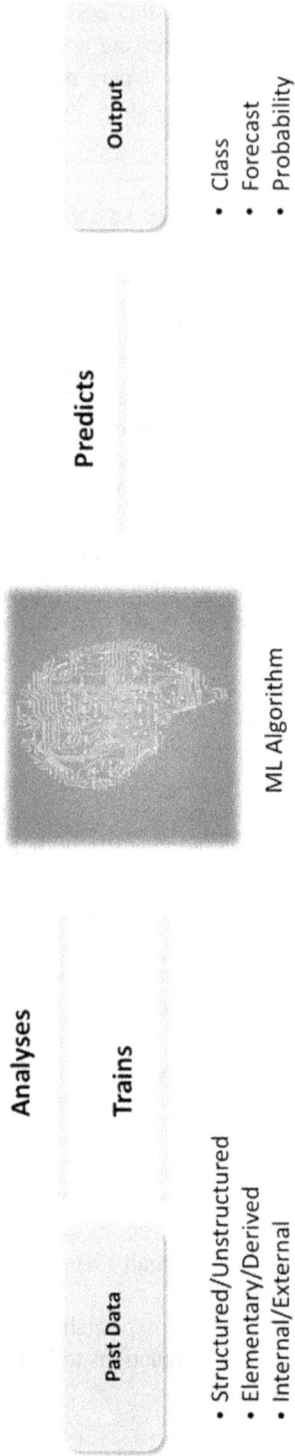

FIGURE 18.3 ML algorithms – data as input and prediction as output.

To understand the applicability of various ML algorithms in different industrial contexts such as finance, economics, or healthcare, a closer look at the algorithms would help.

$$Y = \frac{e^z}{1 + e^z} = \frac{e^{(\beta_0 + \beta_1 * X)}}{1 + e^{(\beta_0 + \beta_1 * X)}}$$

where X represents the feature vector $\{x1, x2, x3, ...xn\}$ β_1= weight matrix, β_0 = bias terms Y = probability of classification.

a. **Logistic Regression:** It is commonly used for estimating the probability that an instance belongs to a particular class. Logistic regression computes the weighted sum of the input features (plus a bias term) but instead of giving direct output, it returns logistic of the function.

This method is used for classification problems where dependent variables is a categorical variable. It can be used for binary classification with sigmoid function and multiclass classification using SoftMax Function.

b. **Support Vector Machines:** In SVM, a hyperplane is selected to best separate the points in the input variable space by their classes as described in Figure 18.4. SVM is capable of linear and nonlinear classification, regression, and outliers detection problems.

This algorithm is widely used in multi-dimensional data analysis as it outperforms other ML algorithms where number of features are very high.

c. **Decision Tree:** This algorithm uses node identification and splitting mechanism to group the variables and build the tree structure for predicting the probabilities for a class or forecast output. There are various algorithms such as ID3, C4.5, and CART, etc., which are used to construct the decision trees based on the purpose and type of target variables (Figure 18.5).

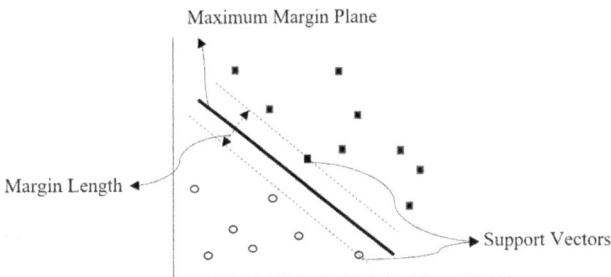

FIGURE 18.4   Key concepts of svm algorithm.

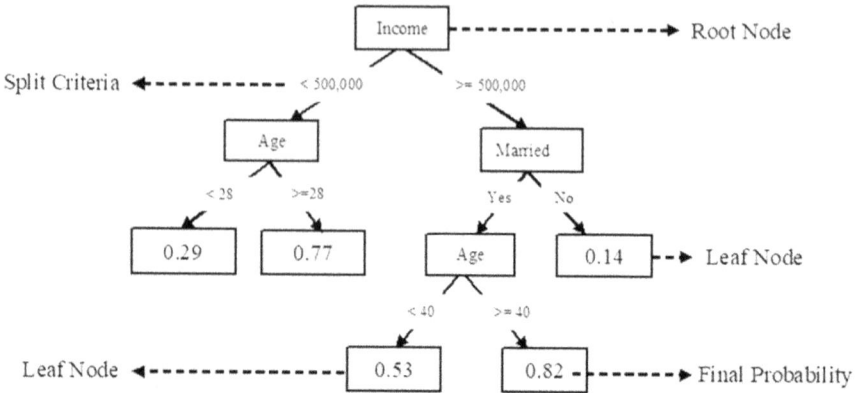

FIGURE 18.5   Decision tree structure.

Popular methods to identify and split the node structure are entropy, information gain, Gini Index, and Chi-Square. This algorithm can be used to solve various classification and regression problems; e.g., Figure 18.5 illustrates the possible structure of decision tree while predicting the probability of taking credit by an individual, given the data set with attributes about income, age, and marital status for a set of individuals.

d. **Random Forest (Bagging Method):** This model operates by constructing multiple decision trees during the training phase. These sub-trees are learned to ensure less correlation in their outcomes. The decision of the majority of the trees is chosen by the random forest as the final outcome in classification. In regression problems, outcomes of all regression trees can be averaged to give the final forecast as explained in Figure 18.6. This method proves to be advantageous over simple decision tree models when Model doesn't generalize well on unseen data.

$$Final\ Foreast = \frac{A + B + C + D + E}{5}$$

e. **Boosting Models:** This category of models refers to any ensemble method that uses several weak learners to turn into a strong learner. These learners can

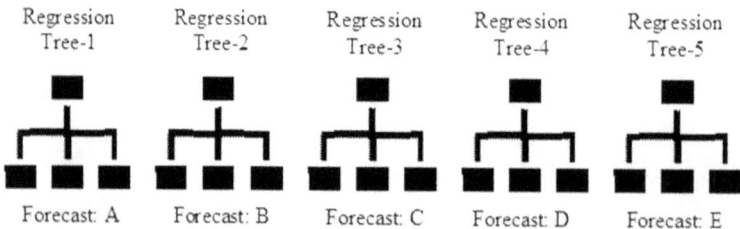

FIGURE 18.6   Solving regression problems using random forest model.

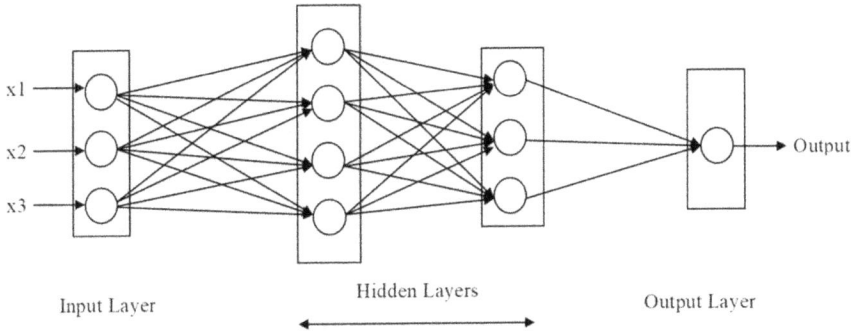

FIGURE 18.7   Fully connected neural network.

be regression model, decision trees, etc. There are a set of algorithms which handle Boosting in different ways; e.g., adaptive boosting, gradient boosting, and XGBoost, etc.

  i. **Adaptive Boost:** It commonly trains predictors sequentially, compute the error of the model on each training example and gives higher importance to examples on which the model made mistakes.
 ii. **Gradient Boost:** This model builds the sequential learners by modeling the residual or error from the previous learner and additively using the newly learned function to build a string learner.
iii. **Extreme Gradient Boosting:** This method is an extension of gradient boosting model and uses Second-order gradients to get the direction of optimizing the loss function. Apart from this, it also uses regularization techniques which generalizes the model well.

 f. **Deep Learning:** This is a completely different approach to solve several data analysis problems such as classification, regression, or anomaly detection. Its exceptional effectiveness at learning patterns in high dimensional space has made it the first choice for analyzing the highly sparse unstructured data such as text, image, and audio, etc. Deep learning algorithms attempt to learn data representation by using a hierarchy of multiple layers as displayed in Figure 18.7.

Neural networks learn the pattern in data with two-way processing mechanism; i.e., forward propagation and backward propagation. Forward propagation process the input nodes with initialized values of weights (W) and Bias (B) and calculates the outcome. Following is the two-step process that is executed at for each node at every hidden and output layer.

$$z^{[l]} = W^{[l]} * x^{[l-1]} + b^{[l]}$$

$$a^{[l]} = g^{[l]}(z^{[l]})$$

where, $x^{[l-1]}$ represents the input parameters from the previous layer $b^{[l]}$ is the bias terms associated with each node in the current layer $W^{[l]}$ represents the weight matrix of all the connections in the current layer and previous layer $g^{[l]}$ is the activation function of choice which can be RelU, Sigmoid, or Tanh $a^{[l]}$ is the output from the node.

As a next intermediate step, a loss function is calculated based on the calculated output and the real output. Further, in backward propagation, a gradient descent approach is taken to minimize the loss function by adjusting the values for W and B by small quantities. Forward and backward propagation steps are repeated iteratively until loss function is converged to a global minimum.

There are few other categories of models which become handy in certain situations. We will discuss these model categories in brief. There is a category of unsupervised models such as clustering. These set of models use distance-based mechanism to identify the cohort group of data points which are similar in their attribute positioning. These models have found a credible place in solving marketing and customer analytics problems. In economic analysis, these models can be extremely useful in target selection scenarios; e.g., targeting the infrastructure projects for PPP mode of development based on various project attributes such as project size, location, and tenure, etc. Anomaly detection is another widely used unsupervised model which uses data grouping and thresholding criteria to capture the unexpected pattern or abnormal data points in a data set. In traditional statistics, univariate anomaly detection is a popular technique to identify the outliers in a column. But machine learning provides advance methods to capture the multivariate anomalies. A few of these methods are cluster-based outlier detection, isolation forest, and autoencoder.

Matrix factorization has been a very sought-after technique in matrix algebra. Machine learning experts have found a tremendous use of this technique in solving many challenging problems; e.g., imputing missing values in a data set or building a recommendation engine using matrix factoring and reformulation. These techniques rely on matrix decomposition methods which converts the original m*n matrix into two different matrices of size m*k and k*n. Each of these matrices is archetype representations of rows and columns in the original matrix. These methods are very useful in handling cross-section data in economics.

18.4 APPLICABILITY OF ADVANCED MACHINE LEARNING METHODS IN ECONOMICS

Machine learning is finding its way to almost all aspects of human life: personal, social, and professional. Economics, also, is not untouched from the evolving impacts of machine learning. The new cognitive methods can radically transform the way data and statistics have been approached over the years by adopting Holistic and empirical methods in place of conventional stepwise and procedural approaches. What triggers the adoption of ML methods in economics? In the analysis, where does the transition starts? These are the key questions that we will discuss in this section.

To understand the whole idea, let's start with a simple example. Imagine a scenario, where the government is faced with a difficulty of consumption slowdown. Household consumption has decreased over the last 3–4 quarters. In such a scenario, there are two big questions in front of the government. 1) What is the reason behind slowdown? 2) What policy measure to be taken to improve consumption? In preparation of policy response, economists gather the recent macroeconomic data and perform the analysis to deduce that reduction in household savings is leading to consumption slowdown as the answer of the first question. Based on several consultations and economics principles, the government decides to reduce the personal income tax to increase the disposable income and, therefore, household savings. Though, both questions are answered. Will it result in the intended outcome? Does the government have infinite resources to sustain with very low/zero income tax for the long term? Possibly. No. Resources are scarce and cannot be distributed or utilized in an unbridled manner. Can we estimate the amount of tax cuts or the specific income groups if targeted well will revive the overall consumption in the economy? This efficiency constraint and policy requirements to be more predictive opens the newer dimension of analysis, i.e., machine learning.

18.4.1 Broad Areas for ML Adoption

Econometrics and traditional approaches of economic analysis, as discussed in the previous section, are sufficient to provide the causal relationships and inference to measure the impact of various factors on an outcome. But they lack the capability for predictive approximation or target selection. The two areas of study, i.e., causal analysis and predictive approximation, as differentiated in (Agrawal, Gans, and Goldfarb, 2019), require a different approach and modeling expectations. But when we use "causal inference" techniques for predictive approximation, the problem arises. Therefore, as highlighted in Figure 18.8, there are two broader areas for the applicability of machine learning in economic data analysis.

Before diving deep into the common challenges with existing econometric analysis techniques and improvements possible using machine learning, let us have a sneak peek in both areas of study and how they differ in their objectives and analytical methodology (Table 18.2).

18.4.2 Challenges in Economic Analysis and Advantages of Machine Learning

There are plenty of evidence that economists have already started using machine learning techniques for both types of analysis in policymaking. We will discuss

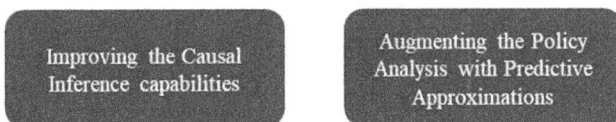

Improving the Causal
Inference capabilities

Augmenting the Policy
Analysis with Predictive
Approximations

FIGURE 18.8 Machine learning application areas.

TABLE 18.2

Requirements and Expectations from Two Different Analysis

Causal Inference	Predictive Approximations
The objective is to identify the positive or negative impacts of factors on outcome	The goal is to predict the approximate outcome. Either class, value, or probability
Identify the relative impact of covariates on the outcome	Relative, as well as absolute impact, is also expected
Inclusion of all possible features is not a necessity.	Maximum number of covariates and confounding variable to be included in Prediction.
The Goodness-of-fit (bias) is not the focus area.	Goodness-of-fit is important as it impacts the accuracy of prediction.
Optimizations are done to minimize the Bias in weights approximation.	Iterative optimizations are done to minimize model bias and Variance.
Model interpretability and transparency is very important.	Model interpretability and transparency can be maintained up to a level depending on the purpose of analysis.

some of these case studies in the next section of this chapter. At this stage, it will be appropriate to understand the challenges faced by Economists using traditional economic modeling techniques and how machine learning or its associated concepts can improve the efficiency as well as the efficacy of policy analysts. Following are the common issues:

1. Inability to take a large number of features into account while modeling
2. Lack in modeling options and over-reliance on regression techniques
3. Handling the nonlinearity in data for better predictions
4. Limitation in reducing "bias" and "variance" problems in models
5. Too many manual interventions to customize the models according to data and objective

"Bias" and "variance" are two types of modeling errors. While bias is the inability of the model to explain the significant variance on the dependent variable, variance is the flaw in generalizing the target function on unseen data.

Referring back to Section 18.2 of this chapter, factor identification and variable selection deal with potential covariates that we would like to study in the analysis. Parametric models such as regression or regression variants grow in complexity as the number of covariates increases. Regression models are based on stringent assumptions and naturally deal with single variate analysis. As the number of feature rises, adhering to the assumptions and customization of models become a fairly time-consuming task, e.g., when taking the two variables in analysis and to ascertain its interaction effects, a regression equation looks like below.

Taking one variable in the analysis,

$$Y = \beta_1 + \beta_2(X_1) + \epsilon$$

Taking more than one variables and its Interaction effects,

$$Y = \beta_1 + \beta_2(X_1) + \beta_3(X_2) + \beta_4(X_1 * X_2) + \epsilon$$

where, Y is the prediction variables
  X_i is the predictor variable
  β_i is intercept and regression coefficient
  ϵ is residual error

Newer machine learning techniques are capable of handling tens and hundreds of variables in one go. Techniques like regression trees, regression forest, as discussed in Section 18.3, can do the multivariate analysis of data and produce the results for causal interpretation as well as prediction without much of a hassle. Decision tree methodology, which is based on the concept of information gain (i.e., change in entropy) do a variable wise analysis to identify the variables which have maximum dissection power in accurately predicting the target continuous variable. Combining the multiple regression trees in using the bagging mechanism leads to the class of models called regression forest. These set of models are less interpretable but outperform regression tree and linear regression models on "bias" and "variance" type of errors.

Handling time series, cross-sectional data, and panel data in economics is overly reliant on regression techniques such as linear regression, Logit, ARIMA, ANOVA, etc. The machine learning field opens the broad horizon of models, as summarized in (Mullainathan and Spiess, 2017), which can be leveraged for various economic tasks based on the purpose of analysis. Figure 18.9 provides a large set of machine learning models that are capable of simplifying a variety of economic analysis activities during economic data analysis.

Economists find a hard time in handling nonlinearity in data. Though, there are certain methods to handle the nonlinear data in traditional econometrics. One popular way is to convert the nonlinear problems in linear construct by leveraging the mathematical transformation such as logarithmic transformation and power functions, e.g., the famous Cobb–Douglas function which is used to model the productivity based on the two factors of production, i.e., capital and labor. Functions are below.

$$Y = AL^\beta K^\alpha$$

where Y is total production A is total factor productivity L is labor input K is capital input α and β are capital and labor output elasticities, respectively.

Parametric Models	Non-Parametric Models
<ul><li>Linear Regression</li><li>Lasso Regression</li><li>Ridge Regression</li><li>SARIMAX Model</li></ul>	<ul><li>Decision Trees</li><li>Support Vector Machine</li><li>k-NN (Nearest Neighbour)</li><li>Matric Factorization based Models</li></ul>
Deep Learning Models	**Bagging and Boosting Models**
<ul><li>Fully Connected Neural Networks</li><li>Convolutional Neural Networks</li><li>Recurrent Neural Network</li><li>Long-Short Term Memory Networks</li></ul>	<ul><li>Random Forest/Regression Forest</li><li>Adaptive Boosting Model</li><li>Gradient Boosting Model</li><li>Ensemble Models</li></ul>

ML

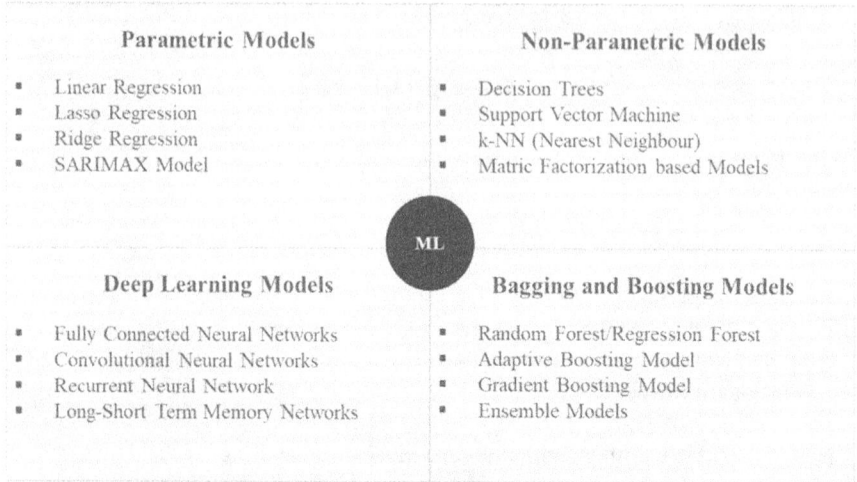

FIGURE 18.9 Different categories of machine learning algorithms.

While modeling the productivity of a sector, industry, or economy, analysts convert nonlinear function in linear regression problem as follows:

$$\ln(Y) = \ln(A) + \alpha \ln(K) + \beta \ln(L)$$

Despite having limited ability to handle nonlinear data, regression functions are constrained to handle the causal reference and prediction problems effectively. These functions, which are linear in their original form, falls short in handling the "bias" and "variance" problems in fitting the function. A model having the elements of "bias" problem cannot be assumed to be comprehensive in its recommendations. On the other hand, model, with variance problems, cannot be trusted as conclusive evidence of a study finding as changing the sample data would provide largely varying results. In this regard, machine learning provide innovative ways to address both of these errors.

In order to minimize the "bias" problem, machine learning provides a host of modeling options to choose from. Each economic analysis problem is unique on its own due to type, variety, and volume of data analysts are going to get to complete the study, e.g., in order to study the impact of equalization levy or digital transaction tax (a form of taxation accruing to foreign companies on their income from home markets where the company is not physically present), economists have a very limited set of data as these set of taxations are still evolving in other countries. However, In order to study the optimal tax structure under the GST regime, a huge volume of data is available. Both of these are unique problems and require different treatment from economists. Machine learning landscape provides two different sets of improvement within modeling criteria to improve the Bias in fitting the functions.

First, flexibility of models to gauge the shape of fit function and adjust to the complexity of data. Models such as Support Vector Machine and deep learning are capable of handling the complex mathematical functions just by changing the minimal configurations. Support Vector Machine Algorithm provides easy-to-configure kernel parameters, which can handle linear, sigmoid, Gaussian, polynomial and many other kernel functions. Similarly, deep learning methods can handle the high level of complexity by adjusting the number of hidden layers and neurons within those layers. (Please check Section 18.4 to get an intuitive understanding of layers and neurons in deep learning models.)

Second is boosting methods. These sets of models, as highlighted in Figure 18.6, are particularly designed to alleviate the bias concern in models. With their ability to construct the strong fit function using weak learners in a sequential manner is what make boosting methods uniquely positioned to handle the bias concern in models. Models such as gradient boosting use gradient techniques to model the errors from previous weak learners and add the learnt function to overall model in an additive manner.

Above discussed methods also control variance problem to an extent. Distinct from these, there are another set of techniques which are proven to be useful in handling the overfitting of models that leads to "variance error"; e.g., regularization techniques and ensemble models built on bagging recommendations.

Risk of overfitting arises when models become too complex or start responding to each training data point instead of patterns in the data set. To handle the erratic behavior of models, regularization techniques add an additional penalty term in the original loss function.

$$Cost\ Function = Loss + Regularization$$

During the fit process, penalty term constraints the feature weights from becoming too high or concentrated towards a handful of independent variables. In practice, there are two common regularization methods.

$$Cost\ Function = Loss + \lambda \sum_{j=1}^{n} \beta_j^2$$

where λ is the regularization rate and β_j is the feature weights.

A. **L1 Regularization:** It adds the multiplier of sum of absolute weights as the additional penalty term to the existing loss functions. The resulting cost function looks as following

$$Cost\ Function = Loss + \lambda \sum_{j=1}^{n} |\beta_j|$$

where λ is the regularization rate and β_j is the feature weights

In regression, this method is referred to as **Lasso regression** and the cost function looks as follows:

$$Cost\ Function = Residual\ Sum\ of\ Square\,(RSS) + \lambda \sum_{j=1}^{n} |\beta_j|$$

B. **L2 Regularization:** This method adds the squared magnitude of feature weights as the penalty term in the existing cost function. The resulting cost function looks like below.

In regression, this method is called **Ridge regression** and the cost function is as follows:

$$Cost\ Function = Residual\ Sum\ of\ Square\,(RSS) + \lambda \sum_{j=1}^{n} \beta_j^2$$

Apart from these, each ML model (from the set of models in Figure 18.6) is not only different from other machine learning model but also provide "bias" and "variance" improvement from over other models. There are few other techniques such as dropout and early stopping which are used in deep learning models to prevent them from overfitting the neural network structure.

Another benefit that machine learning models bring is the automation of complex manual activities. Machine learning algorithms are pre-written methods which can be used and customized by minimum manual intervention. Irrespective of the data and algorithm, any customization on machine learning models can be achieved by altering the settings of parameters. Further evolution in machine learning space has introduced the idea of automated machine Learning which makes the human intervention in the selection and fine-tuning of models to near zero. We shall discuss interesting aspects of automated machine learning in later part of this section.

18.4.3 MAJOR AREAS OF CONCERN FOR LEVERAGING ML IN ECONOMICS

Does machine learning have the answer to all difficulties faced by economists? A key question that requires some analysis and empirical viewpoint. Despite many advantages, there are few gaps between expectations from economists and what machine learning offers. Having said that, we have enough evidence that machine learning developments are underway that help meet both the ends. In this section, we will discuss a few prominent concerns faced by economists and to what extent machine learning help in addressing those concerns.

A. Explanatory Power of Complex ML Models

This is the biggest limitation that restricts economists from applying machine learning models on several economic studies, particularly in the area of causal reference. Separating the correlation from causation is one of the primary objective of economists as their recommendations lead to large-scale policy formations which impacts individuals, societies, businesses, and corporates. Machine learning provides an alternative to solve causation problems but needs to be handled in collabouration with traditional econometric approaches. As far as the current capabilities of machine learning goes, it offers easy-to-interpret models such as logistic regression and decision trees. It also provides moderate to high capabilities in interpreting more complex models such as bagging, boosting, and neural network model. In machine learning, feature importance, and causation interpretation are handled at two levels. 1. At model level (global interpretation) 2. At prediction level (local interpretation). Model-level interpretation offers an overall contribution or dissection power of covariates in classifying or forecasting the dependent variable. Local-level interpretation deals with providing the decision path in the prediction of each data point. State of the art techniques such as "Shapley," which are based on the analogy from game theory and builds on regression concepts, provide a deep level of interpretation for even highly complex models such as neural network. Combined with partial explanations from models and theoretical understanding of economics principles, researchers can leverage machine learning methods for wide-ranging policy problems including causal inference.

B. **Control over Optimization of Models**

A large set of economic analysis exercises are performed in a step-by-step manner. The reasons are two-fold. 1. Econometrics models have limitations in performing all-encompassing analysis. 2. Economists needs to draw inference at each stage of model formation. Machine learning, which handles the first limitation wonderfully, it falls short in meeting the expectation for the second. The reason is the highly automated process of training machine learning models with little or no manual intervention required. This problem can be handled to a certain extent in the ML world. Machine learning models, though, automates the training process but leaves the configuration ability in the control of user; e.g., in order to train a decision tree model, a user has to provide a range of inputs like criteria, split strategy, maximum depth, minimum leaf sample, and many more. Each of these combinations of input values produces a different tree structure. Economists can experiment and compare the results from these different combinations to draw the intermediate inferences to a certain level.

C. **Handling Limited Amount of Experimental Data**

Data sits at the core of any business or economic analysis in today's world. Due to its far-reaching consequences and complex interdependencies among economic indicators, economic studies are driven by theoretical assumptions, proven hypotheses, and clear evidence. By taking a step further, we discover that a large pool of economic exercises is performed on experimental data, survey points, or data collected in a controlled environment. These data sets are not only limited in volume but have different characteristics from data captured through systems or user actions. A simple example of system collected data are transactions, production, orders, etc. While minimizing the uncertainty in data processing is key for survey data sets, maximizing the information exportation is the underlying objective of data captured through automated systems. Minimizing uncertainty and building the appropriate narrative from experimental data is best possible from traditional methods. In handling cases like this, one can stay close to parametric models in machine learning but at the same time utilize ML-based clustering and anomaly detection techniques to control the uncertainty in a survey or experimental data.

D. Expertise in Leveraging ML Capabilities

With the machine learning becoming the indispensable tool for data analysis across industries, a greater emphasis has been given towards inter-disciplinary research. Popular machine learning (ML) methods and tools may require some bit of computer programming skills to define, train, validate, and interpret the ML models. This concern has constrained the researchers in utilizing the full potential of machine learning. However, the rise of citizen data scientists and need for self-service analytics has prompted large technology companies to build automated yet fairly configurable machine learning software and products. These softwares, in the hand of economists, has the potential to completely do away with computer programming or command-based actions. Cloud-based ML products also eliminate the need for infrastructure components such as processor, storage, or Graphic Processing Units (GPUs).

In summary, though ML, on its own, falls short in answering a few questions for an economist, it can augment his ability to achieve the underlying objective in a significant way. There are possible workarounds for most of the ML shortcomings, as discussed in brief above, in order to make the machine learning an all-pervasive tool for economic data analysis and policy study. We will discuss a few examples in the last section of this chapter to understand how economists are using machine learning techniques in various macro and micro economic settings.

18.5 MACHINE LEARNING STUDIES UNDERTAKEN BY ECONOMISTS, INSTITUTIONS, AND REGULATORS

So far, we have seen the reach of machine learning applications and their direct or indirect applicability in economic data analysis. Economists and policy experts in the fields of public policies such as agriculture, education, infrastructure investments, taxation, judiciary, and banking and capital markets are increasingly adopting the use of machine learning in data analysis. In this section, we will go through a few examples and industrial case studies undertaken by various government and regulators around the world.

Bank of England (BoE) and Central Bank of UK took various economic studies to get insights and train predictive models on economic and regulatory data, e.g., as a banking regulator, BoE is expected to monitor the health of Financial Institutions (FI) in the economy and provide necessary guidance and support to financial and operational concerns of banks, NBFCs, and other FIs. In a study (Chakraborty and Joseph, 2017), to achieve the monitoring efficiency of FIs, researchers, at BoE, developed a supervised model to predict the alerts using balance sheet information of banks. The objective behind adopting the machine learning technique for such surveillance was the possibility of incompleteness and uncertainty in the individual measure provided in the balance sheet. Banks used various balance sheet matrices such as leverage, capital, profitability, asset and counter party exposure of banks as independent features and previously collected alerts as Boolean target variable to train the classification models. In comparison, researchers found bagging based random forest model to be highly accurate and effective in predicting the alerts.

In another study, the same group of bankers used macroeconomic time series data from the last 25+ years to predict the change in Consumer Price Inflation (CPI) in the next two years. Projection of accurate inflation scenario, in advance, helps Central Bank in monetary policy decision making such as fixing the repo rate. Researchers used money supply, private debt, unemployment rate, GDP, household income, five-year bond yields, exchange rate, and commodity prices, etc. to predict the change in CPI with the two-year time horizon. In this analysis, the results from a combination of Support Vector Machine and Artificial Neural Network out-performed other models and also the reference models such as Ridge Regression, Auto-Regressive Model with one leg, etc. Surprisingly this unweighted combination of Final model was accurate in for both before and after the financial crisis in 2008. Following is the detail of two models:

- SVM with Gaussian Kernel
- ANN with two hidden layers and RelU activation function

While analyzing the features and feature importance, analysts found two different sets of overlapping important features from both the models, e.g., post financial crisis, SVM gave more importance to money supply and private debt features, while Artificial Neural Network recognized unemployment and gross disposable house-hold income as prevalent contributors in CPI forecasting.

There was another interesting study (McBride and Nichols, 2018); economists from World Bank, about efficient targeting for Social Security programs such as food security and direct cash transfers, etc. Identifying the right beneficiaries and per-forming poverty assessment is an important aspect of economic policy management. A better performing model ensures that government initiatives to provide Social Security benefits reach to the right households or individuals. Accurate targeting ensures less leakage, control on corruption and direct impact on citizens. The analysis was performed at country-level. Researchers used IRIS data set comprising of various predictors such as household demographics: size, age head, type of house: brick wall, cement floor, other products and services: fridge, radio, and fan, etc. They used machine learning techniques to train regression forest and Quantile Regression Forest (QRF) Model and compare their results against benchmark regression and probit models. As a result, researchers found that machine learning-based ensemble models, which automatically selects the variables and perform cross-validation, prove to be no worse than traditional models and, however, improves poverty accuracy and achieves a reduction in under coverage rates.

Studying the unemployment rate in an economy and forming policies for max-imum employment is one of the major focus areas for economist around the world. In a research study (Kutuk and Guloglu, 2019), researchers assessed the transition probabilities from unemployment to employment using household labor force survey data from 2000 to 2016. Survey data contains more than 100 variables containing household characteristics, individual's characteristics, employment status, income, unemployment and inactivity, past work experience, and labor status. For training the model, current employment status (Employed: 1, Unemployed: 0) was assumed to be the dependent variable. Being the binary outcome variable, ML-based classification models were selected. Researchers employed a host of supervised models including random forest, XGBoost, and neural networks and compared their results against the econometric logistic regression model. In the outcome analysis, random forest and XGBoost were found to be performing better than the logistics regression model.

Other than banking regulator, i.e., Central Bank, regulators in the field of capital markets, payments, healthcare, trade and promotion, agriculture, and tax authorities are applying advance analytics and machine learning techniques in 1. Policy administration 2. Prevention of fraud. NASDAQ, the world's largest stock exchange by volume traded as of 2019, has launched the deep learning–based solution to capture the unusual price patterns, trading errors, and cases of market abuse and manipulation. A growing amount of machine learning investment and research in agriculture is helping farmers, and agri-businesses in crop management, yield prediction, water, and soil management. Moreover, accurate predictions and efficient use of natural resources in agriculture help economists in controlling macroeconomic indices such as agriculture sector growth, food inflation, employment, and impact on per-capita income. In the majority of agriculture use cases, data collection steps are driven by image and sensor technologies followed by advance analytics and machine learning processing, e.g., in a bid to predict the yield of winter wheat, a group of researchers in the study (Pantazi et al., 2016) used soil data from prototype sensors, and Satellite NDVI (normalized difference vegetation index) to train Artificial Neural Network and Kohonen Network models. Kohonen Networks are a type of Artificial Neural Network which uses competitive learning rather than loss-based optimization techniques.

18.6 CONCLUSION

Given the huge potential and a growing interest in industrial adoption, machine learning techniques will continue to evolve. The efforts from large technology companies, open source community of statisticians and software professionals are expected to make machine learning a tool for solving any data-related business problem. In economic data analysis, despite a few remaining hurdles, machine learning techniques already outweigh the traditional econometrics methods in speed, efficiency, and comprehensiveness. Having a widespread use in private and public sector organizations, academic research, and technology innovations, machine learning, as a field of study, is ripe to be included in various learning streams such as economics, public policies, and medicine research, etc.

There are different elements (Figure 18.10) of machine learning education: statistical data processing, data modeling, model programming, enterprise scale model deployment and consumption, etc. Each of the elements covers certain

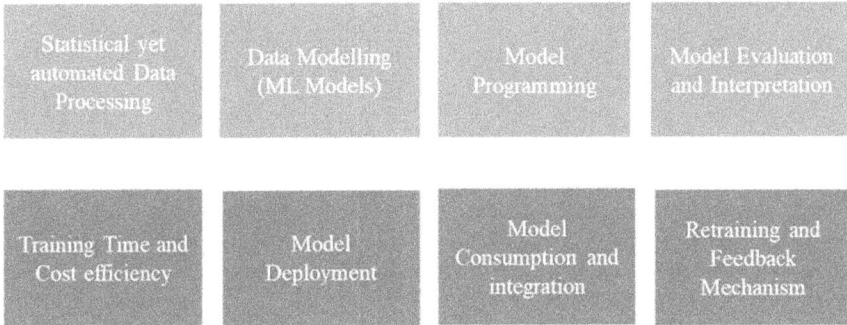

FIGURE 18.10   Elements of machine learning as a field of study.

machine learning aspects in detail; e.g., model evaluation and interpretation deal with various methods and tools available to evaluate and interpret the machine learning models. Enterprise model deployment provides the necessary knowledge of frameworks and platforms to deploy the machine learning models as a software application in a scalable technology environment. In this chapter, we covered details of data modeling elements in the context of economic data analysis. However, from holistic economics and public policy research viewpoint, a balanced approach, which involves a deep understanding of first four elements (In the First row of Figure 18.10), and moderate view of rest of the components (In the Second row of Figure 18.10), is warranted.

REFERENCES

Agrawal, A., Gans, J., and Goldfarb, A. (2019) 'The impact of machine learning on economics', *The Economics of Artificial Intelligence*, (January), pp. 507–552. doi: 10.72 08/chicago/9780226613475.003.0021.

Chakraborty, C. and Joseph, A. (2017) 'Staff Working Paper No. 674 Machine learning at central banks', (674). Available at: www.bankofengland.co.uk/research/Pages/workingpapers/default.aspx.

Kutuk, Y. and Guloglu, B. (2019) 'Prediction of transition probabilities from unemployment to employment for Turkey via machine learning and econometrics', (August). doi: 10.24954/JORE.2019.29.

McBride, L. and Nichols, A. (2018) 'Retooling poverty targeting using out-of-sample validation and machine learning', *World Bank Economic Review*, 32(3), 531–550. doi: 10.1093/wber/lhw056.

Mullainathan, S. and Spiess, J. (2017) 'Machine learning: An applied econometric approach', *Journal of Economic Perspectives*, 31(2), 87–106. doi: 10.1257/jep.31.2.87.

Pantazi, X.E., et al. (2016) 'Wheat yield prediction using machine learning and advanced sensing techniques', *Computers and Electronics in Agriculture*, 121, 57–65. doi: 10.1 016/j.compag.2015.11.018.

19 Industry 4.0

Machine Learning in Video Indexing

R. Amsaveni[1] and M. Punithavalli[2]
[1]Research Scholar, R&D Centre, Bharathiar University, Coimbatore, India
[2]Professor, Department of Computer Applications, Bharathiar University, Coimbatore, India

CONTENTS

DOI: 10.1201/9781003175865-19

19.1　INTRODUCTION

Video is one of the fundamental dynamic media to pass on messages viably. It resulted in improved PC networking innovation, and video is currently available to everybody through different online media networking stages. Video is more powerful than text or audio messages since it commands individuals' notice effectively, draws in the focus of watchers, and is anything but difficult to forget. Likewise, video can grasp the wide range of various types of information including text, audio, music, photographs, and so forth.

To retrieve a multimedia file from an extensive database is a significant fact. Indexing plays a critical role in recovering the required data. It has to describe, store, and organize before the process is executed. This helps to find a resource quick and secure manner. Here video file plays an essential role in this work. In multimedia, a data video is a necessary form of data. It has the following features, much more rich content, vast raw data, and a tiny preceding structure. These features provide quite difficult for indexing and retrieval. In the past, they was a small amount of database in the video, so extraction provided more manageable tasks, and it is entirely based on keywords interpreted manually. But recently, it has large databases and is much more difficult one to retrieve. Hence it required content-based indexing and retrieval method for automatic scrutinize with low human resources. Video indexing is a technique for providing an index related to video content for easy access from the frames of interest. In the database, video is stored beside an index created by the video indexing technique. The video searching is based on each video's index content to ensure that the video matches the keyword searchable and its relevance guaranteed, related to the word count of searchable keywords in video index (Podlesnaya and Podlesnyy). The video searching procedure checks the index appended substance with every video to guarantee that video coordinating with the searching keyword and its significance is guaranteed. The word includes searching for a keyword in the video index. Machine learning offers able tools for huge indexing components for video retrieval. A strategy's performance depends on the calculation being used, yet additionally on the data's attributes. Subsequently, it is imperative for particular data and a specific task to distinguish the job's correct procedure. Assessing how various methods act in indexing video is of much value.

Automatic video depiction age has as of late been getting mindfulness after quick advancement in the picture inscription age. Naturally producing a video depiction is more motivating than a picture because of its transient elements of casings. A large portion of the algorithms depended on the Recurrent Neural Network (RNN). As of late attentional systems, they have also applied to cause the model to figure out how to zero in on individual video casings while creating each word in a depicting sentence. A tale algorithm on a succession-to-arrangement strategy with fleeting consideration instrument introduced.

19.2   IMPORTANCE OF VIDEO INDEXING

A video may have a hearable channel just as a visual channel. The accessible information from videos incorporates the accompanying:

1. Video metadata, which are named messages introduced in recordings, typically including title, summary, date, performers, creator, broadcast term, report size, video configuration, copyright, etc.
2. Audio data from hear-capable channel
3. Records: Speech records can be obtained by talk affirmation and engraving writings can be scrutinized using optical character affirmation techniques
4. Visual data contained in the photos themselves from the visual channel

If the video is associated with a site page, there usually are site page messages related to the video. In this, we center the visual substance of videos and give an overview of visual substance-based video ordering and recovery. The significance and fame of video ordering and recovery have prompted a few review papers recorded, along with the distribution years and points. All in all, each article covers just a subset of the issues in video ordering and recovery. Today video data became vastly found because of new modern and technologies. Many users upload and download videos on the Internet, so the data has become huge. This fast development of video information also requires solid, creative, and available frameworks to consider ordering and recovery. These frameworks should be accessible from meager, transferrable, and operational interfaces to help clients control and quest for video content.

Presently, we don't have adaptable combination platforms to provide to extracted features from videos, with the goal that they could be indexed and searched. The task of indexing separated functions from videos is a troublesome task because of the various idea of the highlights and the transient elements of videos. Video search is recognized as one of the assessment task (Koniusz et al., 2017). The general intention sooner rather than later is that a video search framework will exist that is practically identical to the cutting edge of text search engines, for example, those from Google, Yahoo, and so forth. Videos are all the more impressive and open media that can catch and present data. As of late, large video databases were made due to the headways in numerous video-giving devices and the Internet. A dependable framework is expected to robotize the procedure of this vast quantity of data. Presently video capturing is a straightforward procedure, yet the related video retrieval is the troublesome procedure. For instance, on YouTube, new videos are consistently transferred to the site for more than one day. Thus, it is likewise hard to search for a little bit of text in large videos. Indexing is a data formation method to effectively recover records from the database documents dependent on individual traits on which the indexing has finished. Indexing is a database framework that is like what we find in books (Figure 19.1).

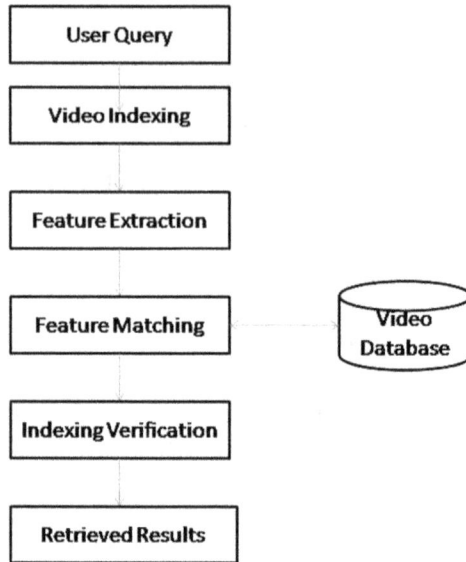

FIGURE 19.1   Basic structure of video indexing.

Indexing is characterized based on its indexing characteristics. Indexing can be described in the following types: Main Index, Secondary Index, Grouping Index, and Multilevel Index. The index is an approach to discover and sort records inside a database table quicker. This makes find data more quickly and efficiently. The user cannot see the files. They are just to speed up searches and queries. We realize that data are stored as records. Each record has a required field that causes it to be perceived particularly.

19.3   VIDEO STRUCTURE ANALYSIS

Large videos are organized by a plunging progression of video cuts, scenes, shots, and casings. Video structure investigation targets fragmenting a video into various underlying components with semantic substance, including shot limit recognition, essential casing mining, and scene dissection.

A. Shot Boundary Detection

A shot is a sequential arrangement of casings caught by a camera activity that happens among start and stop tasks, which point to the shot limits. There are solid substance relationships between edges in a shot. In this manner, shots are viewed as the basic units to sort out the substance of video groupings and the natives for more elevated-level semantic explanation and recovery errands. By and large, shot limits delegated cut. The change between progressive shots is sudden and steady advances that incorporate break up, blur in, become dim, wipe, and so on, extending over various edges. Cut recognition is simpler than a progressive change location.

B. Key Frame Extraction

There are incredible redundancies among the casings in a similar shot; this way, certain edges that best mirror the shot substance are chosen as key edges to speak to the shot compactly. The separated key edges ought to contain however much striking substance of the shot as could be expected and stay away from however much repetition as could reasonably be expected. The highlights utilized for key casing extraction incorporate tones (especially the shading histogram), edges, shapes, optical stream, MPEG-7 movement descriptors. For example, transient movement power and spatial conveyance of movement action, MPEG discrete cosine coefficient and movement vectors, camera action, and highlights from picture varieties brought about by camera movement.

C. Scene Segmentation

Scene segmentation is otherwise called story unit segmentation. A scene is a gathering of touching shots that are lucid with a specific subject or topic by and large. Scenes have more significant level semantics than shots. Scenes are distinguished or divided out by gathering progressive shots with comparable substance into an important semantic unit. The gathering might found on data from texts, pictures, or the video's audio track.

19.4   HOW DATA MINING AND MACHINE LEARNING HELP VIDEO INDEXING

The task of video data mining is utilizing the separated features to discover structural examples of video contents, behavior pattern of moving objects, content qualities of a scene, event designs and their associations, and another video semantic information, to accomplish video intelligence applications, for example, video retrieval. The decision of a methodology for video data mining relies on the form. Current systems incorporate the accompanying in 1. Object Mining, 2. Special Pattern Detection, 3. Pattern Discovery, and 4. Video Association Mining.

Machine learning plans to build up the PC algorithms that can understand from model information sources and make data-driven predictions on complex test data. Indexing and retrieving the video is a very challenging problem among computer vision researchers because of the vast amount of data available on the internet. The overall point of convergence of machine learning is depicting the informed models' information and theory for use on unnoticeable future information (Chen et al., 2005). The conventionality of the information depiction broad influences the show of machine understudies on the information. A helpless information depiction is presumably going to diminish the presence of even a pushed, included machine understudy. In contrast, a fair information depiction can incite unrivaled for a tolerably less convoluted machine understudy (Figure 19.2).

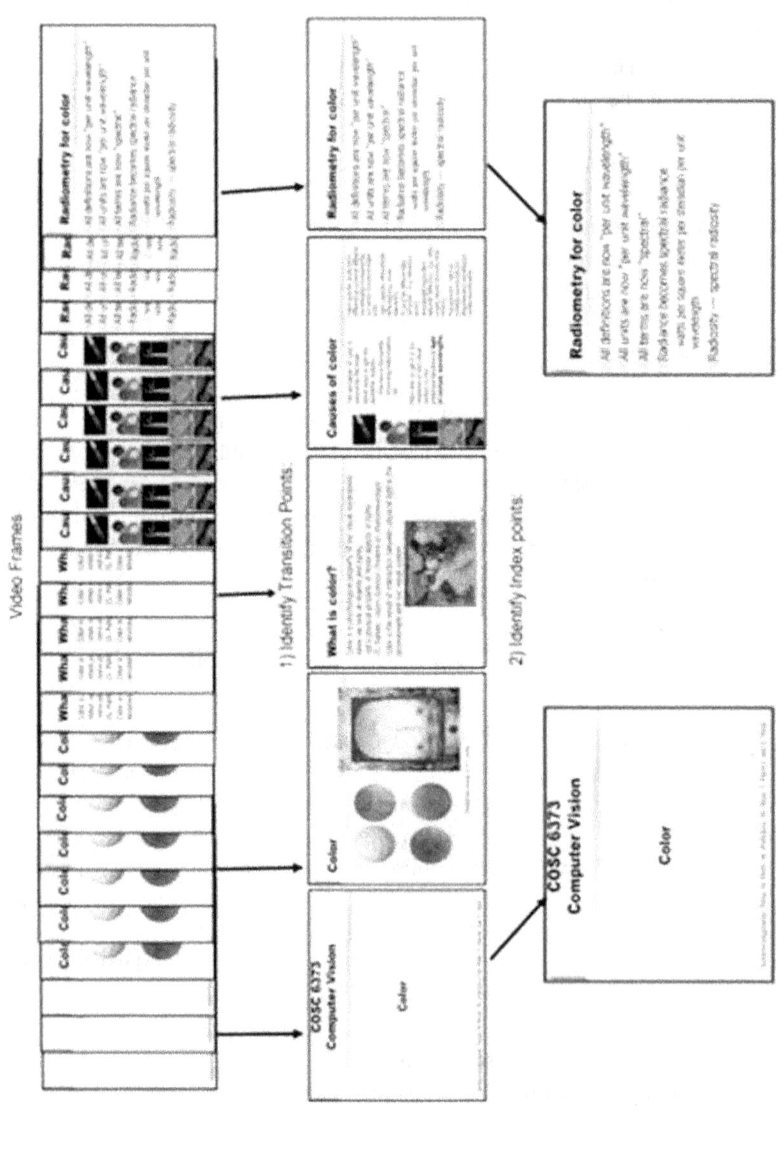

FIGURE 19.2 Video frame indexing.

The video indexing framework encourages the client to have adequate access, search, and perusing capacities to the ideal sight and (sound video) content. A wide assortment of sound and video extending from sound/picture, news communicates, TV projects, and ads are being recorded and put away in large volumes worldwide and made accessible online for clients get to. Arranging and indexing such tremendous assortments of data physically is exceptionally unfeasible for the mixed media data stream.

19.5 ANALYSIS OF MACHINE LEARNING CONCEPTS FOR VIDEO INDEXING

The video indexing method utilizes machine learning that can use every imaginable component; for example, the number of words in a slide, n-grams, right, or text with huge text dimensions (Yang et al., 2011). Among the cutting edge machine learning approach, gathering models, for example, random forest and capturing were discovered proficient and handy to utilize. They likewise give likelihood circulations that empower the client to pick an ideal number of index focuses (Figure 19.3).

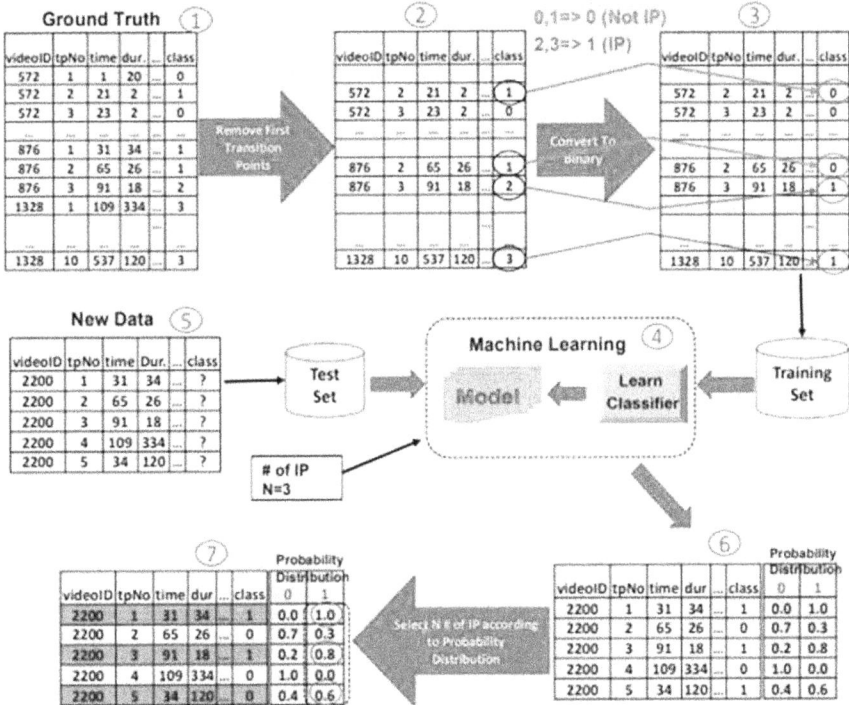

FIGURE 19.3 Machine learning approach of indexing video.

19.5.1 SUPERVISED LEARNING

Supervised learning is the most mainstream worldview for machine learning. It is the most straightforward to comprehend and the least difficult to execute. It is fundamentally the same as showing a youngster with the utilization of blaze cards. Given data as models with names, we can take care of a learning algorithm these model name combines individually, permitting the algorithm to expect the mark for every model, and providing it criticism concerning whether it expected the correct answer or not. After some time, the approach will figure out how to surmise the specific idea of the connection between models and their marks. When wholly prepared, the supervised learning approach will have the option to watch another, at no other time, see the model and predict a proper name for it. Supervised learning is predominantly for the Predictive Model's employments and named data (Deshmukh Bhagyashri, 2014). The common algorithms are as follows:

- Naive Bayes
- Decision Trees
- Linear Regression
- Random Forest
- Support Vector Machines (SVM)
- Ensemble Method (Figure 19.4)

Spam Classification: If you utilize a bleeding-edge email structure, chances are you've encountered a spam channel. That spam channel is a coordinated learning framework. These structures locate the ideal approach to manage the pre-emptive

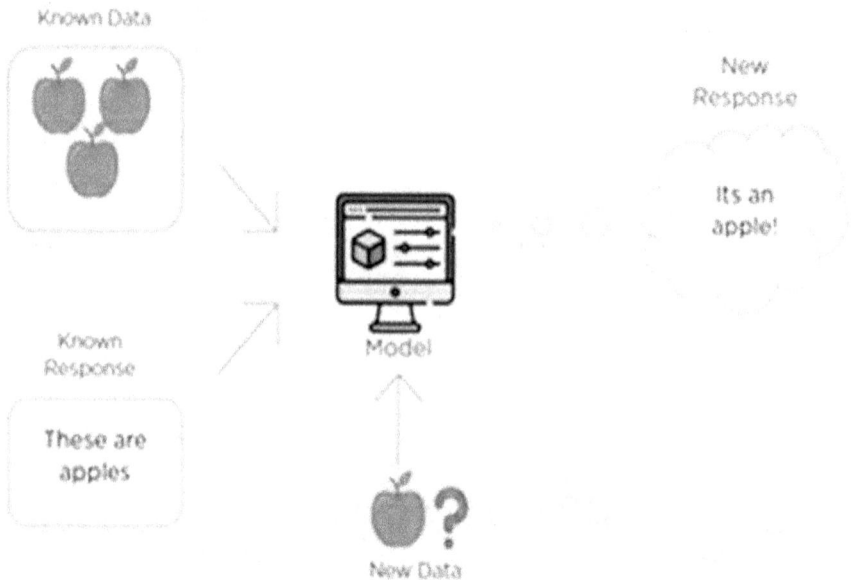

Known Data

New Response

Its an apple!

Known Response

Model

These are apples

New Data

FIGURE 19.4 Supervised learning approach.

channel through risky messages to ensure their customer isn't upset. Massive measures of these other than a show with the target that a customer can give new stamps to the framework can learn customer tendency.

Face Recognition: Do you use Facebook? Your face has probably been used in an overseen learning algorithm set up to see your face. Having a structure that snaps an image, finds faces, and ponders who is in the photo (proposing a tag) is an overseen system. It has different layers to it, seeing faces and sometimes later specific them; it so far managed regardless.

19.5.1.1 Naive Bayes Model

A Naive Bayes method of a classifier is a machine learning model that is used for gathering undertakings. The center of the classifier relies upon the Bayes speculation. The Naive Bayes model isn't difficult to produce and is very useful for enormous data sets. Alongside straightforwardness, Naive Bayes likewise considered to have beaten all the exceptionally refined arrangement techniques (Figure 19.5).

Naïve Bayes classifiers are essentially adaptable, requiring various limits straight in the number of segments (highlights/markers) in a learning issue. Most ridiculous probability preparing should be possible by reviewing a shut structure verbalization, which takes straight time instead of over the top iterative speculation as utilized for different classifiers.

19.5.1.2 Decision Trees

The benefit of the decision tree algorithm is that it has computational unpredictability in the info's number of vertices. The time taken to process chart and subgraph isomorphisms is accordingly autonomous of both the size of the model diagrams and the number of model charts. For a picture or video information base that will contain countless images, and will commonly be questioned by notorious

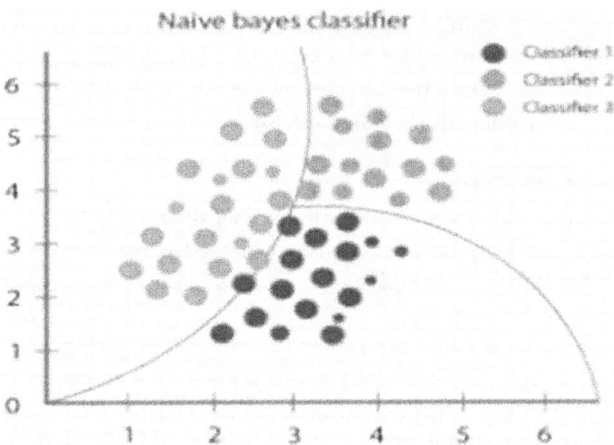

FIGURE 19.5 Naive Bayes classifier.

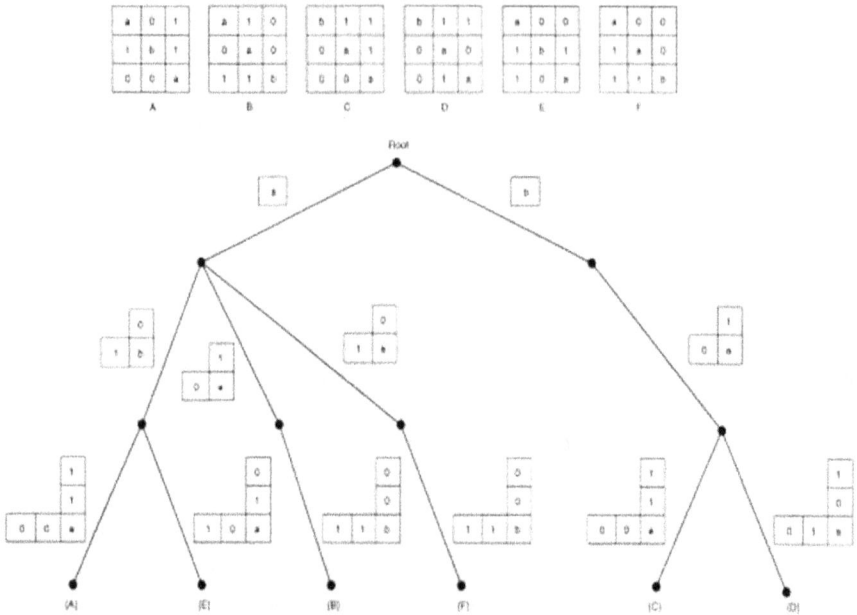

FIGURE 19.6 Decision tree.

inquiry, this computational intricacy is an unmistakable bit of leeway. Looking at O(n2) algorithm's multifaceted computational nature to that of the past best algorithm O(,mnn2), it shows how quickly this algorithm can order the info.

Decision tree learning is a reasonable demonstration of approaches used in experiences, information mining, and machine learning. It utilizes a choice tree (as a discerning model) to go from perceptions about a thing (tended to in the branches) to choices about the thing's genuine worth (tended to in the leaves). Tree models where the target variable can take a discrete game plan of properties called order trees; in these tree structures, leaves address class names, and branches address conjunctions of features that lead to those class names (Gayathri and Mahesh, 2018). Decision trees where the target variable can take decided characteristics (generally affirmed numbers) are called relapse confidence trees (Figure 19.6).

19.5.1.3 Linear Regression

As the name shows this indisputably, direct backslide can't be an approach for displaying the relationship between an impoverished variable "y" and another or continuously free factors implied as "x" and imparted in a vertical structure (Figure 19.7).

The word *linear* shows that the needy variable is straightforwardly relative to the autonomous factors. Different things are to be kept in mind. It must be consistent as though x is expanded/diminished; at that point, Y also changes directly. Numerically the relationship is based and communicated in the perfect structure as

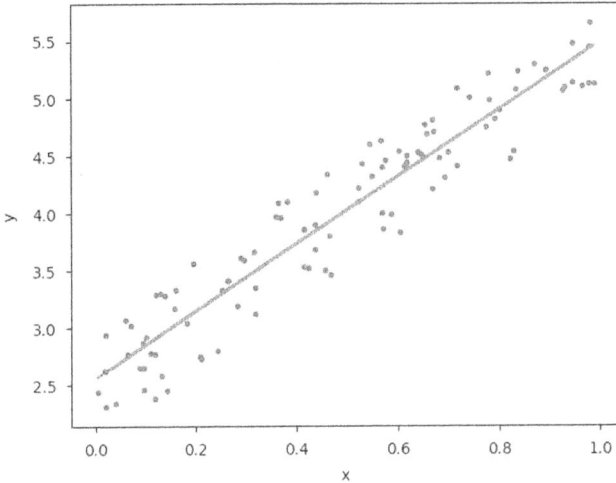

FIGURE 19.7 Linear regression.

$$y = Ax + B \tag{19.1}$$

Here A and B are viewed as consistent variables. The objective holed up behind the Supervised Learning utilizing direct relapse is to locate the specific estimation of the Constants "A" and "B" with the assistance of the informational collections. At that point, these qualities, i.e., the Constants' estimation, will be useful in anticipating the advantages of "y" later on for any expenses of "x." Presently, the situations where there is a solitary and free factor named as basic straight relapse. At the same time, if there is the opportunity of more than one independent variable, at that point, this cycle is called multiple linear regression (Jeong et al., 2012).

19.5.1.4 Random Forest

Random forest is viewed as one of the most adoring machine learning algorithms by data researchers because of its moderately high exactness, vigor, and convenience.

The motivation behind why random forests and other ensemble strategies are phenomenal models for specific data science assignments is that they don't require as much pre-preparing contrast with different techniques and can function admirably on clear cut and numerical information data. A first decision tree isn't healthy. However, random forest, which runs numerous decision trees and totals their yields for prediction, delivers an exceptionally hearty, high-performing model and can even command over-fitting (Figure 19.8).

19.5.1.5 Support Vector Machine (SVM)

Support Vector Machine (SVM) is a regulated machine learning algorithm that can be used for both requests or break confidence challenges. Regardless, it is, all around, utilized in portrayal issues. In the SVM algorithm, we plot each datum thing as a point in n-dimensional space (where n is various features you have) to assess

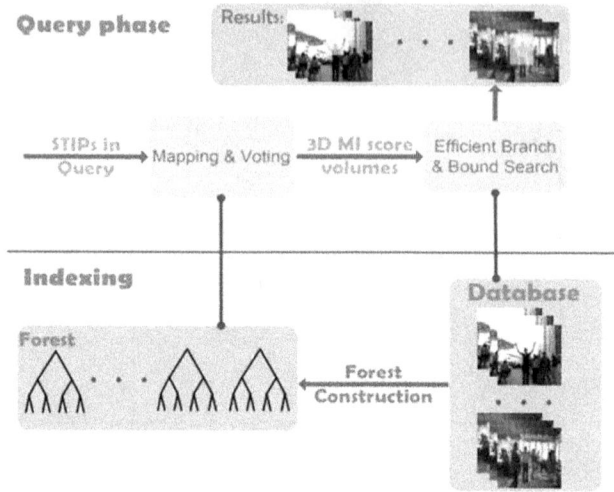

FIGURE 19.8   Random forest.

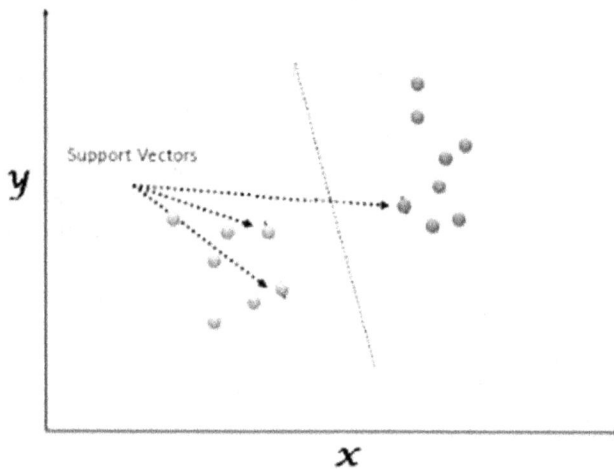

FIGURE 19.9   Support vector machine.

each fragment, examining a particular methodology. We perform a portrayal by finding the hyper-plane that isolates the two classes very well (look at the under portrayal) (Figure 19.9).

This is considered to be used in solving both regression and classification problems. Generally, a Support Vector is used as a classifier so that we can discuss SVM as how it is a classifier. Like other machines, it doesn't have gears, valves, or different electronic parts. It does what it can with ordinary devices to do: it takes the input, does manipulation the information, and then provides the output.

19.5.1.6 Ensemble Method

Ensemble learning improves machine learning results by joining a couple of models. This strategy allows the making of better prescient execution to stand out from a single model (Cortes and Vapnik, 1995). That is the explanation of troupe strategies set first in various regarded machine learning contentions, for instance, the Netflix Competition, KDD 2009, and Kaggle. The methodologies are meta-algorithms that join a couple of machine learning procedures into one prescient model to decrease distinction (packing), inclination (boosting), or improve expectations (stacking). Outfit methods can be isolated into two things.

Supporting group techniques where the base understudies are delivered continuously (for instance, AdaBoost). The basic motivation of the accompanying methods is to mishandle the dependence between the base understudies. The overall execution can be supported by gauging effectively mislabeled models with higher weight.

Most group systems use a solitary base learning algorithm to convey homogeneous base understudies, for instance, understudies of a comparable sort, provoking similar troupes. Furthermore, a couple of methodologies use heterogeneous understudies, for example, understudies of different sorts, moving heterogeneous gatherings. Altogether, for gathering methods to be more careful than any of its people, the base understudies should be as exact as could be normal considering the present situation and as various as could sensibly be normal (Figure 19.10).

In ensemble models, there are many popular machine learning algorithms such as support vector machines, decision trees, Naive Bayes, random forest, among others.

The benefit of the decision tree algorithm is that it has computational unpredictability in the info's number of vertices. The time taken to process chart and subgraph isomorphisms is accordingly autonomous of both the size of the model diagrams and the number of model charts. For a picture or video information base that will contain countless images, and will commonly be questioned by notorious inquiry, this computational intricacy is an unmistakable bit of leeway. Looking at $O(n2)$ algorithm's multifaceted computational nature to that of the past best algorithm $O(_{\,}mnn2)$, it shows how quickly this algorithm can order the info.

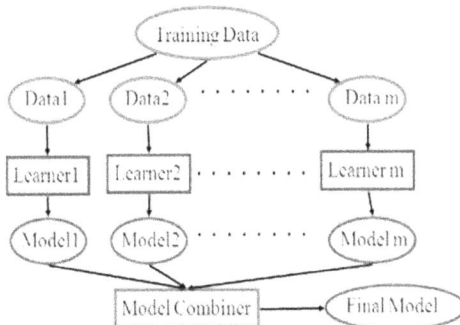

FIGURE 19.10 Ensemble methods.

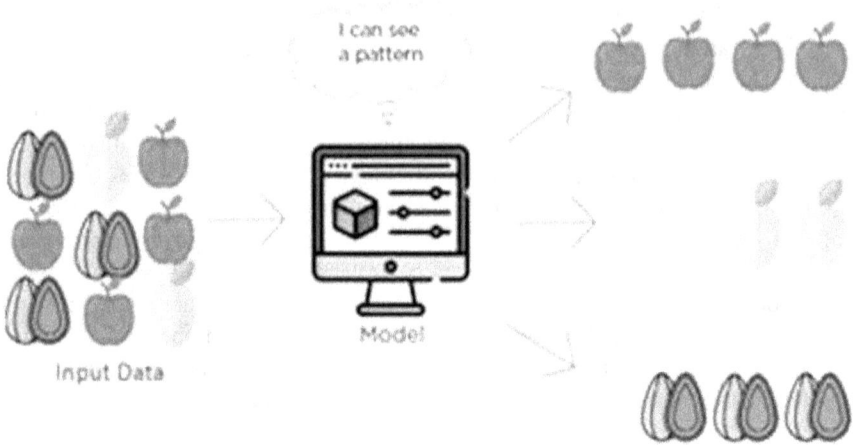

I can see
a pattern

Model

Input Data

FIGURE 19.11   Unsupervised learning.

19.5.2 UNSUPERVISED LEARNING

Unsupervised learning is mostly something despite regulated Learning. It incorporates no imprints. All things being equal, our algorithm would be dealt with a lot of information and given the devices to appreciate the information's properties. Starting there, it can sort out some way to a social occasion, bundle, just as sort out the information in a way with the ultimate objective that a human (or another savvy algorithm) can come in and appreciate the recently made information (Figure 19.11).

Unsupervised learning is transcendently used for the Descriptive Model. The essential kinds of unsupervised learning algorithms fuse clustering algorithms and association rule learning algorithms. A rundown of common algorithms recorded are as follows:

- K-Means Clustering
- Association Rules

The more basic snippet of data in this world is unlabeled (Rumelhart et al., 1988). Having sharp algorithms that can take our terabytes and terabytes of unlabeled data and appreciate it is an enormous wellspring of anticipated preferred position for specific undertakings. That without any other person could help support an advantage in various fields.

For example, imagine a circumstance in which we had an expansive database of every assessment paper whenever coursed. We had an unsupervised learning algorithm that recognized how to package these in a particularly like this that you were reliably mindful of the energy improvement inside a specific locale of investigation. As of now, you start to begin an assessment experience yourself, coordinating your work into this structure that the algorithm can see. As you study your work and take notes, the algorithm makes proposals to you about related positions, works you may wish to suggest, and works that may even help you push

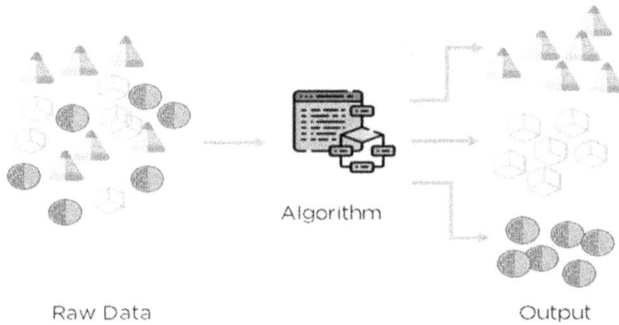

Raw Data   Algorithm   Output

FIGURE 19.12 Unsupervised learning algorithm mechanism.

that space of examination forward. With such a contraption, your benefit can be immensely supported (Figure 19.12).

Since unsupervised Learning relies on the information and its properties, we can say that independent Learning is information-driven. The outcomes from a performance learning task are obliged by the information and the way it is facilitated. You may see a few zones of unsupervised learning crop up.

Recommender Systems

If you've used YouTube or Netflix at some point, you've likely encountered a video proposal structure. These frameworks are generally speaking set in the independent space. We know things about narratives, maybe their length, their sort, etc. We see the watch history of various clients. Considering clients that have seen equal narratives like you and a short period later appreciated the experience of various records that you in a little while can't see, a recommender structure can see this relationship in the information and brief you with such a suggestion.

Purchasing Habit

Your buying propensities are likely contained in an information base some spot, and that information is being bought and sold enough at this moment. These buying affinities can be used in performance learning algorithms to assemble customers into relative purchasing pieces. This urges relationship to market to these amassed areas and can even look like recommender structures.

Gathering User Logs

Less client going up against, yet, at the same time essential, go through performance learning to add to client logs and issues. This can help the relationship with seeing fundamental issues to issues their customers face and correct these issues, through improving a thing or figuring out a FAQ to administer normal issues. Regardless, it is something that is expertly done, and on the occasion that you've at whatever point given an issue a thing or introduced a bug report, likely, it was figured out how to an unsupervised learning algorithm to pack it with other essentially vague issues.

19.5.2.1 K-Means Clustering

K-means gathering is maybe the most un-astounding and striking performance machine learning algorithms. Regularly, independent algorithms make gathering's from data sets using just data vectors without recommending known or named results. To manage the learning information, the K-recommends algorithm in information mining starts with the basic party of emotionally picked centroids, which are used as the beginning concentrations for each social event, and accordingly performs iterative (repetitive) tallies to prompt the spots of the centroids

It closes making and pushing packs by a similar token:

- The centroids have counterbalanced – there is no adjustment in their attributes, considering the way that the clustering has been dynamic.
- The depicted number of highlights has been developed (Figure 19.13).

The framework follows a basic and direct way to deal with overseeing depict a given informative variety through a particular number of packs (perceive k social occasions) fixed from the prior. The standard thought is to portray k centers, one for every get-together. These centroids ought to be set in a cautious way considering assorted district causes an alternate result.

Consequently, the better decision is to put them; notwithstanding, much as could sensibly be conventional far away from each other. The resulting stage is to take each guide having a spot toward a given instructive record and extra it to the nearest centroid. Absolutely when no point is looming, the shrouded advancement is done, and an early groupage is done. As of now, we need to re-figure k new centroids as bary purpose of union of the social events happening considering the past progression (Hu et al., 2011). After we have these k new centroids, another coupling ought to be done between comparable enlightening combination living spaces and the nearest new centroid. A circle has been made. Due to this circle, we may see that the k centroids change their district step by step until no more changes are done. At the day's end, centroids don't move anymore.

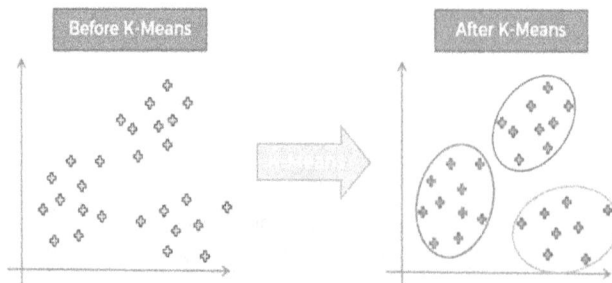

FIGURE 19.13 K-means clustering.

19.5.2.2 Association Rules

An association rule is named to be the learning issue. This is the spot you would locate the particular principles that will depict your information's huge fragments. Model: People who buy X are also the individual who will work by and large buy Y. It is every so often insinuated as "Market Basket Analysis," as it was the essential application zone of association mining. The fact is to discover the relationship of things happening together more much of the time than you'd envision from haphazardly testing all the possible results (Saravanan and Srinivasan, 2012). The commendable story of Beer and Diaper will help in understanding this better. The story goes this way: young American men who go to the stores on Fridays to buy diapers tend also to get a container of blend.

Association rules are made by totally separating information and looking for a little while in case/by then plans. By then, dependent upon going with two boundaries, the huge associations are viewed:

- Support: Support shows the amount of time the in case/by then relationship appears in the information base.
- Confidence: Confidence tells about the events these associations have been viewed as proof.

Association rule mining is a technique that plans to look as frequently as conceivable happening models, connections, or relationships from data sets found in various kinds of information bases, such as social information bases, esteem based data sets, and different sorts of chronicles.

19.5.3 Reinforcement Learning

Reinforcement learning is genuinely momentous when veered from supervised and unsupervised Learning. Where we can without a truly momentous stretch see the relationship among managed and solo (the nearness or nonappearance of engravings), the relationship to support learning is somewhat murkier. Two or three people try to annex reinforcement learning nearer to the two by depicting it as such a preparation that depends upon a period a discretionary movement of names, regardless, my examination is that makes things all the more baffling. Recognize a reinforcement learning algorithm into any condition, and it will present a huge load of bumbles above all (Kate et al., 2015). In as much as we offer a sort of clue to the algorithm that assistants high lead's with a positive sign and repulsive practices' with a negative one, we can fortify our algorithm to incline toward fabulous practices' over unpleasant ones. After some time, our learning algorithm figures out some approach to submit fewer bumbles than it used to (Figure 19.14).

Reinforcement learning is lead driven. It has impacts from the fields of neuroscience and psych research. If you've considered Pavlov's pooch, by at that point, you may, as of now, be comfortable with sustaining a topic master, anyway a characteristic one. To truly understand this learning, we ought to seclude a good model and take a gander at demonstrating an executive to play the game, Mario. For

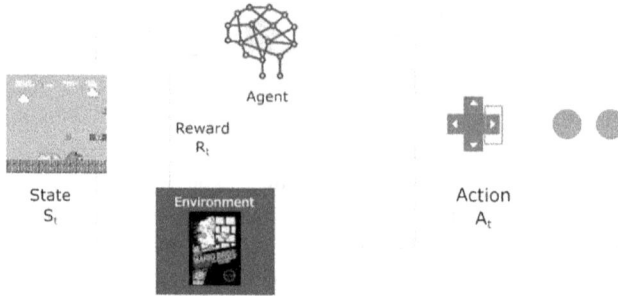

FIGURE 19.14 Reinforcement learning.

any issue, we need a prepared proficient and a condition likewise as an approach to manage interface the two through an investigation circle. To interface the operator to the earth, we give it a huge load of moves that it can have that affect nature. To interface the ground to the director, we have it interminably issue two signs to the topic master: a refreshed state and a prize (our support signal for lead).

Where Is Reinforcement Learning in the Real World?

Video Games: One of the most comprehensively saw spots to see fortress learning is in learning to play. Take a gander at Google's stronghold learning application, AlphaZero, and AlphaGo, which figured out some approach to play the game Go. Our Mario model is besides a typical model. Right now, I don't have the foggiest idea concerning any creation grade game that has a fortress learning master passed on as its game AI. In any case, envision that this will soon be an engaging choice for game designers to utilize.

Industrial Simulation: For some mechanical applications (think back to back advancement systems), it is critical to have our machines figure out some approach to finish their assignments without hardcoding their strategies. This can be a more reasonable and more secure choice; it can even be less inclined to disappointment. We can comparatively assist our machines by utilizing less influence to set aside our cash. More than that, we can begin this all inside an entertainment to not waste some money if we may break our machine (Tuna, 2015).

Resource Management: Reinforcement learning is useful for examining complex conditions. It can deal with the need to change specific necessities. Take, for instance, Google's data living spaces. They utilized fortress learning to fit the need to fulfill our capacity necessities; in any case, do it as proficiently as could be ordinary considering the current circumstance, reducing immense expenses. How might this affect the ordinary individual and us? More reasonable data are hoarding costs for us and less of an effect on nature we as a whole offer.

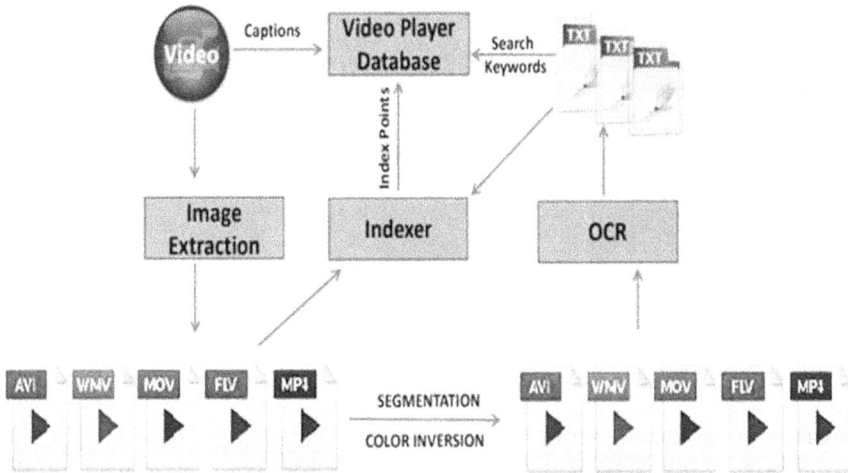

FIGURE 19.15   Videos framework: indexing analyzes frames.

19.6   APPLICATIONS OF MACHINE LEARNING APPROACH FOR VIDEO INDEXING

Video ordering, confining the video into basic segments, can essentially improve the accessibility – machine learning for indexing records to give point-based division. Specific text-based indexing algorithms were made to see point change in the video. These algorithms join neighboring video bundles with high substance similarity to shape subject pieces, which are tended to by indexing focuses. Exactly when everything is said in done, it isn't clear which recall for a video slide is enormous for recognizing subject change (Figure 19.15).

A video indexing approach utilizing machine learning can use every single authentic part, for example, the number of words in a slide, n-grams, title, or text with enormous substance estimations. Among the top-level machine learning algorithms, outfit models, for example, random forest and bagging, were discovered valuable and reasonable to utilize. They moreover give likelihood spreads, which draws in the customer to pick an ideal number of record focuses. Few of the applications are dealt further.

19.6.1   News Classification

News characterization is another benchmark use of a machine learning approach (ubuntupit, 2020). Presently, the volume of information has grown hugely on the web through video. Video order is the essential zone where sound-based philosophies are found rather than in writings and video approach. The usage of weakly supervised machine learning methods can hugely diminish the computational cost. Up until this point, no work has been represented on the utilization of the Multiple Instance Learning (MIL) approach on news video ordering. The MIL issue was the first point by point for the task of digit affirmation. Here ordering is done by the reports with pertinent catchphrases found in talk and the kind of "ticker text" on the visuals. Here, video can be recorded with a lot of catchphrases, which give the semantics of the video-divide around the time-point. News video ordering builds up yield from Optical Character Recognition (OCR) on the visual content, face recognizer, and speaker recognizing evidence (Repp et al., 2008). Hence, there are a couple of techniques for machine learning, i.e., support vector machine, Naive Bayes, k-nearest neighbor, etc. Also, there is a couple of "news characterization programming" that are open.

19.6.2 VIDEO SURVEILLANCE

A little video record contains more information diverged from text files and other media reports, such as sound and pictures (ubuntupit, 2020). Hence, isolating important information from video, i.e., the robotized video perception framework, has become a hot exploration issue. With this regard, video observation is one of the impelled use of a machine learning approach. Reconnaissance video indexing and retrieval used to (1) consolidate perceived video contents (yield from a video examination module) with visual words (figured over all the crude video outlines) to enhance the video indexation in a complementary manner; utilizing this plan, user can make questions about objects of intrigue in any event when the video investigation yield isn't accessible; (2) support an intelligent component age (at present shading histogram and direction) that gives an office for users to make inquiries at various levels as indicated by the from the earlier accessible data and the health outcomes from retrieval; (3) build up an importance input module adjusted to the indexing plan and the particular properties of observation videos for the video reconnaissance context.

19.6.3 SPEECH RECOGNITION

Speech recognition discourse acknowledgment is the path toward changing verbally communicated words into text. It is besides called programmed discourse acknowledgment, PC talk affirmation, or talk to message (ubuntupit, 2020). This field is benefitted by the movement of the machine learning approach and broad information. This development should be used in this video ordering. The talk is removed from the soundtrack and is taken care of as metadata in a condition of amicability with the video. During recovery, a watchword is changed over to a phoneme string, and this phoneme string is looked for in the video metadata. Alternatively, this engine can record the soundtrack and change it to the video. The talk affirmation framework using the machine learning approach defeats in a better way than The framework utilizing a typical procedure. Since, in a machine learning approach, the framework is set up before it goes for endorsement. What makes a difference is generally in the way the talk information is interpreted and recorded. There is no language word reference used in the phoneme-based limit, and a constant arrangement of phonemes addresses the talk information.

19.6.4 SERVICES OF SOCIAL MEDIA

Online media utilizes the machine learning way to deal with oversee make beguiling and remarkable highlights; for example, individuals you may know, proposition, and respond alternatives for their customers. These highlights are only a delayed consequence of the machine learning strategy. Do you consider how they utilize the machine learning way to deal with a draw in you in your social record? For instance, Facebook continually notices your exercises like those you visit, your tendencies, working atmosphere, and study place. Additionally, machine learning dependably acts subject to experience. Along these lines, Facebook gives you a suggestion subject to your exercises.

19.6.5 MEDICAL SERVICES

Machine learning strategies, contraptions are utilized comprehensively in the region of the associated clinical issue. To perceive an illness, treatment coordinating, related clinical assessment, and assumption for the infirmity circumstance (ubuntupit, 2020). Utilizing machine learning-based programming in the human organization's issue gets progress in our clinical science. A video observing framework with wearable cameras is utilized for early diagnostics of Dementia. A video acquiring setup is organized, and the methods are made for ordering the recorded video (Tsutsumi and Nakajima, 2001). The uproar of expansive media material and its manner yield testing issues for this substance's modified ordering. Video plans will be used by clinical practicing, who are enthusiastic about explicit events (cooking, washing, scrutinizing), explicitly put (kitchen, garden, parlor) in the family and besides in outdoor conditions. To make their work less complex, the course of action parts should be listed and summarized.

19.6.6 AGE/GENDER IDENTIFICATION

The recently forensic related task has become a hot examination issue in the domain of exploration. Various specialists are attempting to convey an incredible and capable framework to develop an upgraded framework. In this unique circumstance, age, or sexual direction, unmistakable verification is a huge endeavor for some instances. Age or sex ID should be conceivable using a machine learning and AI algorithm, for instance, using an SVM classifier. Many machine learning programming applications are utilized to recognize clients' age and sex who pass by dependent on online face examinations and consequently begins playing. It tends to be utilized to figure age and sexual orientation alongside that can likewise discover numerous appearances in an image and gauge each face's age. The late machine learning approach of the Convolutional Neural Network is generally utilized for age and sexual orientation acknowledgment and preparation (Figure 19.16).

Neural organizations were instructed to separate age and sex by video close to 80% even more definitely; it predicts age and sex, and makes a ton of 1,000 numbers (quality vector) that astoundingly property each person and licenses them to be perceived from others by using video assessment.

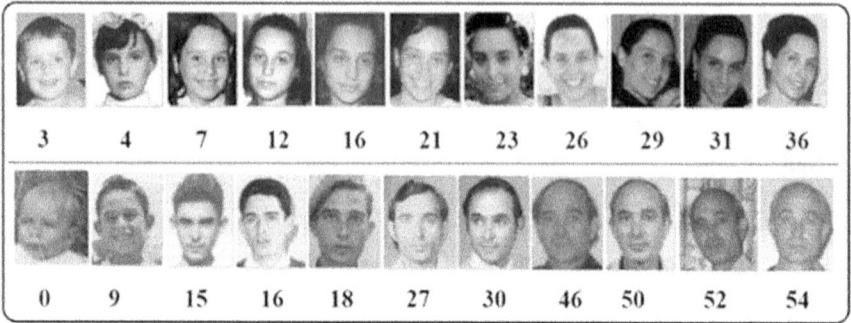

FIGURE 19.16   Sample age detection mechanism.

19.6.7 Information Retrieval

The primary machine learning and AI approach is data retrieval. It is the way toward eliminating the information or composed data from the unstructured data. Since, eventually, data accessibility has been developed greatly for online web diaries, districts, and electronic life. It anticipates a key occupation in a colossal data locale. In a machine learning approach, a lot of unstructured data is taken for input and, all things considered, eliminates the information from the data. The arranged article is being followed for raised level examination. In this examination, the focus is on distinguishing individuals and not considering the affirmation of their astounding activities. Human acknowledgment is a problematic task from a machine vision perspective as it is affected by a full extent of possible appearance as a result of changing articulated present, pieces of clothing, lighting, and establishment, yet prior data on these limitations can improve the area execution.

19.6.8 Language Identification

Language recognition (Language Guessing) is the path toward recognizing such a style. Apache OpenNLP, Apache Tika, is the language perceiving programming. There are a couple of approaches to manage to isolate the word. Among these, the machine learning and man-made cognizance approach are capable. Furthermore, in a customary world, communicating in language likewise is recognizing by utilizing the ordering mechanism. And besides, in an ideal world, conveying in language also is recognizing by using the ordering instrument. Ordering with different reports recorded from various Indian coordinates in English and Bangla is one of the critical Indian lingos.

Various scholarly tasks, incorporating imparted inconspicuous language verification, are straightforward for individuals yet simultaneously going after for PCs. One way to deal with advancing toward such a task is to reflect the human cerebrum. The top tier in the field is called machine Learning and is all things considered successfully used for different endeavors in speech and language understanding, computer vision, and re- gardless, beating individuals in explicit tasks (Figure 19.17).

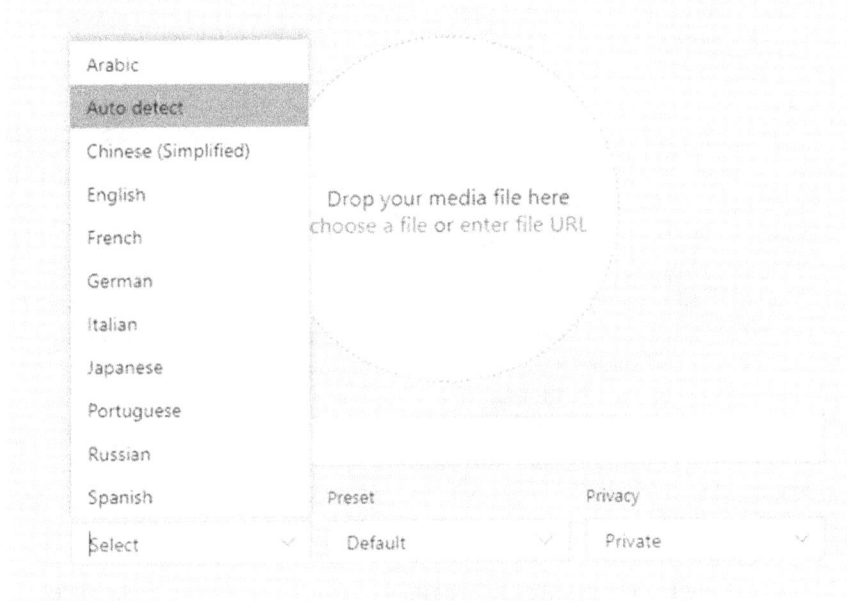

FIGURE 19.17   Sample language identification using video indexing.

19.6.9   ROBOT CONTROL

A machine learning algorithm is used in a grouping of the robot control structure. For instance, a few sorts of examinations have been attempting to manage a steady helicopter flight and helicopter aerobatics starting late. A robot driving for more than 100 miles inside the desert was won by a robot that used machine learning to refine its ability to see out of reach things. This ought to be conceivable by giving the support check after each second for this video mentioning wants an amazing strategy to give further. The Android application will open a site page with a video screen for knowledge and control of the robot and camera. Android Smartphone and Raspberry pi board are associated with Wi-Fi. An Android Smartphone sends a removed sales, which Raspberry pi board gets and in a way the robot moves. The video streaming is done using the MJPG decoration program that gets mjpeg information and sends it through an HTTP meeting.

19.7   CASE STUDIES

Case study 1: Indexing using visual cues, transcription, and OCR

Indexing permits the watcher to rapidly find an ideal spot in the introduction or talk without the need to burrow around physically. This is priceless for more extended presentations and talks where the watcher might need to return to critical minutes or underlying learning themes in the video (epiphan, 2020).

Machine learning can index a being broadcast video utilizing a couple of various techniques:

Audio transcription: Audio can be genuinely deciphered to make indexable content information. Notwithstanding, this technique costs gigantic time and human effort.

Visual/audio cues: Alternatively, a recorded talk or live event can be filed subject to visual or sound signs, for instance, crowd adulation worship, a slide change, or another speaker on the stage (epiphan, 2020).

Optical character recognition: Optical Character Recognition, or OCR, is an advancement that allows you to change over a collection of records, for instance, checked paper files, PDF reports, or computerized pictures into accessible content information (epiphan, 2020). This information would then have the option to be filed, allowing clients to conveniently discover express information inside a report or media record.

Machine learning can help motorize all of these video ordering strategies, helping with saving gigantic costs by diminishing the prerequisite for manual interpretation. Human administrators can rather use their occasion to affirm/change over content, thus assisting the item with learning words and any language issues.

Machine learning possibilities:

- Convert sound into text, and rundown key bright lights in the VOD subject to the interpreted substance.
- Convert overlays, lower thirds, and other on-screen text into available data with OCR and regularly record key focus in the video.
- Learn clear visual and sound finishes paperwork (for example, applause, the disclosure of a mediator's face) and typically make a document territory when signs are perceived in the video (Figure 19.18).

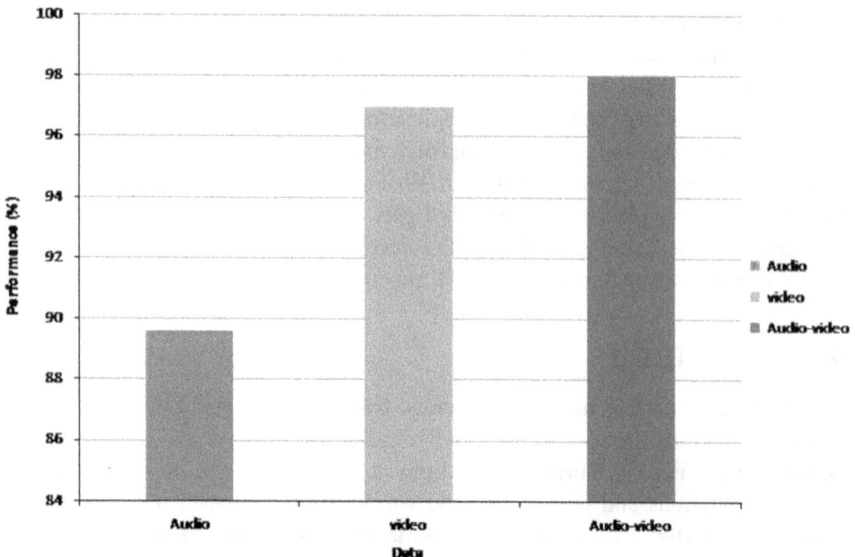

FIGURE 19.18   Performance of audio and video indexing.

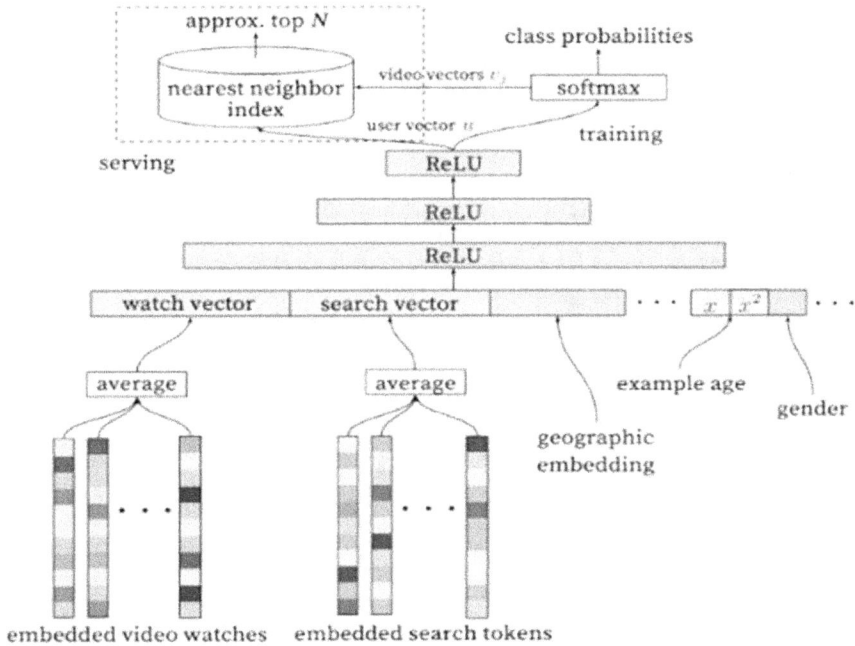

FIGURE 19.19   Machine learning for YouTube video indexing methods.

Case study 2: View duration and session time based on YouTube videos

YouTube re-jigged the algorithm to support see span (a.k.a. watch time), and time spent on the platform by and large (a.k.a. meeting time). This caused another flood of irritating strategies: like setting aside a pointless measure of effort to convey on a video's guarantee. Even though to be reasonable, YouTube has consistently told individuals that snakey enhancement rehearses don't ensure anything and simply concentrate on making great videos. Remunerating videos that held watchers for longer measures of time (some content makers decipher this as "longer videos," however that is not the situation) implied that makers needed to reduce the time they spent creating every video (HootSuite, 2020). They couldn't stand to make visits, excellent, and work escalated videos that were additionally long (Figure 19.19).

19.8   SUMMARY

Indexing is a data structure technique to productively recover records from the database documents dependent on specific properties on which the indexing has been completed. The video indexing system encourages users to have productive access, search, and perusing capacities to the ideal mixed media (sound video) content. The video indexing and retrieval system gives the user the ability to index and recover the video data in an effective way. In this chapter, a machine learning-based approach for indexing videos was discussed. This approach analyzes the various technique of machine learning algorithms.

REFERENCES

Chen, S.-C., Shyu, M.-L., and Zhang, C., "Innovative shot boundary detection for video indexing," *Video Data Management and Information Retrieval*, pp. 217–236. IGI Global, 2005.

Cortes, C. and Vapnik, V., "Support-vector networks," *Machine Learning*, 20(3), 273–297, 1995.

Deshmukh Bhagyashri, D., "Review of content-based video lecture retrieval," *International Journal of Research in Engineering and Technology*, 3(11), 306–312, 2014.

epiphan, https://www.epiphan.com/blog/machine-learning-applications/, 7 Jul 2020.

Gayathri, N. and Mahesh, K., "A systematic study on video indexing," *International Journal of Pure and Applied Mathematics*, 118(8), 425–428, 2018.

HootSuite, https://blog.hootsuite.com/how-the-youtube-algorithm-works/, 16 Jul 2020.

Hu, W., Xie, N., Li, L., Zeng, X., and Maybank, S., "A survey on visual content-based video indexing and retrieval," *IEEE Transactions on Systems, Man, and Cybernetics, Part C (Applications and Reviews)*, 41(6), 797–819, 2011.

Jeong, H.J., Kim, T.-E., and Kim, M.H., "An accurate lecture video segmentation method using sift and adaptive threshold," in Proc. 10th Int. Conf. Advances Mobile Comput., pp. 285–288, 2012. [Online]. Available: http://doi.acm.org/10.1145/2428955.2429011.

Kate, L.S., Waghmare, M.M., and Priyadarshi, A., "An approach for automated video indexing and video search in large lecture video archives," in 2015 International Conference on Pervasive Computing (ICPC), pp. 1–5. IEEE, 2015.

Koniusz, P., Yan, F., Gosselin, P.H., and Mikolajczyk, K., "Higher-order occurrence pooling for bags-of-words: Visual concept detection," *IEEE Transactions on Pattern Analysis and Machine Intelligence*, 39(2), 313–326, 2017.

Podlesnaya, A. and Podlesnyy, S., "Deep learning-based semantic video indexing and retrieval" Proceedings of SAI Intelligent Systems, Springer, 2016.

Repp, S., Gross, A., and Meinel, C., "Browsing within lecture videos based on the chain index of speech transcription," *IEEE Transactions on Learning Technologies*, 1(3), 145–156, 2008.

Rumelhart, D.E., Hinton, G.E., and Williams, R.J., "Learning representations by back-propagating errors," *Cognitive Modeling*, 5, 533–536, 1988.

Saravanan, D. and Srinivasan, S., "Video image retrieval using data mining techniques," *Journal of Computer Applications* 5(01), 39–42, 2012.

Tsutsumi, F. and Nakajima, C., "Hybrid approach of video indexing and machine learning for rapid indexing and highly precise object recognition," in Proceedings 2001 International Conference on Image Processing (Cat. No. 01CH37205), vol. 2, pp. 645–648. IEEE, 2001.

Tuna, T., "Automated lecture video indexing with text analysis and machine learning (Doctoral dissertation)," 2015.

ubuntupit, https://www.ubuntupit.com/top-20-best-machine-learning-applications-in-real-world/, 20 Dec 2020.

Yang, H., Siebert, M., Lühner, P., Sack, H., and Meinel, C., "Automatic lecture video indexing using video OCR technology," in *Proceedings of International Symposium on Multimedia (ISM)*, pp. 111–116, 2011.

20 A Risk-Based Ensemble Classifier for Breast Cancer Diagnosis

*B. Malar, Priyadarshini Srirambalaji,
and T.S. Vanitha*
Department of Applied Mathematics and Computational
Sciences, PSG College of Technology, Coimbatore, India

CONTENTS

20.1 INTRODUCTION

With 1 in 22 women predicted to develop breast cancer, this disease is an increasing challenge in India (Bailey, 2013). The five-year survival rate stands at 60% for Indian women. According to WHO's latest assessment, the cancer cases are said to multiply five times over the next decade (by 2025) in India. The results also show that women are more likely to fall prey to it than men (Basu et al., 2019). The data collected from the www.breastcancerindia.com website shows that one-fourth of all female cancer cases are breast cancers. Although over a million cancer cases are diagnosed every year in India, over 7 lakh people die due to disease because of late diagnosis. By 2020, the Indian Council of Medical Research projections show that India is at the risk of developing over 17.3 lakh new cases of cancer and having over 8.8 lakh deaths due to the disease. The most important and threatening fact is that the oncologist-patient ratio in our country is 1:2,000 (Sushmi, 2016). These facts motivate us to develop a system to assist oncologists/onco-surgeons in diagnosing breast cancer from fine-needle aspiration (FNA) data. The main focus of the chapter is to design a decision support system using FNA data and an efficient machine learning algorithm.

Given a data set that contains a set of n instances each has a set of d inputs and an outcome, supervised machine learning algorithms focus on finding a mapping from input to output. The machine learning models are evaluated and analyzed by applying models on the test set and predicting them. Models are evaluated using metrics such as accuracy to area-under-the-ROC curve. Thus, the objective of a machine learning algorithm is to improve the generalization performance on a test set for a task. An ensemble of classifiers (Alpaydin, 2004) is one such algorithm to increase the classifying ability of classifiers by strategically combining the predictions of multiple base classifiers and constructing models. It reduces the chance of predicting data points wrongly. Furthermore, it improves the stability and accuracy of the ensemble classifier.

To improve the ensemble accuracy and stability, various techniques have been entrenched. The strategy of treating the training data, the algorithms used and the aggregation methods followed vary in across these techniques. Bagging (Breiman, 1996), boosting (Freund and Schapire, 1997), and cascading (Gama and Brazdil, 2000; Malar and Nadarajan, 2020; Viola and Jones, 2001) fall under the category of popular ensembling techniques.

This chapter proposes a risk-based ensemble classifier for cancer diagnosis. The key notion of the proposed work is to develop an ensemble machine learning algorithm to construct an efficient model by combining all the weak learners and predict future data accurately. The main contributions of the proposed work are three-fold:

1. Propose an efficient predictive model for diagnosing cancer disease using an ensemble model that combines diverse machine learning algorithms like the k-nearest neighbor, Bayesian classifier, decision tree, Support Vector Machine, Linear discriminant analysis, and Isotonic Separation.
2. Prove the efficiency of ensemble classifier empirically and statistically by comparing the top of the line machine learning algorithms with ensemble classifier in terms of F-measure.
3. Improve the performance of the ensemble classifier using risk analysis is also done on the class label chosen through majority voting from the ensemble classifier.

The contributions of this chapter are arranged as follows. In section 2 the reviews of the literature related to the ensemble classifier are captured. In section 3 the background details of base classifiers are highlighted. Section 4 details the proposed risk-based ensemble classifier. Section 5 demonstrates and analyzes the experimental and statistical results of base classifiers and the proposed risk-based ensemble classifier. Finally, in section 7 the summary and scope for future works conclude the chapter.

20.2 RELATED WORKS

Recently, ensemble learners have become well known to address time and space complexities in learning abundant data using an amalgamation of multiple learners. Numerous ensemble algorithms are omnipresent across a variety of applications. Stacking amalgamates multiple classifiers using meta classifiers (Alpaydin, 2004). Based on the predictions of multiple classifiers, test data is predicted based on majority voting (Alpaydin, 2004). Bagging (Breiman, 1996) combines multiple weak learners using the deterministic method. Boosting (Freund and Schapire, 1997) learns a model by increasing the probability of data points that are misclassified. Cascade architecture (Gama and Brazdil, 2000; Malar and Nadarajan, 2020; Viola and Jones, 2001) has also been deployed for solving the scalable optimization problem in isotonic separation (Malar and Nadarajan, 2020) and Support Vector Machine (SVM) (Graf et al., 2004). The underlying principle of an SVM is a constrained convex optimization problem that is used for isolating support vectors from the data set (Christopher, 1998; Joachims, 1998; Joachims, 2002; Catanzaro et al., 2008). Finally, online algorithms take data in chunks and construct and update models. These algorithms have been proposed on SVM and isotonic separation (Malar and Nadarajan, 2020). These works motivate to use ensemble technique to enhance the classification performance of the ensemble classifiers using risk analysis.

20.2.1 PROBLEM STATEMENT

Given a data set $D = \{(\mathbf{x}_i, y_i)\}$ with n instances in which each instance $\mathbf{x}_i$ is an input vector of size d, $\mathbf{x}_i = (x_{i1}, x_{i2}, \dots, x_{id}) \in \mathfrak{R}^d$, and an output label $y_i \in \{0, 1\}$. Given a set of training instances, the significance of the risk-based ensemble classifier is to develop a model that is an ensemble of multiple classifiers and predict test data using risk analysis in such a way that the model obtained from the risk-based ensemble classifier increases accuracy.

20.3 BACKGROUND

This section discusses the theory behind the base classifiers and their description.

20.3.1 K-NEAREST NEIGHBOR

The objective of this simple classifier is to classify a new, unseen instance based on attributes and training data set. The strategy is to measure the Euclidean distance between the test instance and training data. We find K training points that are closest to the test or query instance and the query instance is assigned to a class with a majority of its K-closest neighbors. In the case of ties, predictions are done by the human expert. K-Nearest neighbor algorithm uses the neighborhood as the prediction value of the new query instance (Boutin, 2008).

20.3.2 Naïve Bayes Classifier

It is a straightforward probabilistic classifier to detect class labels and deploys Bayes theorem for classification. In the Bayesian framework, the probability that a given data belongs to either of the class, benign or malignant, is calculated by using the Bayes theorem given as follows:

$$\hat{y} = \begin{cases} malignant & if \ P(malignant|X) > P(benign|X) \\ benign & otherwise \end{cases} \tag{20.1}$$

$$\text{Posterior probability } P(C|X) = \frac{P(X|C)P(C)}{P(X)} \ where \ C \in \{malignant, \ benign\} \tag{20.2}$$

$$\text{Marginal probability } P(X) = \sum_{i=1}^{k} P(X|C_i)P(C_i) \tag{20.3}$$

Where k is the number of possible classes, $P(C_i|X)$ is the posterior probability that x belongs to the class C_i, $P(x|C_i)$ is the probability of x given that x belongs to C_i. For our classification task, the posterior probabilities of malignant and benign are as follows:

$$P(malignant|X) = \frac{P(X|malignant)P(malignant)}{P(X)} \tag{20.4}$$

$$P(benign|X) = \frac{P(X|benign)P(benign)}{P(X)} \tag{20.5}$$

$$P(X) = P(X|malignant)P(malignant) + P(X|benign)P(benign) \tag{20.6}$$

The likelihood or the conditional probability is calculated as given below:

$$P(X|C_k) = \prod_j P(x_j|C_k) \tag{20.7}$$

The Bayesian classifier is obtained by assuming that the attributes are conditionally independent.

20.3.3 ISOTONIC SEPARATION

The model of isotonic separation is found in Chandrasekaran et al. (2005), Jacob et al. (2007), Ryu et al. (2007), Malar et al. (2012, 2019), and Malar and Nadarajan (2013).

Given D, learning a concept in isotonic separation is to find an isotonic function from the data. Isotonic separation relabels the data points in the non-isotonic data set and minimizes the number of misclassifications to convert the data set into isotonic. This scenario can be formulated as a linear programming problem (LPP), which minimizes the total misclassification penalty.

$$
\begin{aligned}
&\min \quad \alpha \Sigma_{\forall \mathbf{x}_i, y_i \in \{1\}} (1 - \hat{y}_i) + \beta \Sigma_{\forall \mathbf{x}_i, y_i \in \{0\}} \hat{y}_i \\
&\text{subject to the constraints} \\
&\hat{y}_i - \hat{y}_j \geq 0 \ \textit{for} \ (i, j) \in R \quad \text{(isotonic constraint)} \\
&0 \leq \hat{y}_i \leq 1 \ \textit{for} \ \forall \, \mathbf{x}_i \in D \quad \text{(boundary constraint)}
\end{aligned}
\tag{20.8}
$$

where $\hat{y}_i$ is a label assigned to a data point during relabeling for transforming the data set into isotonic. α and β are penalties assigned to misclassifications $\Sigma_{\forall \mathbf{x}_i, y_i = 1} (1 - \hat{y}_i)$ and $\Sigma_{\forall \mathbf{x}_i, y_i = 0} \hat{y}_i$ denote the number of misclassifications in each class. Let $Y^* = \{\hat{y}_i | x_i \in D\}$ be a solution obtained from traditional solution techniques. Let A_1^* and A_0^* be not only sets of boundary corner points for each class but also these points become the isotonic separator and the model at the end of training in isotonic separation.

$$
\begin{aligned}
A_1^* &= \{i | \hat{y}_i = 1 \ \textit{and} \ \nexists \hat{y}_j \in Y^*, \ i \neq j, \ \hat{y}_j = 1 \ \textit{and} \ (i, j) \in R\} \\
A_0^* &= \{i | \hat{y}_i = 0 \ \textit{and} \ \nexists \hat{y}_j \in Y^*, \ i \neq j, \ \hat{y}_j = 0 \ \textit{and} \ (j, i) \in R\} \\
B &= A_1^* \cup A_0^*
\end{aligned}
\tag{20.9}
$$

where $A_1^* \neq \emptyset$ and $A_0^* \neq \emptyset$.

Test data $h, \mathbf{x}_h = (x_{h1}, \ x_{h2}, \dots, x_{hd})$ is predicted based on the weighted distance between test data h and boundary points obtained as a model.

$$
\begin{aligned}
D_{h1} &= \beta \min \{\Sigma_{k=1}^d \max(x_{ik} - x_{hk}, 0) \mathbf{x}_i \in A_1^*\} \\
D_{h0} &= \alpha \min \{\Sigma_{k=1}^d \max(x_{hk} - x_{ik}, 0) \mathbf{x}_i \in A_0^*\} \\
\hat{y}_h &= \begin{cases} 1 & \text{if } D_{h1} < D_{h0} \\ 0 & \text{otherwise} \end{cases}
\end{aligned}
\tag{20.10}
$$

20.3.4 RANDOM FOREST

Random forest (Sousa and Cardoso, 2011; Gonzalez et al., 2015) is a supervised learning technique that can best be described as an ensemble of decision tree classifiers. To generate each of the individual decision trees, at each node, a random selection of attributes is taken into consideration to determine the split. During the prediction, the output of each tree is counted as a vote and the class is assigned on the principle of majority voting.

20.3.5 SUPPORT VECTOR MACHINE

Support Vector Machine (SVM) (Christopher, 1998) is a classification technique that separates instances in a d dimensional space into two regions using a maximum margin hyperplane. Given a data set D, this algorithm creates a line or hyperplane which separates the data into two classes namely benign and malignant. According to the SVM algorithm, we define the points that are closest to the line from both the classes as support vectors. The distance between the line and the support vectors is called the margin. Our goal is to find the optimum hyperplane with a maximum margin. To estimate the parameters w and w_0 such that

$$
\begin{aligned}
W^T X_i + W_0 &\geq 1 \quad \forall \ y_i \in +1 \\
W^T X_i + W_0 &\leq -1 \quad \forall \ y_i \in -1
\end{aligned}
\tag{20.11}
$$

which can be rewritten as $y_i(W^T X_i + W_0) \geq 1 \quad \forall \ y_i \in \{+1, \ -1\}$. Our task is to minimize ‖w‖ in order to maximize the margin. The standard quadratic optimization problem is defined as

$$
\begin{aligned}
&\min \frac{1}{2} \|w\|^2 \\
&s.\,t.\,c \ \ y_i(W^T X_i + W_0) \geq 1 \quad \forall \ y_i \in \{+1, \ -1\}
\end{aligned}
\tag{20.12}
$$

To convert this into an unconstrained problem using Lagrange multipliers α_i,

$$
L_P = \frac{1}{2} \|W\|^2 \ + \sum_{i=1}^{N} \alpha_i (y_i(W^T X_i + W_0) - 1)
\tag{20.13}
$$

This L_p should be minimized by finding partial derivatives of w, w_0, and maximized with $\alpha^t \geq 0$. It is solved by making use of the Karush–Kuhn–Tucker condition. This implies that the parameters are given by

$$
W = \sum_i \alpha_i y_i X_i \quad \forall \ \alpha_i \neq 0
\tag{20.14}
$$

$$
W_0 = \sum_i \alpha_i y_i X_i
\tag{20.15}
$$

The kernel trick is a method of using a linear model in the new space that corresponds to a non-linear model in the original space using suitably chosen basis functions. The kernel functions are

- Linear function
- Polynomial function
- Radial-basis function

20.3.6 LINEAR DISCRIMINANT ANALYSIS

Linear Discriminant Analysis (LDA) (Alpaydin, 2004) is a classification technique based on the statistical properties of the data set and uses the Bayes Theorem for making predictions. As seen in Naïve Bayes, while using Bayes theorem, we make use of the probability $P(x|C_i)$ which is the probability of x given that x belongs to the class C_i. However, in practice, it is infeasible to obtain this probability and is easier to assume the probability distribution of x and thereby calculate $P(x|C_i)$ theoretically. LDA assumes that each attribute follows the Gaussian distribution, which has the same variance. Using these assumptions, the estimates for mean and variance of each attribute is obtained for each class.

Given a new example x', LDA returns the probability of x' belongs to each class and thus assigns x' to the class with the highest probability. Bayes theorem states that:

$$P(C_k|X) = \frac{P(X|C_k)P(C_k)}{P(X)} \tag{20.16}$$

where,
$P(C_k)$ is the prior probability of the class k,
$P(X|C_k)$ is the probability function for x belonging to class k.
According to assumptions made in the LDA setting, we have:

$$f_k(x) = \frac{1}{\sqrt{2\pi\sigma_k}} \exp\left(-\frac{1}{2\sigma^2}(x - \mu_k)^2\right) \tag{20.17}$$

Substituting (2) in (1), and applying log, we obtain the following equation known as the discriminant function:

$$\underbrace{\delta_k(x)}_{discriminant} = x\frac{\mu_k}{\sigma^2} - \frac{\mu_k^2}{2\sigma^2} + \log(\pi_k) \tag{20.18}$$

The class for which this value is maximum is the predicted class.

We obtain the setting for quadratic discriminant analysis just by tweaking the assumptions made in LDA. Here, while retaining the fact that each attribute follows Gaussian distribution, we let them each take their variance. Thus the discriminant function is changed to $\delta_k(x) = -\frac{1}{2}(x - \mu_k)^T \Sigma_k^{-1}(x - \mu_k) + \log(\pi_k)$ which is quadratic as the name suggests.

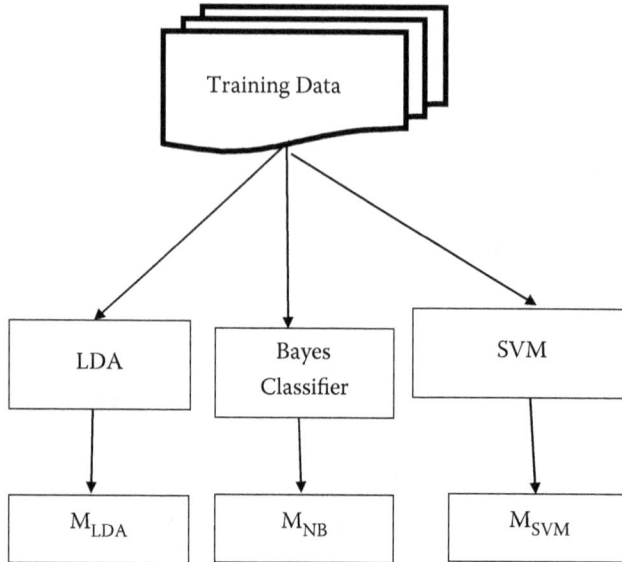

FIGURE 20.1   Training of the proposed risk-based ensemble classifier.

20.3.7   PROPOSED RISK-BASED ENSEMBLE CLASSIFIER

Given the predictions $\hat{y}_1$, $\hat{y}_2$, ..., $\hat{y}_k$, of k base classifiers, N_1, N_2, N_3, ..., N_k, the ensemble classifier combines a series of classifiers to create an improved composite classification model, N^* using the majority voting method. Training data are modeled using Naïve Bayes, Random forest, Linear SVM, Polynomial SVM, Radial SVM, Linear Discriminant Analysis (LDA), and Quadratic Discriminant Analysis (QDA) as the base classifiers as shown in Figure 20.1, and models are obtained. Given a new test data (X) to classify, the ensemble classifier counts the vote for each class and assigned the class label by considering loss functions which are formulated based on risk due to misclassification.

$$Cj = \sum_{c=1}^{k} 1(\hat{y}_c = j) \tag{20.19}$$

$$P(Cj|X) = \frac{Cj}{K} \tag{20.20}$$

Let α_m be the action that assigns data point X to class m and δ_{ik} be the loss or risk involved due to the action α_i of assigning a data point to ith class when it belongs to the kth class. For every data point to be predicted, expected loss $R(\alpha_m|X)$ is calculated for each class m and a data point is predicted as a class with minimum loss. Test data is assigned to the class with a minimum expected risk. The testing phase is shown in Figure 20.2.

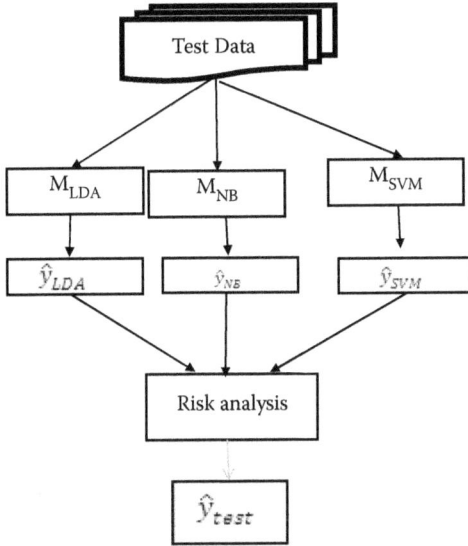

FIGURE 20.2 Testing phase of the proposed risk-based ensemble classifier.

$$R(\alpha_m|X) = \sum_{j=1}^{k} P(Cj|X)\delta_{mj} \quad 1 \le m \le k \tag{20.21}$$

$$\hat{y} = \min_j R(\alpha_j|X) \quad 1 \le m \le k \tag{20.22}$$

20.4 EXPERIMENTAL ANALYSIS

To prove the efficiency of the risk-based ensemble classifier, experiments are conducted on the Wisconsin Breast cancer data set and the results are reported.

20.4.1 DATA SETS

The Wisconsin Breast Cancer data set (WBCD) (Merz and Murphy, 1998) consists of 699 data points that were obtained from the University of Wisconsin Hospitals are taken for the study. Among these data points, 458 are diagnosed as benign and 241 are diagnosed as malignant, respectively. There are nine attributes for each data point namely, uniformity of cell size, uniformity of cell shape, clump thickness, marginal adhesion, mitoses, bland chromatin, epithelial cell size, bare nuclei, and normal nucleoli. All values are in the range of 0 to 10, denoting the abnormal state of the tumor (0-low 10-high).

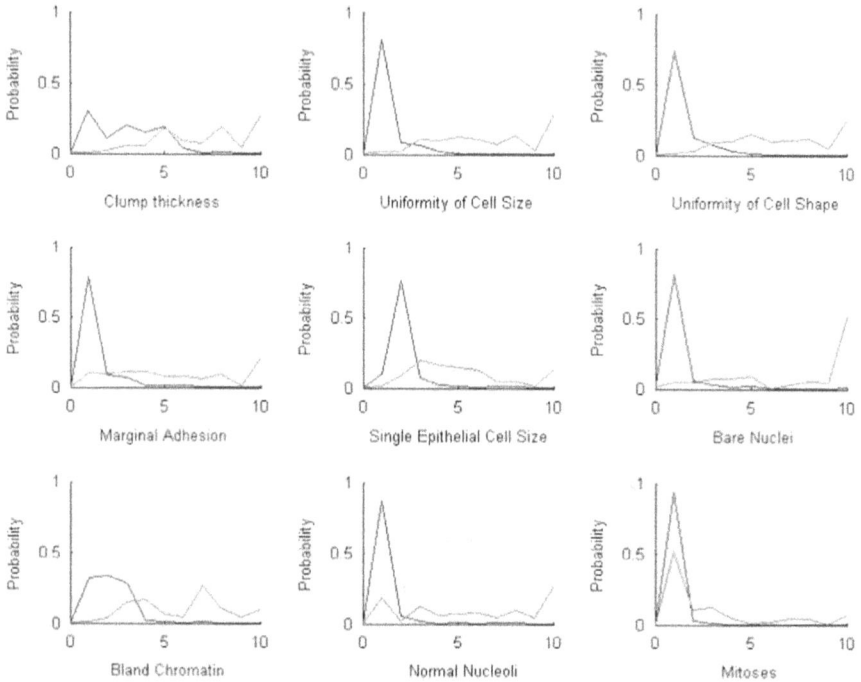

FIGURE 20.3 Feature-wise histograms for the breast cancer data.

20.4.2 EXPERIMENTAL SETUP

Experiments of base classifiers and the risk-based ensemble classifiers are conducted using the breast cancer data set and the impact of each feature in the malignant and benign cancer is presented as histograms (Han, 2005) in Figure 20.3. The red curve denotes the probability of malignancy (Range from 1 to 10) of a particular feature. The blue curve denotes the probability of benign for a feature. It is observed that the probability of malignancy is less when a feature takes smaller values and becomes more for bigger values. Similarly, the probability of benign is more for smaller values and less for bigger values.

Average performance measures are calculated using accuracy, Precision, Recall, F-measure, ROC, and AUC (Fawcett, 2006). The given classifier and a patient's lump features results in four possible outcomes during prediction. For instance, a malignant patient is diagnosed as malignant, it is counted as true positive (TP), it is counted as false negative (FN) when a malignant patient is diagnosed as benign by the classifier. Another instance, when a benign patient is diagnosed as benign, it is counted as true negative (TN). When a benign patient is diagnosed as malignant, it is counted as a false positive (FP). Testing error terms are calculated by using the terminologies as given below. Accuracy of the classifier is defined as the total number of correctly predicted patients (both malignant and benign) divided by the total number of patients. Precision is the fraction of true positive predictions (/true negative predictions) to a total number of positive predictions (negative predictions) and recall is defined as the fraction of true positives predictions (/ true negative predictions) to a total number of positives (/negatives) in the data set.

$$Accuracy = \frac{TP + TN}{TP + TN + FP + FN}$$

$$Precision = \frac{TP}{TP + FP}$$

$$Recall \frac{TP}{TP + FN}$$

$$F - measure = \frac{2 * Preciison * Recall}{Precision + Recall}$$

Since the data set has class skew i.e., imbalanced classes, Receiver Operating Characteristic (ROC) (Fawcett, 2006) is used to evaluate the classifier. The measures associated with ROC are as follows:

$$True\ Positive\ Rate = \frac{TP}{TP + FN}$$

$$False\ Positive\ Rate = \frac{FP}{TN + FP}$$

A ROC graph demonstrates the relative conflict between false positive rate and true positive rate. The average accuracy, precision, recall, and F-measure of base classifiers and the proposed risk-based ensemble classifier is shown in Table 20.1. Results show that the proposed risk-based ensemble classifier gives significant outcome in terms of accuracy, precision, and recall.

The corresponding algorithm shows better results, which are indicated in bold.

Figures 20.4 and 20.5 demonstrate the ROC curves of all the base classifiers and the proposed risk-based ensemble classifier. Results show that the random forest is superior to all other classifiers. Results from Figure 20.5 show that risk-based ensemble classifier performs better than base classifiers and random forest. To find the significance of the models using the paired t-test and one-way ANOVA test for F-measure and AUC measure, a statistical analysis is done.

20.4.3 STATISTICAL ANALYSIS

To validate the significance of the proposed risk-based ensemble classifier (Klotz, 2006; Dawson, 1997) statistical analysis is done. One-way ANOVA is conducted

TABLE 20.1

Comparative Study of Different Measures Using Base and Ensemble Classifiers

Model	Accuracy	Precision	Recall	F-Measure	AUC
Naïve Bayes	0.96	0.97	0.97	0.97	**0.99**
Random Forest	0.97	0.99	0.97	**0.98**	**0.99**
SVM Linear	0.96	0.97	0.97	0.97	**0.99**
SVM Polynomial	0.97	**0.99**	0.96	**0.98**	**0.99**
SVM Radial	0.96	**0.99**	0.95	0.97	**0.99**
LDA	0.96	0.96	0.98	0.97	0.97
QDA	0.95	0.98	0.94	0.96	0.98
Isotonic Separation	0.92	0.87	0.91	0.89	0.92
Risk-Based Ensemble	**0.98**	**0.99**	**0.99**	0.97	**0.99**

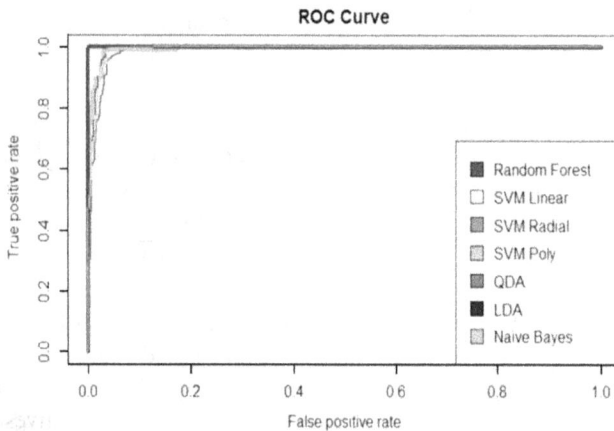

FIGURE 20.4 ROC curve of base classifiers.

by setting the null hypothesis as there is no significant difference between the proposed risk-based ensemble classifier and base classifiers in terms of AUC, and the alternate hypothesis as there is a significant difference in AUC between the classifiers. Results from Table 20.2 show that there are significant differences between all the base classifiers and the risk-based ensemble at a 95% confidence level. To find the statistical validity between every pair of algorithms paired t-test is conducted and the results are presented in Table 20.3.

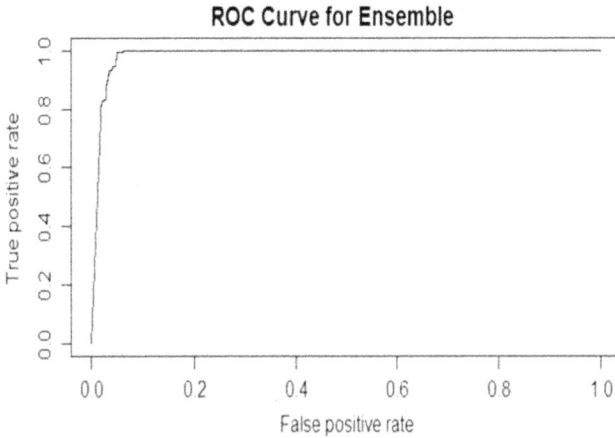

FIGURE 20.5   ROC curve for the proposed. Risk-Based Ensemble Classifier

TABLE 20.2
One-Way ANOVA between the Base and the Proposed Classifier Based on AUC

	DF	Sum of Squares	Mean Squares	F Value	Probability (>F)
Model	6	0.001226	0.0002043	2.007	0.0778
Residuals	63	0.006410	0.0001018	–	–

Signif.codes:0'***'0.001'**'0.01'*'0.05'.'0.1''1

TABLE 20.3
Results of Paired t-Tests

	Isotonic Separation	LDA	Naïve Bayes	QDA	Random Forest	SVM Linear	SVM Poly	RBE
LDA	0.003	–						
Naïve Bayes	0.002	1						
QDA	0.004	1	1					
Random Forest	0.0008	1	1	1				
SVM Linear	0.002	1	1	1	1			
SVM Polynomial	0.002	1	1	1	1	1		
SVM Radial	0.001	1	1	1	1	1	1	
Risk-Based Ensemble	0.001	0.001	0.002	0.001	0.001	1	1	

The statistical and experimental results show that there is a significant difference between isotonic separation and the other models.

20.4.4 FINDINGS

The proposed risk-based ensemble classifier predicts data by combining the models of diverse classifiers. This ensemble includes machine learning algorithms that model data with an assumption of normality (LDA, QDA, Naïve Bayes), algorithms that model linearly separable (SVM) and non-separable data (SVM with kernel functions), algorithms that model ordered data (Isotonic separation), and algorithms that model discrete features (random forest). So, this is capable of modeling data that comes from any distribution. Furthermore, the expected risk is calculated using a penalty for each misclassification. So, the performance of the proposed risk-based ensemble classifier works well.

20.5 CONCLUSION

The proposed risk-based ensemble classifier is a mixture of ensemble classifier and risk analysis. An ensemble classifier is a combination of diverse classifiers that handle and kind of data. The proposed classifier is evaluated using breast cancer data and experimental and statistical results show that it outperforms other algorithms. It can be extended by conducting experiments on different data sets and analyzed.

REFERENCES

Alpaydin, E. (2004). *Introduction to Machine Learning*. The MIT Press.
Bailey, L. (2013). The growing problem of breast cancer in India. https://global.umich.edu/newsroom/
Basu, A., Ghosh, D., Mandal, B., Mukherjee, P., & Maji, A. (2019). Barriers and explanatory mechanisms in diagnostic delay in four cancers – A health-care disparity? *South Asian Journal of Cancer*, 8, 221–225. http://journal.sajc.org/text.asp?2019/8/4/221/269700
Bhattacharyya, M., Nath, J., & Bandyopadhyay, S. (2015). MicroRNA signatures highlight new breast cancer subtypes. *Gene*, 556(6), 192–198. 10.1016/j.gene.2014.11.053.
Boutin, M. (2008). A summary of KNN and other non-parametric classification techniques (including pseudo-code). https://www.projectrhea.org/rhea/index.php/KNN_Algorithm_OldKiwi
Breiman, L. (1996). Bagging predictors. *Machine Learning*, 24(2), 123–140.
Catanzaro, B., Sundaram, N., & Keutzer, K. (2008). Fast Support Vector Machine training and classification on graphics processors. In *Proceedings of the 25th International Conference on Machine Learning*, Helsinki.
Chandrasekaran, R., Ryu, Y.U., Jacob, V., & Hong, S. (2005). Isotonic separation. *Informs Journal Computing*, 17(4), 462–474.
Christopher, J.C.B. (1998). A tutorial on support vector machines for pattern recognition. *Journal of Data Mining and Knowledge Discovery*, 2, 121–167.
Dawson, R.J.M. (1997). Turning the tables: A t-table for today. *Journal of Statistics Education*, 5(2), 1–6, DOI: 10.1080/10691898.1997.11910530.
Fawcett, T. (2006). An introduction to ROC analysis. *Pattern Recognition Letters*, 27(8), 861–874.

Freund, Y. & Schapire, R.E. (1997). A decision theoretic generalization of on line learning and an application to boosting. *Journal of Computer and System Sciences*, 55(1), 119–139.

Gama, J. & Brazdil, P. (2000). Cascade generalization. *Machine Learning*, 41(3), 315–343

Gonzalez, S., Herrera, F., & Garcia, S. (2015). Monotonic random forest with an ensemble pruning mechanism based on the degree of monotonicity. *New Generation Computing*, 33(4), 367–388.

Han, J. (2005). *Datamining Concepts and Techniques*. Morgan Kaufmann Publishers Inc., San Francisco, CA, USA.

Graf, H.P., Cosatto, E., Bottou, L., Durdanovic, I., & Vapnik, V. (2004). Parallel support vector machines: the cascade SVM, Technical report, 521–528.

Jacob, V., Krishnan, R., & Ryu, Y.U. (2007). Internet content filtering using isotonic separation on content category ratings. *ACM Transactions on Internet Technology*, 7(1), 1–19.

Joachims, T. (1998). Text categorization with support vector machines: Learning with many relevant features. In *Proceedings of 1998 European Conference on Machine Learning (ECML)*.

Joachims, T. (2002). SVM light support vector machine. http://svmlight.joachims.org/.

Khan, M.U., Aziz, S., Bilal, M., & Aamir, M. (2019). Classification of EMG signals for assessment of neuromuscular disorder using empirical mode decomposition and logistic regression. In International Conference on Applied and Engineering Mathematics (ICAEM), 237–243. 10.1109/ICAEM.2019.8853684

Klotz, J.H. (2006). *A Computational Approach to Statistics*, Department of Statistics, University of Wisconsin at Madison.

Malar, B. & Nadarajan, R. (2013). Evolutionary isotonic separation for classification: Theory and experiments. *Knowledge and Information Systems*, Springer-Verlag, 10.1007/s10115-012-0579-5

Malar, B. & Nadarajan, R. (2020). An online isotonic separation with cascade architecture for binary classification. *Expert Systems with Applications*, 57, 113466.

Malar, B., Nadarajan, R., & Gowri Thangam, J. (2019). A hybrid isotonic separation algorithm for training. *Knowledge and Information Systems*, Springer-Verlag, 10.1007/s10115-012-0579-5

Malar, B., Nadarajan, R., & Sai Sundara Krishnan, G. (2012). Isotonic separation with an instance selection algorithm using softest: Theory and experiments. *WSEAS Transactions on Information Science and Applications*, 9(11), 350–367.

Merz, C.J. & Murphy, P.M. (1998). UCI Repository of Machine Learning Databases. Department of Information and Computer Sciences, University of California, Irvine.

Ryu, Y.U., Chandrasekaran, R., & Jacob, V.S. (2007). Breast cancer detection using the isotonic separation technique. *European Journal of Operational Research*, 181, 842–854.

Ryu, Y.U. & Yue, W.T. (2005). Firm bankruptcy prediction; Experimental comparison of isotonic separation and other classification approaches. *IEEE Transactions on System Man and cybernetics, Part A: Systems and Humans*, 35(5), 727–737.

Singh, P., Jain, N., & Maini, A. (2015). Investigating the effect of feature selection and dimensionality reduction on phishing website classification problem, In 1st International Conference on Next Generation Computing Technologies (NGCT), 388–393. 10.1109/NGCT.2015.7375147

Sousa, R.G. & Cardoso, J.S. (2011). Ensemble of decision trees with global constraints for ordinal classification. In *Proceedings of 11th International Conference on Intelligent Systems Design and Applications*, pp. 1164–1169.

Sushmi, D. (2016, February 4). India has just 2,000 oncologists for 10 million patients. *The Times of India*. https://timesofindia.indiatimes.com/india

Vellasques, E., Soares de Oliveira, L., Jr, A., Koerich, A., & Sabourin, R. (2008). Filtering segmentation cuts for digit string recognition. *Pattern Recognition*, 41, 3044–3053. 10.1016/j.patcog.2008.03.019

Viola, P. & Jones, M. (2001). Rapid object detection using a boosted cascade of simple features. In *Proceedings of CVPR* 3, 4.

Xu, Y., Zomer, S., & Brereton, R. (2006). Support vector machines: A recent method for classification in chemometrics. *Critical Reviews in Analytical Chemistry*, 36, 177–188. 10.1080/10408340600969486

21 Linear Algebra for Machine Learning

P. Dhanalakshmi

Associate Professor and Head, Department of Applied
Mathematics, Bharathiar University, Coimbatore, India

CONTENTS

DOI: 10.1201/9781003175865-21

NOTATIONS We start by providing the notations used in this chapter:

R, R^m real numbers, m-tuples of reals
$\mu, \lambda, \mu_1, \mu_2, \ldots \mu_m$ scalars
x,y,u,v   vectors
$(V, +, \cdot)$ vector space
m_{ij} row i and column j of matrix M
$\mathbb{R}^{p \times q}$ the real-valued matrices of order $p \times q$
$\hat{B} = (b_1, b_2, \ldots b_q), \hat{C} = (c_1, c_2, \ldots c_q)$ ordered basis
$\hat{e} = (e_1, e_2, \ldots e_q)$ the standard basis for R^n
$0 = [0, \ldots, 0]^T$ zero vector
L_w lower triangular matrix
U_p upper triangular matrix
$|A|$ determinant of the matrix
A^T transpose

21.1   INTRODUCTION

Machine learning is one of the core branches of artificial intelligence (AI). It is a technique of data analysis that mechanizes analytical model building [1–3]. The main intent of machine learning is to plan an algorithm that can extricate information from the data, recognize patterns, and build decisions with minimal human involvement. The focused advantage of machine learning is its computational speed and accuracy of the system. There are four components in machine learning: problem framing, data analysis, model building, and application, as shown in Figure 21.1.

Problem framing is focusing on the problem definition. It determines the type of alternative considered to address the problem, important observations, and the accomplishment of the solution. The data available for building the model is handled by the data analysis part [4]. This includes handling missing data, normalization, dimensionality reduction, etc. One among the appropriate linear regression methods, logistic regression, time series analysis, etc. is employed in the model building stage used to fit the training data. The model tuned in this phase is expected to the entire hidden data. Finally, the model's parameter is selected to fit the data and actual performance on the construction procession has been analyzed. Mathematical concepts and foundations are very essential to all the components in the machine learning system. Simply, machine learning is incomplete without mathematics.

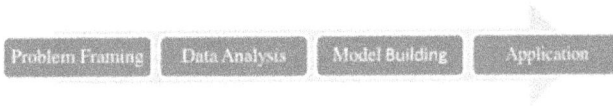

FIGURE 21.1   Components in machine learning.

Mathematics in machine learning

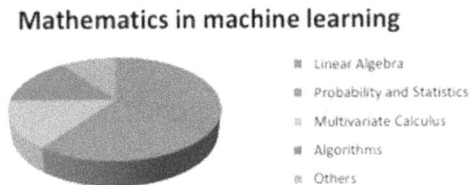

- Linear Algebra
- Probability and Statistics
- Multivariate Calculus
- Algorithms
- Others

FIGURE 21.2   Mathematics in machine learning.

21.2   LINEAR ALGEBRA – BASICS AND MOTIVATIONS

The aim of this chapter is to provide the basic mathematical concepts required for computer science learners. Linear algebra plays a prominent role in the under-standing of machine learning. Figure 21.2 will help to understand linear algebra and statistics are how important and powerful in machine learning. Hence, there is a necessity to understand the fundamental concepts of linear algebra to learn machine learning [5]. Linear algebra is used in data preprocessing, data transformation, and model evaluation. It is the study of lines and planes, vector spaces, and mappings that are essential for linear transforms. The basic concepts are discussed in this section.

21.2.1   VECTORS

Vectors and matrices are expressions of data. A numerical data is represented as a vector whereas the dataset is characterized as the matrix. A *vector* is an ordered finite list of numbers. They are usually written as a vertical array of numbers surrounded by square or curved brackets. The number of elements it contains is called the *size* of the vector. A vector of size m is called an m-vector. The set of all real numbers is written as R. The set of all m-real numbers is written as R^m. For example, In a plane, a 2-vector is used to represent a position, and a 3-vector can be used to represent the color of an image giving the RGB intensity values between 0 and 1. The vectors (0,1,0), (0,0,0) represent green and black colors, respectively. Two vectors of the same size can be *added* to form another vector of the same size by adding the corresponding elements. *Vector subtraction* is also defined similarly. Another operation *scalar multiplication* is defined as every element will get mul-tiplied by the scalar; e.g., when a vector x represents a displacement and if $\mu > 0$, then μx is a displacement in the same direction of x and if $\mu < 0$, then μx is a displacement in the opposite direction of x.

21.2.2 Vector Space

A **vector space** $W = (V, +, *)$ is a real-valued vector space of a set V under the operations

$$+ : V \times V \rightarrow V$$
$$* : \mathbb{R} \times V \rightarrow V$$

where

    i. $(V, +)$ satisfy the Abelian group
    ii. Distributive property:
        1. $\forall \mu \in \mathbb{R},\, x,\, y \in V$: $\mu * (x + y) = \mu * x + \mu * y$
        2. $\forall \mu \in \mathbb{R},\, x \in V$: $(\mu + \varphi) * x = \mu * x + \varphi * x$

    iii. Associative property: $\forall \mu,\, \varphi \in \mathbb{R},\, x \in V$: $\mu * (\varphi * x) = (\mu\varphi) * x$
    iv. There is an identity element with respect to the operation: $\forall x \in V$: $1 * x = x$

The set of all elements $x \in V$ are called *vectors*. The identity element under **addition of vectors** operation+ is the 0-vector $0 = [0, \ldots, 0]^T$. The operation $*$ is a **scalar multiplication,** where the scalars μ belong to the real number set $\mathbb{R}$.

If $x_1, x_2, \ldots x_m$ are m-vectors and $\mu_1, \mu_2, \ldots \mu_m$ are scalars, then $\mu_1 x_1 + \ldots + \mu_k x_k$ is the combination of $x_1, x_2, \ldots x_m$ vectors, linearly. If there exists no trivial linear combination satisfying $\sum_{i=1}^{k} \mu_i x_i = 0$ with one $\mu_i \neq 0$, the set of vectors $x_1, \ldots, x_k$ are called **linearly dependent** and if for trivial solutions $\mu_1 = \ldots = \mu_k = 0$ the vectors $x_1, \ldots, x_k$ are called **linearly independent**. The linear independence/dependence are the vital concepts of linear algebra. Instinctively, a set of vectors that are linearly independent have no repetition, i.e., by removing any vectors from the set, something will be lost. In particular, for a vector space W, the sets of vectors A are called special vectors since they have the feature that any vector $v \in W$ can be written in the frame of the linear combination of vectors in the set A.

21.2.3 Vector Subspace

Consider the vector space $W = (V, +, *)$ and U be a subset of V; i.e., $U \subseteq V, U \neq 0$. Then the subset $U = (\mho, +, *)$ is called **vector (linear) subspace of W** if U satisfies the conditions of vector space under the operations $+$ and $*$ limited to $U \times V$ and $\mathbb{R} \times U$. Then such vector subspace can be written as $U \subseteq V$. To prove $(\mho, +, *)$ is a subspace of V it is enough to express

    1. $U \neq 0$, specifically $0 \in U$.
    2. Closure property: (i) $\lambda \in R,\, u \in U$, and $\lambda u \in U$.

(ii) $x \in U,\, y \in U,\, x + y \in U$.

21.2.4 SPAN

For the vector space $W = (V, +, \cdot)$, consider $A = \{x_1, \dots, x_k\}$ be the set of vectors. Then every vector $v \epsilon V$ is manifesting terms of the linear combination of the set of vectors in A, then such set A is called *a **generating set** of W. The smallest set of A which contains the linear combinations form a **span** of A. If A spans W, we can write $W = span[A]$ or $W = span[x_1, \dots, x_k]$. The generating sets generate the vector (sub)spaces, i.e., the vectors of the generating set can be used to represent every vector of W in the linear combination.

21.2.5 BASIS

The generating set A of the vector space V is called ***minimal*** if there exists set $\bar{A}$ such that $\bar{A} \subseteq A \subseteq V$ and spans the vector space V. Equivalently, the collection of all linearly independent generating sets of W is called minimal and it is known to be a ***basis*** of W.

21.2.6 LINEAR MAPPING

The vector spaces V *and* W under the mapping $\tau \colon V \to W$ are called a ***linear (vector space) homomorphism*** if

$$\forall\, x,\, y \epsilon W \; \forall\, \mu,\, \varphi \epsilon \mathbb{R} \colon \tau(\mu x + \varphi y) = \mu\tau(x) + \varphi\tau(y)$$

21.2.7 MATRIX

For $p, q \epsilon \mathbb{N}$, a real-valued (p, q)***matrix*** **M** is an p·q- computing of elements $m_{ij}, i = 1, \dots, p, j = 1, \dots, q$, which is arranged in an orderly manner comprised of p rows and q columns:

$$M = \begin{bmatrix} m_{11} & m_{12} & \cdots & m_{1q} \\ m_{21} & m_{22} & \cdots & m_{2q} \\ \vdots & \vdots & & \vdots \\ m_{p1} & m_{p2} & \cdots & m_{pq} \end{bmatrix}, \quad m_{ij} \epsilon \mathbb{R}.$$

By convention $(1, q)$, is called ***row matrix (vectors)*** and $(p, 1)$ is called ***column matrix (vectors)***. $\mathbb{R}^{p \times q}$ denotes the real-valued matrices of order $p \times q$.

21.2.8 MATRIX REPRESENTATION OF LINEAR MAPPINGS

Consider $\hat{B} = (b_1, b_2, \dots b_q)$ be an ordered basis of the vector space U. Every element $u \epsilon U$ can be written in the form of $u = \alpha_1 b_1 + \dots \alpha_q b_q$ in a unique way with respect to $\hat{B}$. Then the vector $[\alpha]_{\hat{B}} = \begin{pmatrix} \alpha_1 \\ \vdots \\ \alpha_q \end{pmatrix} \in R^q$, is the **coordinate vector** re-

presentation of u with respect to $\hat{B}$ with the *coordinates* of u be $\alpha_1, \ldots \alpha_n$. The standard representation of U with respect to $\hat{B}$, $\Gamma : U \to R^q$ is given by $\Gamma_{\hat{B}}[\alpha] = [\alpha]_{\hat{B}}$.

21.2.9 TRANSFORMATION MATRIX

For the vector spaces V and W, consider the ordered bases $\hat{B} = (b_1, b_2, \ldots b_p)$ and $\hat{C} = (c_1, c_2, \ldots c_q)$, respectively. Consider the linear mapping $\Gamma : V \to W$. For $i \in \{1, \ldots, q\}$,

$$\Gamma(b_j) = \alpha_{1j} c_1 + \ldots \alpha_{pj} c_q = \sum_{i=1}^{q} \alpha_{ij} c_i$$

be the unique representation of $\Gamma(b_j)$ w.r.t. $\hat{C}$. Thus the matrix A_Γ of order $p \times q$ with the elements given by $A_\Gamma(i, j) = \alpha_{ij}$ is called the **transformation matrix** of Γ.

21.2.10 DETERMINANT

A determinant means a scalar-valued function used to analyze the system of linear equations in a mathematical way. Determinants are defined only for the matrices having the same number of rows and columns (square matrices) $M \in R^{q \times q}$. I.e.

$$\det(M) = \begin{vmatrix} m_{11} & m_{12} & \cdots & m_{1q} \\ m_{21} & m_{22} & \cdots & m_{2q} \\ \vdots & \vdots & \ddots & \vdots \\ m_{q1} & m_{q2} & \cdots & m_{qq} \end{vmatrix}.$$ The **determinant** of matrix $M \in R^{q \times q}$ means

function with the square matrix as input and that maps onto a real or complex number. The determinant of an $q \times q$ matrix M can be defined with the following formula:

$$\det(M) = \sum_{i_1, i_2, \ldots i_q} \pm m_{i1} m_{i2.} \ldots m_{iq}$$

with the terms are summed over all permutations $(i_1, i_2, \ldots i_q)$ and the sign + and -, respectively, for the permutation is even or odd.

21.2.11 EIGENVALUE

For the matrix $M \in R^{q \times q}$, $\mu \in R$ is called an **eigenvalue** of M and $x \in R^q \setminus \{0\}$ as its equivalent **eigenvector** when it is satisfying **eigen equation** $Mx = \mu x$.

21.2.12   RANK

The maximum number of columns of a matrix $M \in \mathbb{R}^{p \times q}$, which are linearly independent, equals the maximum number of linearly independent rows, and it is simply called **rank**(M).

21.2.13   DIAGONAL MATRIX

A *diagonal matrix* is a matrix whose entries other than the diagonal elements are zero, i.e., they are of the form

$$D = \begin{bmatrix} c_1 & \cdots & 0 \\ \vdots & \ddots & \vdots \\ 0 & \cdots & c_n \end{bmatrix}.$$

In linear algebra, the diagonal matrix occurs in many areas because of its simple procedure to permit rapid computation of determinants, powers, and inverses. For example, the determinant value of the diagonal matrix is nothing but the product of its diagonal entries; the power value D^k can be calculated by raising the power of each diagonal element to k and in a similar way, the inverse of the diagonal matrix is the reciprocal of diagonal elements of all the nonzero elements.

21.2.14   DIAGONALIZABLE

A matrix $M \in \mathbb{R}^{q \times q}$ is called *diagonalizable* if there exists an invertible matrix $P \in \mathbb{R}^{q \times q}$ such that $D = P^{-1}MP$ is a diagonal matrix, i.e., The sequential procedure will describe in brief about diagonalizing a matrix $M \in \mathbb{R}^{q \times q}$ in the means of same linear mapping yet on a further basis and it happens to be a basis that contains the eigenvectors of M. Consider $M \in \mathbb{R}^{q \times q}$, let $\mu_1, \ldots, \mu_q$ and let $p_1, \ldots, p_q$ denote the set of scalars and vectors in $\mathbb{R}^q$, respectively. Fix $P = [p_1, \ldots, p_q]$ and $D \in \mathbb{R}^{q \times q}$ be the diagonal matrix with values $\mu_1, \ldots, \mu_q$. Now it shows that

$$MP = PD$$

if and only if $\mu_1, \ldots, \mu_q$ are the eigenvalues of M and $P = [p_1, \ldots, p_q]$ its corresponding eigenvectors. This statement holds because

$$MP = M[p_1, \ldots, p_q] = [Mp_1, \ldots, Mp_q],$$

$$PD = M[p_1, \ldots, p_q] \begin{bmatrix} \mu_1 & \cdots & 0 \\ \vdots & \ddots & \vdots \\ 0 & \cdots & \mu_q \end{bmatrix} = [\mu_1 p_1, \ldots, \mu_q p_q]$$

$Mp_1 = \mu_1 p_1 \ldots Mp_q = \mu_q p_q$. Accordingly, the columns of P necessarily are eigenvectors of M. The diagonalization definition requires the matrix $D \in \mathbb{R}^{q \times q}$ is invertible, i.e., P must be of full rank. Here it desires to hold q eigenvectors $p_1, \ldots, p_q$, which are linearly independent, i.e., the p_i form a basis of $\mathbb{R}^q$.

21.3 MATRIX DECOMPOSITIONS

A lot of problems in machine learning can be solved using matrix algebra and vector calculus. This section aims to precede in brief about the matrix decomposition techniques. A key for decomposing a matrix is nothing but factorization of a number, like factoring the composite number 15 in terms of prime numbers 5 * 3. This is why matrix decomposition is often called matrix factorization. In general, describing a matrix by means of factors of different interpretable matrices is the ultimate aim of matrix decomposition. It is an approach to simplify complex matrix operations that can be achieved on the dissolved matrix instead of the original matrix. Hence it is a foundation of linear algebra in data processing, even for finding the value of determinant and calculating inverse. There is a range of techniques to reduce a matrix into its constituent part. The most generally used decomposition approaches are Lower-Upper (LU)Decomposition, QR Decomposition, Cholesky Decomposition, Eigenvalue decomposition, Singular Value decomposition (SVD), etc. This section includes a brief discussion on the above-mentioned decompositions with a numerical example.

21.3.1 THE LU DECOMPOSITION

A matrix A of order $m \times n$ can be decomposed into two triangular matrices, L_w and U_p, where L_w is a lower triangular matrix of order $m \times m$ with the diagonal elements equal to one and U_p stands for an upper triangular matrix. For instance,

$$A = \begin{bmatrix} 1 & 0 & 0 & 0 \\ * & 1 & 0 & 0 \\ * & * & 1 & 0 \\ * & * & * & 1 \end{bmatrix} \begin{bmatrix} * & * & * & * & * \\ 0 & * & * & * & * \\ 0 & 0 & * & * & * \\ 0 & 0 & 0 & 0 & * \end{bmatrix}.$$ Computers are used to solve the system of n-

number of linear equations with n-number of variables by LU decomposition while it plays a vital step in finding inverse or determinant of a matrix, since $A = L_w U_p$ speeds up a solution of $Ax = b$ by row reduction method, provided that L_w and U_p are known.

Algorithm: Consider $Ax = b$ then $L_w U_p x = b$, and by denoting $U_p x$ by y, then x can be found out easily by solving the set of equations $L_w y = b$ and $U_p x = y$, because L_w and U_p are triangular.

Example: Consider $\begin{pmatrix} 4 & 3 \\ 6 & 6 \end{pmatrix} = \begin{pmatrix} l_{11} & 0 \\ l_{21} & l_{22} \end{pmatrix} \begin{pmatrix} u_{11} & u_{12} \\ 0 & u_{22} \end{pmatrix}$ yields $l_{21} = 1.5, \ l_{21} = 1.5, \ l_{21} = 1.5$

and $l_{21} = 1.5$. Thus, $\begin{pmatrix} 4 & 3 \\ 6 & 6 \end{pmatrix} = \begin{pmatrix} 1 & 0 \\ 1.5 & 1 \end{pmatrix} \begin{pmatrix} 4 & 3 \\ 0 & 1.5 \end{pmatrix}$.

21.3.2 THE QR DECOMPOSITION

The QR decomposition (factorization) is also a part of linear algebra, which is used to factor a matrix into matrices of orthogonal elements, and it forms a basis for a triangular component and a triangular matrix. In adaptive signal processing, the QR decomposition is often used in conjunction with a triangular solver. If A is a matrix with linearly independent columns of order $m \times n$, then the factorization of A can be expressed as $A = QR$. Here, Q is a $m \times n$ matrix and columns of Q form an orthonormal basis for column A and R is an $n \times n$ invertible upper triangular matrix with positive diagonal. If A is a matrix with $|A| \neq 0$, then this factorization is unique. Since there are many ways to compute QR factorization, one such among them is the Gram-Schmidt procedure.

Algorithm: Let us consider the Gram-Schmidt approach along with the vectors in the process as columns of the matrix A; i.e., $A = [a_1|a_2|...|a_n]$. It follows that

$$u_1 = a_1, \quad e_1 = \frac{u_1}{\|u_1\|}, \quad u_2 = a_2 - (a_2 \cdot e_1)e_1, \quad e_2 = \frac{u_2}{\|u_2\|}, \quad u_{k+1} = a_{k+1} - (a_{k+1} \cdot e_1)e_1$$

$$- ... - (a_{k+1} \cdot e_k)e_k, \quad e_{k+1} = \frac{u_{k+1}}{\|u_{k+1}\|}$$

with $\|\cdot\|$ is defined as L_2 norm. Then the resulting QR factorization is

$$A = [a_1|a_2|...|a_n] = [e_1|e_2|...|e_n] \begin{bmatrix} a_1 \cdot e_1 & a_2 \cdot e_1 & ... & a_n \cdot e_1 \\ 0 & a_2 \cdot e_2 & ... & a_n \cdot e_2 \\ \vdots & \vdots & \ddots & \vdots \\ 0 & 0 & ... & a_n \cdot e_n \end{bmatrix} = QR. \text{ Then it is quite}$$

easy to find QR factorization, once we find $e_1, ..., e_n$.

Example: Consider $A = \begin{bmatrix} 1 & 1 & 0 \\ 1 & 0 & 1 \\ 0 & 1 & 1 \end{bmatrix}$ with the column vectors $a_1 = (1, 1, 0)^T$, $a_2 = (1, 0, 1)^T$, $a_3 = (0, 1, 1)^T$, where the notation $(1, 1, 0)^T$ is used for simplicity to denote the vectors are column vectors. By the above defining the Gram-Schmidt procedure, it follows that

$$u_1 = a_1 = (1, 1, 0)^T, \quad e_1 = \frac{u_1}{\|u_1\|} = \frac{1}{\sqrt{2}}(1, 1, 0) = \left(\frac{1}{\sqrt{2}}, \frac{1}{\sqrt{2}}, 0\right),$$

$$u_2 = a_2 - (a_2 \cdot e_1)e_1 = (1, 0, 1) - \frac{1}{\sqrt{2}}\left(\frac{1}{\sqrt{2}}, \frac{1}{\sqrt{2}}, 0\right) = \left(\frac{1}{2}, -\frac{1}{2}, 1\right),$$

$$e_2 = \frac{u_2}{\|u_2\|} = \frac{1}{\sqrt{\frac{3}{2}}}\left(\frac{1}{2}, -\frac{1}{2}, 1\right) = \left(\frac{1}{\sqrt{6}}, -\frac{1}{\sqrt{6}}, \frac{2}{\sqrt{6}}\right),$$

$$u_3 = a_3 - (a_3 \cdot e_1)e_1 - (a_3 \cdot e_2)e_2 = (0, 1, 1) - \frac{1}{\sqrt{2}}\left(\frac{1}{\sqrt{2}}, \frac{1}{\sqrt{2}}, 0\right)$$

$$- \frac{1}{\sqrt{6}}\left(\frac{1}{\sqrt{6}}, \frac{1}{\sqrt{6}}, \frac{2}{\sqrt{6}}\right) = \left(-\frac{1}{\sqrt{3}}, \frac{1}{\sqrt{3}}, \frac{1}{\sqrt{3}}\right),$$

$$e_3 = \frac{u_3}{\|u_3\|} = \left(-\frac{1}{\sqrt{3}}, \frac{1}{\sqrt{3}}, \frac{1}{\sqrt{3}}\right).$$

$$\text{Thus, } Q = [e_1|e_2|e_3] = \begin{bmatrix} \frac{1}{\sqrt{2}} & \frac{1}{\sqrt{6}} & -\frac{1}{\sqrt{3}} \\ \frac{1}{\sqrt{2}} & -\frac{1}{\sqrt{6}} & \frac{1}{\sqrt{3}} \\ 0 & \frac{2}{\sqrt{6}} & \frac{1}{\sqrt{3}} \end{bmatrix}, \; R = \begin{bmatrix} a_1 \cdot e_1 & a_2 \cdot e_1 & a_3 \cdot e_1 \\ 0 & a_2 \cdot e_2 & a_3 \cdot e_2 \\ 0 & 0 & a_3 \cdot e_3 \end{bmatrix} = \begin{bmatrix} \frac{2}{\sqrt{2}} & \frac{1}{\sqrt{2}} & \frac{1}{\sqrt{2}} \\ \frac{1}{\sqrt{2}} & \frac{3}{\sqrt{6}} & \frac{1}{\sqrt{6}} \\ 0 & 0 & \frac{2}{\sqrt{3}} \end{bmatrix}.$$

21.3.3 THE CHOLESKY DECOMPOSITION

Based on linear algebra's concept, the Cholesky decomposition (or factorization), is a decomposition of Hermitian's matrix, a matrix with a positive eigenvalue into the product of a lower triangular matrix and its conjugate transpose, which gives an efficient numerical solution; i.e., every symmetric and positive definite matrix A can be decomposed into $A = LL^T$. Here, L is a unique lower triangular matrix and it is called a Cholesky factor of A. The matrix L can be used to interpret as a generalized square root of A. When it is applicable, the Cholesky decomposition is approximately twice more efficient than the LU decomposition for solving the set of linear equations.

Algorithm: Consider a 3×3 matrix.

$$A = \begin{pmatrix} a_{11} & a_{21} & a_{31} \\ a_{21} & a_{22} & a_{32} \\ a_{31} & a_{32} & a_{33} \end{pmatrix} = \begin{pmatrix} l_{11} & 0 & 0 \\ l_{21} & l_{22} & 0 \\ l_{31} & l_{32} & l_{33} \end{pmatrix} \begin{pmatrix} l_{11} & l_{21} & l_{31} \\ 0 & l_{22} & l_{32} \\ 0 & 0 & l_{33} \end{pmatrix} = LL^T = \begin{pmatrix} l_{11}^2 & l_{21}l_{11} & l_{31}l_{11} \\ l_{21}l_{11} & l_{21}^2 + l_{22}^2 & l_{31}l_{21} + l_{32}l_{22} \\ l_{31}l_{11} & l_{31}l_{21} + l_{32}l_{22} & l_{31}^2 + l_{32}^2 + l_{33}^2 \end{pmatrix}.$$

It seems quite easy to solve for the diagonal elements (l_{kk}) of L with the calculation pattern $l_{11} = \sqrt{a_{11}}$, $l_{22} = \sqrt{a_{22} - l_{21}^2}$ and $l_{33} = \sqrt{a_{33} - (l_{31}^2 + l_{32}^2)}$ and in general $l_{kk} = \sqrt{a_{kk} - \sum_{j=1}^{k-1} l_{kj}^2}$. For the elements below the diagonal $(l_{ik}, \text{ where } i > k)$, $l_{21} = \frac{1}{l_{11}} a_{21}$, $l_{31} = \frac{1}{l_{11}} a_{31}$ and $l_{32} = \frac{1}{l_{22}}(a_{32} - l_{31}l_{21})$ a general expression is of the form $l_{ik} = \frac{1}{l_{kk}}\left(a_{ik} - \sum_{j=1}^{k-1} l_{ij}l_{kj}\right)$.

Example:

i. : Consider $A = \begin{pmatrix} 25 & 15 & -5 \\ 15 & 18 & 0 \\ -5 & 0 & 11 \end{pmatrix}$ by the above algorithm $L = \begin{pmatrix} 5 & 0 & 0 \\ 3 & 3 & 0 \\ -1 & 1 & 3 \end{pmatrix}$

ii. : Consider $A = \begin{pmatrix} 18 & 22 & 54 & 42 \\ 22 & 70 & 86 & 62 \\ 54 & 86 & 174 & 134 \\ 42 & 62 & 134 & 106 \end{pmatrix}$ by the above algorithm

$$L = \begin{pmatrix} 4.24264 & 0.00000 & 0.00000 & 0.00000 \\ 5.18545 & 6.56591 & 0.00000 & 0.00000 \\ 12.72792 & 3.04604 & 1.64974 & 0.00000 \\ 9.89949 & 1.62455 & 1.84971 & 1.39262 \end{pmatrix}$$

21.3.4 THE EIGENVALUE DECOMPOSITION

In linear algebra, eigenvalue (spectral) decomposition is the decomposition of a matrix into its canonical form, where the matrix is characterized in terms of its eigenvalues and eigenvectors. The decomposition of a matrix $M \in \mathbb{R}^{q \times q}$ can be expressed as $M = PDP^{-1}$ in this equation $P \in \mathbb{R}^{q \times q}$ and diagonal matrix D has its diagonal entries as its corresponding values. The eigenvalue decomposition is possible only if the original matrix is diagonalizable. Since the diagonal matrix D can efficiently be raised to a power, it is effortless to find a power of matrix $M \in \mathbb{R}^{q \times q}$ via the eigenvalue decomposition with the intention that $M^k = (PDP^{-1})^k = PD^kP^{-1}$. Calculating D^k is simple because of this operation which we can apply individually to any diagonal element. In sequence, if the eigenvalue decomposition of M exists, then the determinant $|M|=$ the product of elements presented in the diagonal of D.

Algorithm: Consider an eigenvector of the square matrix M of order q as an eigenvector u that satisfies the following equation $Mu = Pu$. By defining the matrices composed of eigenvalues and eigenvectors it leads $MP = PD$. By applying similarity transformation between P and D, it gives $M = PDP^{-1}$.

Example: Let $M = \begin{bmatrix} 2 & 1 \\ 1 & 2 \end{bmatrix}$. To compute the eigenvalues and eigenvectors, consider the characteristic polynomial of M as $\det(M - \mu I) =$

$\det\left(\begin{bmatrix} 2-\mu & 1 \\ 1 & 2-\mu \end{bmatrix}\right) = (2-\mu)^2 - 1 = \mu^2 - 4\mu + 3 = (\mu - 3)(\mu - 1)$. Thus the eigenvalues of M are $\mu_1 = 1$ and $\mu_2 = 3$ (the solutions of the characteristic polynomial of M) and the normalized (associated) eigenvectors are inherited

via $\begin{bmatrix} 2 & 1 \\ 1 & 2 \end{bmatrix} p_1 = 1 p_1$, $\begin{bmatrix} 2 & 1 \\ 1 & 2 \end{bmatrix} p_2 = 3 p_2$ yields $p_1 = \frac{1}{\sqrt{2}} \begin{bmatrix} 1 \\ -1 \end{bmatrix}$, $p_2 = \frac{1}{\sqrt{2}} \begin{bmatrix} 1 \\ 1 \end{bmatrix}$. M can be diagonalized while the eigenvectors p_1, p_2 form a basis of $\mathbb{R}^2$. Thus we can evaluate the matrix P to diagonalize M. The eigenvectors of M in P such that

$P = [p_1, p_2] = \frac{1}{\sqrt{2}} \begin{bmatrix} 1 & 1 \\ -1 & 1 \end{bmatrix}$. Hence it can be acquired that $MP = \begin{bmatrix} 1 & 0 \\ 0 & 3 \end{bmatrix} = D$.

Equivalently, we get $\begin{bmatrix} 2 & 1 \\ 1 & 2 \end{bmatrix} = \frac{1}{\sqrt{2}} \begin{bmatrix} 1 & 1 \\ -1 & 1 \end{bmatrix} \begin{bmatrix} 1 & 0 \\ 0 & 3 \end{bmatrix} \frac{1}{\sqrt{2}} \begin{bmatrix} 1 & -1 \\ 1 & 1 \end{bmatrix}$.

21.3.5 THE SINGULAR VALUE DECOMPOSITION (SVD)

The main aim of the SVD or central matrix decomposition method is to factorize a real or complex-valued matrix. Since SVD can be applied to all matrices (including rectangular matrices), it has been called the "fundamental theorem of linear algebra." The singular value decomposition gives a way to compress data without affecting too much information. It is recalled that if a square matrix is diagonalizable, which means that it can be factored as $M = PDP^{-1}$ where P is an invertible matrix, D is a diagonal matrix. If M factors as the product of P, D, and P^{-1}, then the transformation of multiplication by M can be done in three steps:

- Multiply by P^{-1}, which takes the basis of columns of P and transforms it into the standard bases along the axes.
- Multiply by D, which scales the standard basis vectors along the axes by the corresponding eigenvalues.
- Multiply by P, which turns the standard basis vectors back into the basis given by the columns of P.

So to be diagonalizable means that the transformation just looks like scaling in certain special directions. The scaling factors are the eigenvalues and the special directions are the eigenvectors and these form the columns of P. A special case of this is when the matrix M is symmetric. Real symmetric matrices are diagonalizable, and, in fact, the special directions can be taken to be an orthonormal set. So, then the columns of P are orthonormal and the matrix is orthogonal. Then P^{-1} is just P^T, revealing that any symmetric matrix can be factored as $M = PDP^T$, where P is the orthogonal matrix and D is the diagonal matrix.

Algorithm: Let $M^{p \times q}$ (where $p \neq q$) be a matrix of rank $r \in [0, \min(p, q)]$. Then the SVD of M can be expressed in the form as $M = U \Sigma V^T$, where $U \in \mathbb{R}^{p \times p}$ and $V \in \mathbb{R}^{q \times q}$ represent orthogonal matrices with column vectors u_i, $i = 1, ..., p$ and v_j, $j = 1, ..., q$ and Σ is a $p \times q$ diagonal matrix. The diagonal entries of Σ (say θ_i, $i = 1, ..., r$) are called the singular values, u_i and v_j are called the singular left and right vectors, respectively. Together, the singular values are in an orderly manner, i.e., $\theta_1 \geq \theta_2 \geq \theta_r \geq 0$. Further, Σ is the singular value matrix and is unique, but it needs some attention. Furthermore, it can be observed that the $\Sigma \in \mathbb{R}^{p \times q}$ is rectangular and its order is the same as the order of M. By the aforementioned statement, that Σ has a diagonal submatrix that contains the singular values and needs additional zero paddings. Particularly, if $p > q$, then the matrix Σ has a diagonal structure up to row q and then consists of 0^T

row vectors from $q + 1$ to p below so that $\Sigma = \begin{bmatrix} \theta_1 & 0 & 0 \\ 0 & \ddots & 0 \\ 0 & 0 & \theta_q \\ 0 & \cdots & 0 \\ \vdots & \ddots & \vdots \\ 0 & \cdots & 0 \end{bmatrix}$ and if $p \times q$, the

matrix Σ has a diagonal structure up to column p and columns that consist of 0

from p + 1 to q $\Sigma = \begin{bmatrix} \theta_1 & 0 & 0 & 0 & \cdots & 0 \\ 0 & \ddots & 0 & 0 & \cdots & 0 \\ 0 & 0 & \theta_p & 0 & \cdots & 0 \end{bmatrix}$.

Example: To find SVD of $M = \begin{bmatrix} 1 & 0 & 1 \\ -2 & 1 & 0 \end{bmatrix}$, compute the singular right vectors v_j, the singular values θ_k and the singular left vectors u_i. In first,

$$M^T M = \begin{bmatrix} 1 & -2 \\ 0 & 1 \\ 1 & 0 \end{bmatrix} \begin{bmatrix} 1 & 0 & 1 \\ -2 & 1 & 0 \end{bmatrix} = \begin{bmatrix} 5 & -2 & 1 \\ -2 & 1 & 0 \\ 1 & 0 & 1 \end{bmatrix}$$ is evaluated to calculate the

singular values and singular right vectors v_j by the eigenvalue decomposition of $M^T M$ provides

$$M^T M = \begin{bmatrix} \frac{5}{\sqrt{30}} & \frac{-2}{\sqrt{30}} & \frac{1}{\sqrt{30}} \\ 0 & \frac{1}{\sqrt{5}} & \frac{2}{\sqrt{5}} \\ \frac{1}{\sqrt{30}} & \frac{2}{\sqrt{5}} & \frac{1}{\sqrt{6}} \end{bmatrix} \begin{bmatrix} 6 & 0 & 0 \\ 0 & 1 & 0 \\ 0 & 0 & 0 \end{bmatrix} \begin{bmatrix} \frac{5}{\sqrt{30}} & \frac{-2}{\sqrt{30}} & \frac{1}{\sqrt{30}} \\ 0 & \frac{1}{\sqrt{5}} & \frac{2}{\sqrt{5}} \\ \frac{-1}{\sqrt{6}} & \frac{-2}{\sqrt{6}} & \frac{1}{\sqrt{6}} \end{bmatrix} = PDP^{-1},$$

and thus the singular right vectors as the columns of P such that

$$V = P = \begin{bmatrix} \frac{5}{\sqrt{30}} & \frac{-2}{\sqrt{30}} & \frac{1}{\sqrt{30}} \\ 0 & \frac{1}{\sqrt{5}} & \frac{2}{\sqrt{5}} \\ \frac{1}{\sqrt{30}} & \frac{2}{\sqrt{5}} & \frac{1}{\sqrt{6}} \end{bmatrix}.$$

The square roots of the eigenvalues of $M^T M$ are the singular values θ_i, can directly be obtained from D. Since rank(M) = 2, there we have only two nonzero singular values: $\theta_1 = \sqrt{6}$ and $\theta_2 = 1$. The singular value matrix must be in the order as the order of M, and it is in the form $\Sigma = \begin{bmatrix} \sqrt{6} & 0 & 0 \\ 0 & 1 & 0 \end{bmatrix}$. In order to find the singular left vectors compute the image of the singular right vectors under M and divide them by their corresponding singular value to normalize.

$$u_1 = \frac{1}{\theta_1} M v_1 = \frac{1}{\sqrt{6}} \begin{bmatrix} 1 & 0 & 1 \\ -2 & 1 & 0 \end{bmatrix} \begin{bmatrix} \frac{5}{\sqrt{30}} \\ \frac{-2}{\sqrt{30}} \\ \frac{1}{\sqrt{30}} \end{bmatrix} = \begin{bmatrix} \frac{1}{\sqrt{5}} \\ \frac{-2}{\sqrt{5}} \end{bmatrix}, \quad u_2 = \frac{1}{\theta_2} M v_2 = \frac{1}{1} \begin{bmatrix} 1 & 0 & 1 \\ -2 & 1 & 0 \end{bmatrix} \begin{bmatrix} 0 \\ \frac{1}{\sqrt{5}} \\ \frac{1}{\sqrt{30}} \end{bmatrix} = \begin{bmatrix} \frac{2}{\sqrt{5}} \\ \frac{1}{\sqrt{5}} \end{bmatrix},$$

$$U = [u_1, u_2] = \frac{1}{\sqrt{5}} \begin{bmatrix} 1 & 2 \\ -2 & 1 \end{bmatrix}.$$

Note: The SVD and the eigenvalue decomposition are closely related in some manners; i.e., the singular left and right vectors of M are eigenvectors of $M^T M$. The singular values of M which are not always zero are equal to the square roots of the eigenvalues of $M^T M$ which is also not equal to zero and both are equal to the nonzero eigenvalues of $M^T M$. For a real symmetric matrix with dimension $p \times q$, the SVD and eigenvalue decompositions are one and the same. But the small difference between the eigenvalue decomposition and the SVD is domain and codomain can be vector spaces of different dimensions in SVD. In general, the SVD, the left- and right-singular vector matrices are not inverses of each other but in the eigenvalue decomposition, the basis change matrices P and P^{-1} are inverses of each other. Based on the SVD procedure, the diagonal matrix entries Σ are all real and nonnegative and are not always satisfied for the diagonal matrix in the eigenvalue decomposition.

21.3.5.1 Geometric Interpretation of SVD

The SVD has a simple geometric interpretation to describe a transformation of matrix M. Under the linear transformation of M, the unit sphere in R^p is transformed into a filled or hollow ellipsoid in R^q, if the rank of the matrix is less than the dimension. In particular, it transforms the unit circle into an ellipse. The matrix Σ in the SVD is a $p \times q$ matrix with the diagonal entries are zeros except for m nonzero rows; i.e., it is a $p \times q$ matrix with an $m \times m$ diagonal block D and every other block is filled with zeros. Thus, Σ is called a diagonal matrix even it is not square. The diagonal elements of Σ are the singular values and there exist m nonzero singular values due to the reason that the rank of P is m. The columns of the matrix U show directions of the principal axes in order from largest to smallest axes and the columns of V are the unit vectors in R^p that map to the directions of the principal axes of the ellipsoid. In order to show the general feeling of linear transformation from R^p to R^q, Figure 21.3 is provided.

Suppose that under multiplication by P, the unit circle gets transformed into some tilted ellipse. The vectors along the principal axes of the ellipse are the left singular vectors with unit length. Their lengths are called singular values. For example, the vector and the semi-major axis of the ellipse will be S_1, the largest singular value, times g_1. Similarly, the vector along the semi-minor axis of this ellipse will be S_2 times the unit vector g_2. These vectors along the axes of the

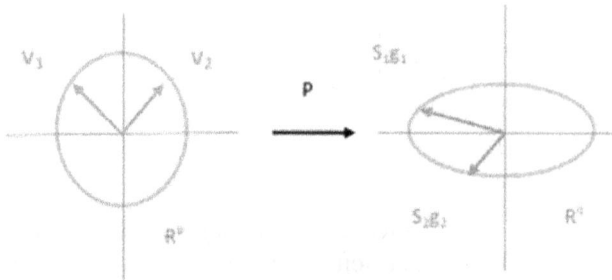

FIGURE 21.3 Linear transformation from R^p to R^q.

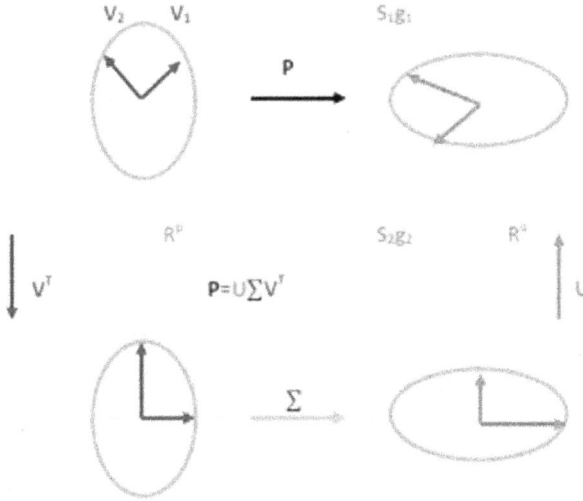

FIGURE 21.4 SVD factorization.

ellipse, colored in green, are images of certain unit vectors in the domain, colored in blue. These corresponding singular right vectors form the columns of V. In higher dimensions, the left singular vectors would align with the principal axes of the ellipsoid from largest to smallest. The image doesn't span all of R^q, if the linear transformation does collapsing it leads the singular values to zero. In such cases, there may not be unique choices for the singular vectors. But the singular values are uniquely defined. Now, let's see how the SVD factorization works. Let us enlarge the factorization in the previous diagram by including two more pictures. The matrix M means to factor in 3 parts, as a linear transformation acting on a vector in R^p and producing a vector in R^q. We will get exactly the same result as in the three-step process: first multiplying the vector by V^T on the left, then by X on the left, and then by U on the left. This is indicated in Figure 21.4 by an alternate path that goes from the top-left picture down to the bottom-left picture, then across to the bottom-right picture, and then up to the top-right picture.

21.3.5.2   Application: Data Compression Using SVD

In our technological world, the storage of large quantities of digital data and efficient transmission has become a major problem. Thus, the SVD plays an important role in compressing digital data hence it requires less storage space speeding up the electronic transmission. The idea in compressing a visual image is to represent it in a numerical matrix from which the image can be recovered whenever it is needed.

If the matrix M has size $m \times n$, then it takes mn entries individually. There is an alternative procedure to calculate the reduced SVD:

$$M = s_1 u_1 v_1^T + s_2 u_2 v_2^T + \ldots + s_k u_k v_k^T,$$

where $s_1 \geq s_2 \geq \ldots \geq s_k$ and it stores s's, u's and v's. Whenever the image is needed, it can be reconstructed from the above linear equation. Since k is the rank of the matrix M, u_j has m entries and v_j has n entries, it requires only storage space $km + kn + k = k(m + n + 1)$. If the singular values $s_{r+1}, \ldots s_k$ are sufficiently small which dropping the corresponding linear equation produces an acceptable **rank r approximation** as

$$M = s_1 u_1 v_1^T + s_2 u_2 v_2^T + \ldots + s_r u_r v_r^T$$

and the consequent image requires only storage space $rm + rn + r = r(m + n + 1)$ instead of mn.

We compare the results for different ranks with an example. The image with 600×399 pixels shown at the upper left in Figure 21.5 is a photo of Bharathiar University and the remaining are its compressed images for various rank r=2, 10, 50, 90, 100, respectively. The original image requires $mn=600.399=239400$. If $r=2$, then the space required for the compressed image is $2(600+399+1)=2000$. If $r=100$, then the storage space required for the compressed image is $100(600+399+1)=100000$, which is about 37% of the original image. This compression saves almost 63% without compromising the original quality of the image.

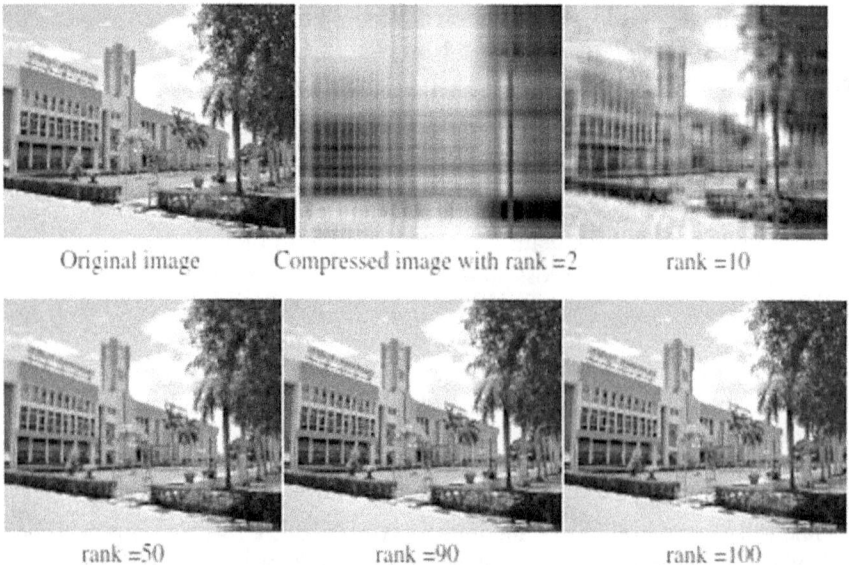

| Original image | Compressed image with rank =2 | rank =10 |

| rank =50 | rank =90 | rank =100 |

FIGURE 21.5 Data compression using SVD.

21.3.5.3   Dimensionality Reduction

Modeling data with many features is not easy, and models built from data that include the most relevant features are superior to data with irrelevant features. It is hard to find which features of the data are relevant and which are not. Methods for automatically reducing the number of columns of a data set are called dimensionality reduction. It is the process of reducing the number of random variables under consideration, by getting a set of principal variables. The two components of dimensionality reduction are separated into feature selection and feature extraction.

Feature selection: To find a subset of the original set of variables, or features to get a smaller subset that can be used to model the problem. It involves three ways: a) filter, b) wrapper, and c) embedded.

Feature extraction: It reduces the data in a high dimensional space to a lower dimension space.

Methods used for dimensionality reduction include Principal Component Analysis (PCA) and Kernel Principal Component Analysis (KPCA). Dimensionality reduction may be both linear or non-linear, depending upon the method used. Principal Component Analysis is discussed below.

21.3.5.4   Principal Component Analysis (PCA)

Principal Component Analysis is the most popular unsupervised dimensionality reduction technique. It is used in machine learning to reduce the dimensions by which projections of high dimensional data for both visualization and training models. The foundation of the PCA method is a matrix factorization method from linear algebra. The easiest way to realize PCA is to imagine a group of green and blue data points dispersed in three-dimensional space. They can be projected onto a two-dimensional surface in various ways, like onto the XY plane, YZ plane, ZX plane. We will get distributions of points in each of these projections that are slightly different. Here, PCA plays a major role in identifying which projections give maximal separation (maximum variance in the data), which is helpful to us. It works on a condition that whereas the data in a higher-dimensional space is mapped to data in a lower-dimensional space, the variance of the data in the lower-dimensional space should be maximum. It involves the following

- Form the covariance matrix of the data
- Calculate the eigenvectors of this matrix
- Find the direction of maximum variance and projects the data along them to reduce the dimension. The principal eigenvectors of the covariance matrix corresponding to the largest eigenvalues are used to reconstruct a large fraction of the variance of the original data.

21.4   LINEAR REGRESSION

Linear regression is habitually coupled to the least squares objective function, and is also referred to as least squares regression. In favor of hand over an optimization-centric aspect for solving systems of equations, least squares regression was introduced [6]. An additional accepted appliance of least squares regression is to design the dependence of a target variable on the feature variables.

Suppose we have a set of data $(x_1, y_1),...,(x_n, y_n)$. This is called training data.

Each x_i is a vector $\begin{bmatrix} x_{i1} \\ x_{i2} \\ \vdots \\ x_{in} \end{bmatrix}$ of measurements, where x_{i1} an instance of the input

variable is X_1, x_{i2} is an instance of the input variable X_2, etc. $X_1, ...,X_p$ are called **features or predictors**.

$y_1, ...,y_n$ are instances of the output variable Y, which is called the **response**.

In linear regression, we assume that the response depends on the input variables in a linear fashion $y = f(X) + \varepsilon$, where $f(X) = \beta_0 + \beta_1 X_1 + ...+\beta_p X_p$.

Here, ε is called the **error term** and $\beta_0, ...,\beta_p$ are called **parameters**.

The values of $\beta_0, ...,\beta_p$ are not known. However, the training data can be used to approximate the values of $\beta_0, ...,\beta_p$. The amount by which the predicted value $f(x_i)$ differs from the actual y_i for each of the pairs $(x_1, y_1),...,(x_N, y_N)$ from the training data is $y_i - f(x_i)$.

Taking square and sum this for i=1... N;

$$\sum_{i=1}^{N} (y_i - f(x_i))^2$$

This is called the **residual sum of squares** and denoted RSS(β) where $\beta = \begin{bmatrix} \beta_0 \\ \beta_1 \\ \vdots \\ \beta_p \end{bmatrix}$.

When the residual sum of squares are as small as possible means that predicted value $f(x_i)$ is to be as close to the actual value y_i as possible for each of the pairs (x_i, y_i), doing this will give us a linear function of the input variables that best fits the given training data. In the case of only one input variable, we get the best-fit line. In the case of two input variables, we get the best-fit plane; and so on, for a higher dimension.

21.4.1 THE LEAST SQUARES METHOD

By minimizing RSS(β), we estimate $\hat{\beta}_0, ...,\hat{\beta}_p$ of parameters $\beta_0, ...,\beta_p$. This method is called *the least squares method*.

$$\text{Let } X = \begin{bmatrix} 1 & x_{11} & x_{12} & \cdots & x_{1p} \\ 1 & x_{21} & x_{22} & \cdots & x_{2p} \\ \vdots & \cdots & \cdots & \cdots & \cdots \\ 1 & x_{N1} & x_{N2} & \cdots & x_{Np} \end{bmatrix} \text{ and } y = \begin{bmatrix} y_1 \\ \vdots \\ y_N \end{bmatrix}$$

$$\text{Then } y - X\beta = \begin{bmatrix} y_1 \\ \vdots \\ y_N \end{bmatrix} - \begin{bmatrix} 1 & x_{11} & x_{12} & \cdots & x_{1p} \\ 1 & x_{21} & x_{22} & \cdots & x_{2p} \\ \vdots & \cdots & \cdots & \cdots & \cdots \\ 1 & x_{N1} & x_{N2} & \cdots & x_{Np} \end{bmatrix} \begin{bmatrix} \beta_0 \\ \beta_1 \\ \vdots \\ \beta_p \end{bmatrix}$$

$$= \begin{bmatrix} y_1 \\ \vdots \\ y_N \end{bmatrix} - \begin{bmatrix} \beta_0 + \beta_1 x_{11} + \ldots \beta_p x_{1p} \\ \vdots \\ \beta_0 + \beta_1 x_{N1} + \ldots \beta_p x_{Np} \end{bmatrix}$$

$$= \begin{bmatrix} y_1 - f(x_1) \\ \vdots \\ y_N - f(x_N) \end{bmatrix}$$

$$so \ (y - X\beta)^T (y - X\beta) = \Sigma_{i=1}^{N} \left(y_i - f(x_i) \right)^2 = RSS(\beta)$$

$$so \ RSS(\beta) = (y - X\beta)^T (y - X\beta)$$

consider the vector of the partial derivative of RSS(β):

$$\begin{bmatrix} \frac{\partial RSS(\beta)}{\partial \beta_0} \\ \frac{\partial RSS(\beta)}{\partial \beta_1} \\ \vdots \\ \frac{\partial RSS(\beta)}{\partial \beta_p} \end{bmatrix} = \begin{bmatrix} -2[1 \ldots 1](y - X\beta) \\ -2[x_{11} \ldots x_{N1}](y - X\beta) \\ \vdots \\ -2[x_{1p} \ldots x_{Np}](y - X\beta) \end{bmatrix} = -2 \begin{bmatrix} 1 & 1 & 1 & \cdots & 1 \\ x_{11} & x_{21} & x_{31} & \cdots & x_{N1} \\ \vdots & \cdots & \cdots & \cdots & \cdots \\ x_{1p} & x_{2p} & x_{3p} & \cdots & x_{Np} \end{bmatrix} (y - X\beta)$$

$$= -2X^T(y - X\beta)$$

If we take the second derivative of RSS(β): $\frac{\partial^2 RSS(\beta)}{\partial \beta_k \partial \beta_j} = 2a_{jk}$ where $a_{jk} = x_{1j}x_{1k} + \ldots + x_{Nj}x_{Nk}$

The matrix of second derivatives of RSS(β) is $2X^T X$. It is called the **Hessian matrix**.

By the second derivative test, if the Hessian of RSS(β) at a critical point is positive definite, then RSS(β) has a local minimum there. If we set the vector of derivative to **0**, we get $\beta = (X^T X)^{-1} X^T y$.

Thus we solved the vector of parameters $\begin{bmatrix} \beta_0 \\ \beta_1 \\ \vdots \\ \beta_p \end{bmatrix}$ which minimizes the residual sum

of squares RSS(β), so $\begin{bmatrix} \hat{\beta}_0 \\ \hat{\beta}_1 \\ \vdots \\ \hat{\beta}_p \end{bmatrix}$

21.4.2 LINEAR ALGEBRA SOLUTION TO LEAST SQUARES PROBLEM

We can arrive at the solution for the least squares problem by using linear algebra.

Let $X = \begin{bmatrix} 1 & x_{11} & x_{12} & \cdots & x_{1p} \\ 1 & x_{21} & x_{22} & \cdots & x_{2p} \\ \vdots & \cdots & \cdots & \cdots & \cdots \\ 1 & x_{N1} & x_{N2} & \cdots & x_{Np} \end{bmatrix}$ and $y = \begin{bmatrix} y_1 \\ \vdots \\ y_N \end{bmatrix}$ as before, from our training data.

We want a vector β such that $X\beta$ is close to y. In other words, we want a vector β such that the distance $\|X\beta - y\|$ between $X\beta$ and y is minimized. A vector β that minimizes $\|X\beta - y\|$ is called a **least squares solution** of $X\beta = y$.

X is an N by (p+1) matrix. We want a $\hat{\beta}$ in $\mathbb{R}^{p+1}$ such that $X\hat{\beta}$ is closest to y. Note that $X\hat{\beta}$ is a linear combination of the columns of X, so $X\hat{\beta}$ lies in the span of columns of X which is a subspace of $\mathbb{R}^N$ denoted by *col X*. So we want the vector in *col X* that is closest to y. This projection y onto the subspace *col X* is that vector, $proj_{col\ X}y = X\hat{\beta}$ for some $\hat{\beta}$ in $\mathbb{R}^{p+1}$.

Consider $y - X\hat{\beta}$. Note that $y = X\hat{\beta} + (y - X\hat{\beta})$.

$\mathbb{R}^N$ can be broken into two subspaces *col X* and $(col\ X)^{\perp}$, where $(col\ X)^{\perp}$ is the subspace of $\mathbb{R}^N$ consisting of all its as orthogonal vectors to the vectors in *col X*. Any vector in $\mathbb{R}^N$ can be written uniquely as $z + w$ where $z \in col\ X$ and $w \in (col\ X)^{\perp}$.

Since $y \in \mathbb{R}^N$, and $y = X\hat{\beta} + (y - X\hat{\beta})$, with $X\hat{\beta} \in col\ X$, the second vector $y - X\hat{\beta}$ must lie in $(col\ X)^{\perp}$.

$\Rightarrow$ $(y - X\hat{\beta})$ is orthogonal to the columns of X.

$$\Rightarrow \quad X^T(y - X\hat{\beta}) = 0$$

$$\Rightarrow \quad X^Ty - X^TX\hat{\beta} = 0$$

$$\Rightarrow \quad X^TX\hat{\beta} = X^Ty$$

Thus, it turns out that the set of least squares solutions of $X\beta = y$ consists of all and only the solutions to the matrix equation $X^T X\beta = X^T y$.

If $X^T X$ is positive definite, then the eigenvalues of $X^T X$ are all positive. So 0 is not an eigenvalue of $X^T X$. It follows that $X^T X$ is invertible. Then we can solve the equation $X^T X\hat{\beta} = X^T y$ for $\hat{\beta}$ to get $\hat{\beta} = (X^T X)^{-1}X^T y$, which is the same result as earlier.

21.5   LINEAR ALGEBRA IN MACHINE LEARNING

As we ascertain to attain more acquaintance about technologies, the influential components like machine learning, robotics, data science, and artificial intelligence having specific words/terms that are common to these technologies. A few of these terms include support vector machines (SVM), Lagrange multipliers, kernel PCA, and ridge regression. So, it becomes very important for every individual who is learning machine learning or data science to first move towards the requisites with what linear algebra is. It is required to recognize how to use them when solving problems using ML or when making more sense of the enormous data available using data science.

21.5.1   SHINING IN MACHINE LEARNING COMPONENTS

Vector and matrix are key data structures in linear algebra. In machine learning, we fit a model on a data set. This is the table-like set of numbers where each row represents an observation and each column represents a feature of the observation. When we split the data into inputs and outputs to fit a supervised machine learning model, we have a matrix (X) and a vector (Y). Each row has the same length; i.e., the same number of columns, therefore we can say that the data is vectorized where rows can be provided to a model, one at a time or in a batch, and the model can be pre-configured to expect rows of a fixed width. Eigenvalues and eigenvectors are very important in machine learning which are used to minimize data noise. Eigenvectors are vectors that only change by a scalar factor, and there is no change in their direction at all. The eigenvalues corresponding to eigenvectors is the magnitude by which they are scaled. When the linear transformation is applied to eigenvectors, it is noted that they don't change their direction.

It is quite difficult to visualize the features of sound, textual, or image data. This data is usually represented in 3D. This is where eigenvalues and eigenvectors come into the picture. They can be used to capture all the huge amount that is stored in a matrix. Eigenvalues and eigenvectors are used in facial recognition, too. A photo is another instance of a matrix from linear algebra. Operations on the image, such as shearing, cropping, scaling, and so on are all explicated using the notation and operations of linear algebra. It is the input to improve and shine the awareness or instinct that plays an important role in machine learning. It will be able to provide more perspectives and helps to widen our thinking and make it more steady. It could start using more parameters for different machine learning components.

A linear regression model fits a given data in the following way:

- Start with some arbitrary prediction function
- Utilize it on the independent features of the data to predict the output
- Calculate the difference between the predicted output from the expected output. Apply these calculated values to optimize the prediction function using some approaches like gradient descent.

A loss function is an application of the vector norm in linear algebra which is used to calculate how prediction output differs from expected output. The norm of a vector is simply defined as its magnitude. For example the L1 norm of the vector v= $(v_1, v_2, \ldots v_n)$ is $\|v\| = |v_1| + |v_2| + \ldots |v_n|$ and L2 norm of the vector v= $(v_1, v_2, \ldots v_n)$ is $v = \sqrt{v_1^2 + v_2^2 + \ldots v_n^2}$. The predicted values are stored in vector A and the expected values are stored in vector B. Then the norm of the difference vector A-B is the total loss for the prediction.

Regularization is actually one of the applications of the norm. It is a technique used to prevent models from overfitting. Regularization is a process of modifying the loss function to penalize specific values of the weight on learning. To minimize the cost function, we have to minimize the norm of the weight vector by using L1 or L2 norms discussed above.

21.5.2 ENHANCING MACHINE LEARNING ALGORITHMS

Today, ML algorithms have become an integral part of various industries, including business, finance, and healthcare. The linear algebra will help to develop a more in-depth understanding of the machine learning project that affords special graphical interpretations to work on – images, audio, video, and edge detection. Linear algebra is used to build better supervised as well as unsupervised machine learning algorithms. Machine learning algorithms have classifiers that train a part of the given dataset based on their categories. Another work of classifiers is to do away with errors from the data that has already been trained. It is at this stage that linear algebra comes in to help compute this complex and large dataset. It uses matrix decomposition techniques like Q-R and L-U decompositions to process and handles large data for different projects. Length squared sampling in matrices, singular value decomposition, and low-rank approximation are a few techniques that are widely used in data processing. Logistic regression, linear regression, decision trees, and support vector machines (SVM) are a few supervised learning algorithms that can create from scratch with the help of linear algebra. SVD is typically used in the principal component analysis (PCA), which in turn is widely used for feature extraction and for knowing how significant the relationship among the features is to an outcome. PCA is widely used in computer vision and image compression by reducing the storage space. It reduces computation time.

Using the concept of transpose and matrix multiplication in linear algebra, the covariance matrix of the data matrix containing numerical features are calculated in PCA. In the principal component analysis, we find the directions in the data with the most variation; i.e., the eigenvectors corresponding to the largest eigenvalues of the covariance matrix, and project the data onto these directions. The motive for doing this is that the most second-order information are in these directions. The eigenvectors are called principal components.

Support vector machine is an application of the concept of vector spaces in linear algebra. SVM is a discriminative classifier that works by finding a decision surface. It is a supervised machine learning algorithm. In this algorithm, each data item is plotted as a point in an n-dimensional space with the value of each feature as the coordinate. Classification is done for finding the hyperplane which differentiates the two classes very well. A hyperplane is a subspace vector space whose dimension is less than its corresponding vector space. Kernal transformation used in SVM depends on the idea of transformation from one space to another in linear algebra.

Without knowing the theory and algorithm behind ML, we are using it in our day-to-day life. Some of them are

1. Traffic predictions by using GPS, online transportation network like **UBER,OLA** in the entire cycle of service, ML plays a prominent role.
2. To improve the search results **search engines** use ML.
3. Automatic friend tagging suggestions on **Facebook** is the major common application of ML.
4. ML is an important part of virtual personal assistants like **Siri**, **Alexa, etc**.
5. One of the coolest applications of ML is product recommendations. Google tracks our search history and recommends ads based on search history.

ACKNOWLEDGMENTS

I would like to express my deep gratitude to Honorable Vice Chancellor Prof. Dr. P. Kaliraj, Bharathiar University for providing an excellent opportunity and enthusiastic encouragement to this work. I would also extend my thanks to Prof. Dr. T. Devi, Professor and Head, Department of Computer Applications for her professional guidance and valuable support.

REFERENCES

Ahmed Elgohary, Matthias Boehm, Peter J. Haas, Frederick R. Reiss, Berthold Reinwald, 2019. Compressed linear algebra for declarative large-scale machine learning, Communications of the ACM, 62(5), 83–95.

Charu C. Aggarwal, 2020. Linear Algebra and Optimization for Machine Learning: A Textbook, Springer Nature, Switzerland, 507 pp.

Engin Ipek, 2019. Memristive accelerators for dense and sparse linear algebra: From machine learning to high-performance scientific computing, IEEE Micro, 39(1), 58–61.

Ethem Alpaydin, 2020. Introduction to Machine Learning, 4th edn, The MIT Press, Cambridge, Massachusetts, 643 pp.

Gilbert Strang, 2020. Linear Algebra and Learning from Data, Wellesley Publishers, India, 415 pp.

Jean Gallier, Jocelyn Quaintance, 2019. Linear Algebra for Computer Vision, Robotics, and Machine Learning, University of Pennsylvania, Philadelphia, PA, USA, 753 pp.

22 Identification of Lichen Plants and Butterflies Using Image Processing and Neural Networks in Cloud Computing

P. Ponmurugan[1], K. Murugan[2], and C. Panneerselvam[3]
[1]Department of Botany, Bharathiar University, Coimbatore, India
[2]Department of Zoology, Bharathiar University, Coimbatore, India
[3]Department of Biology, Faculty of Science, University of Tabuk, Tabuk, Saudi Arabia

CONTENTS

22.1 INTRODUCTION

To identify lichen plants and butterflies rapidly without following the conventional methods such as morphological, anatomical, biochemical, and molecular techniques, it is proposed to develop a simple protocol that includes IT-based image processing techniques. The images of lichens and butterflies will be captured, subsequently stored in the database using SQL and ASP.NET servers, followed by image pre-processing, segmentation, feature extraction, and extrapolation performed using MATLAB®. Further identification may be performed by a developing lichen and butterfly finder algorithm using an Artificial Neural Network (ANN). The technology for the identification of lichen and butterfly species developed may be made available in the public domain through cloud computing methods.

22.2 OBJECTIVES OF THE PRESENT STUDY

Attempts were made to collect photographic images of lichen plants and butterflies across India and to classify them based on genus and species level by applying the concept of an image processing technique. The captured images of both lichen plants and butterflies are being stored in the database using SQL and ASP.NET servers. Image pre-processing, segmentation, feature extraction, and extrapolation were performed on both lichen plants and butterflies images using MATLAB® followed by the use of lichen and butterfly finder algorithm and Artificial Neural Network. In case new lichen and butterfly species collected from the Western Ghats were not classified by the database, they were subjected to identify them by the manual cum conventional methods. The collected lichen and butterfly species were identified based on conventional methods of identification for comparison purposes. The technology for the identification of lichen and butterfly species developed through image processing techniques were made available in the public domain through cloud computing methods for easy access.

22.3 BACKGROUND INFORMATION

lichenologists are identifying the indigenous lichen species routinely by their external and internal morphology along with chemical constituents contained in it. Lichen taxonomy is very complex in the general and time-consuming process for identifying collected lichen species, including a skilled workforce. Even then, the lichens suffer in deficiency of characters for segregating them up to species level resulting in several species complexes (Kalidoss et al., 2020). To overcome this lacuna with recent studies, most of the lichenologists around the globe depend on molecular data for identification, to solve the complexity and to understand their evolution in lichen research. India is still following classical taxonomy methods and yet to initiate molecular systematics and IT-based digital techniques (Mariraj et al., 2020). In this context, digital image processing techniques with the implementation mobile application software which follow the process of electronic and communication engineering tools are the new methods for easy identification of lichens on the spot or site, wherein lichens are growing profusely. It consumes less time with accurate results without transferring digital lichen images from conventional camera to computer/data storage system. Once the application software is developed to identify the lichens, it will be made available for public access to rapidly identify economically important plants and insects.

22.3.1 ABOUT LICHENS

Lichens are fascinating, self-supporting symbiotic associations between fungal organisms called mycobionts and photoautotrophic algal partners called phycobionts. There are about 20,000 species of lichens distributed throughout the world. India harbors about 2,300 species. Among different states of India, Tamil Nadu records the highest number of lichens, represented by 785 *taxa,* followed by Karnataka (612 *taxa*), and Andhra Pradesh (656 *taxa*) in southern India. This is due to large tracts of Western Ghats and several biodiversity hotspots in the region, including Eastern Ghats biodiversity hotspots like Yercaud hills, Kolli hills, and Yelagiri malai hills (Ponmurugan et al., 2016). They can grow on rock (saxicolous), soil (terricolous), and bark (corticolous) as habitats across the world. It is estimated that around 557 lichen species are recognized as endemic to India. Lichens are known for unique secondary metabolites of about 1,050 total compounds. Over 550 compounds are unique to only lichens. The derivatives of lichen compounds are fatty acids, macrolytic lactones, zeorins, pulvic acid derivatives, cumarone derivatives, dibenzofurans, depsides, depsidones, terpenoids, anthroquinone derivatives, steroids, carotenoids, and diphenyl ethers (Ayyappadasan et al., 2017).

Bioactive compounds extracted from lichen thallus are being rendered several biological activities and promising anti-microbial agent alternatives to antibiotics. It is observed that lichen bioactive compounds have a large number of medicinal properties. More than 50% of the known lichen species exhibited medicinal values (Vartia, 1973). Most of the lichen compounds exert a broad spectrum of biological actions such as antifungal, antibacterial, antiviral, antimalarial antioxidant, anticancer, anti-inflammatory, anti-arthritis anti-analgesic, anti-pyretic, and antiproliferative activities (Tanas et al., 2010; Shrestha et al., 2015), including anti-snake venom properties (Kalidoss et al., 2020). The secondary metabolites are inevitable chemical substances, which assist lichen identification as well as using chemotaxonomy methods.

22.3.2 ABOUT BUTTERFLIES

Similarly, insects like butterflies are very important in ecological niches towards diversity and conservation (Yago et al., 2010). Among the 17 megadiverse countries of the world, India is one in terms of various colorful varieties of butterflies. Approximately 1,400 species of butterflies are reported in India, in which many of them are endemic to India (Murugan, 2009). It is essential to design and disseminate complete information about the various aspects of the biology and distribution of

Indian butterflies worldwide. Entomologists are being encouraged to study their natural history, ecology of adaptation, population diversity, and distributional data of Indian butterflies. A centralized database and spread of various butterflies in India are needed, which is useful to create awareness towards their conservation in the ecological niche. Butterflies are worldwide in their distribution, and different kinds of butterflies are reported in the butterfly ecosystem (Vukusic et al., 2000).

A butterfly is a flying insect closely related to moths found during day time. It is the last major group of flying insects to appear on the planet. The notable features of butterflies are exhibiting an extraordinary range of colors and patterns and their wing. A butterfly is from the order of Lepidoptera, phylum of Arthropoda, the family of Hedylidae, and kingdom of Animalia. Usually, a butterfly's life is closely connected to flowering plants based on feeding on flowers starting from their larvae (caterpillars), adults, and laying their eggs. A butterfly also helps pollination in angiosperms (flowering plants). They have four long wings covered with few tiny scales. The wings and tiny scales are patterned uniformly and are often brightly colored. The males and females of butterflies are often slightly different from each other in terms of the pattern of wings and their tiny scales (Dennis et al., 2005; Harpel et al., 2015).

22.3.3 IMAGE PROCESSING TECHNIQUES IN LICHEN AND BUTTERFLY IDENTIFICATION

It is documented that India is being considered as one of the mega biodiversity centers across the world. Because India contains diverse ecosystems with a variety of plants and animals including a wide spectrum of microorganisms having novel genes encoding for bioactive secondary compounds. The bioactive secondary compounds obtained from plants and microorganisms such as fungi, bacteria, and actinomycetes have various biological activities (Ayyappadasan et al., 2017). The potential of novel plants and microorganisms needs to be reassessed and cataloged for plant diversity researchers' biomedical scientists to benefit humankind. Studies on biomedical applications of plants and microorganisms available in the country's biodiversity spots are the highest priority in terms of Intellectual property rights. These kinds of studies should be taken up immediately both by the developed countries and developing countries like India, and some extend to underdeveloped countries.

According to Narendran (2001), who suggested many ideas to improve systematic research in India to protect intellectual property rights in doing research upon biomedical applications of plants and microorganisms for the benefit of humankind, to improve systematic research in India, some of the suggestions are needed to increase the sizable number of systematic researchers, preparation of identification manuals and bulletins, increase in funding source from government and private sectors, introduction of taxonomy as well as conservation aspects in syllabus, conducting short-term training programmes and awareness workshops in taxonomy of plants, animals, and microorganisms, improving library facilities for referring previous research, creating research facilities, establishing repositories of specimens and improving identification services, use of the latest tools and techniques, and so on (Arnal Barbedo, 2013). To enhance the research activities among scientists, faculty, and research scholars, information technology tools and techniques should be used towards identifying plant and animal samples, especially insect-like specimens. Of the information technology tools and techniques, an image processing technique is very important in terms of rapid identification of plant and insect-like samples without any confusion and errors.

However, there are some major problems across India in biosystematic research, because of a lack of plant and animal taxonomists and entomologists. In India, plant and animal taxonomic research is confined to India's Botanical Survey (BSI) and Zoological Survey of India (ZSI) and a few research groups in famous universities, R&D centers, and colleges. Another major problem in taking up taxonomic studies is a lack of future job opportunities among young research scholars and funding avenues from the government and private sectors (Arnal Barbedo, 2013). Similarly, inter- and intra-disciplinary coordination and collaborative research among universities, R&D organizations, and colleges involving taxonomists are negligible. Due to lack of proper objectivity and scope of future work including a work plan in researching plant and animal taxonomy is vague. Lack of networking, poor funding support from the government, and nature conservation agencies like Indian Forest Departments among the research groups is completely missing in India. The above issues drive the Indian scientists and faculty members, including research scholars, to select their disciplines in plant and animal taxonomy. Due to poor knowledge in plant and animal taxonomy, identifying samples is tough, leading to lucrative career prospects like the latest subjects of information technology, electronic and communication engineering, biotechnology, microbial technology, and genetic engineering (Hamuda et al., 2016).

In India, there is no proper direction and encouragement in prioritizing research and development work between the macro- and microorganisms. The systematic research in macro flora and fauna and microbial diversity is being continuously neglected. Moreover, the documentation of many macro- and microorganisms and novel microorganisms still remained unexplored due to listing out lack of novelty, enumeration of expected outcome, and social relevance to the society. It is also handicapped in R&D work in India in terms of novel pharmaceutical products development from potential medicinal plants and microbial systems. Among the literature surveyed, the best example is the under-explored lichen studies and many insect groups like butterflies, even though there is a global demand and increase in use to tap these bio-resources using biotechnological applications (Vivian et al., 2001). Hence, there is a greater attention required for biodiversity studies in lichens and butterflies targeting the so-far neglected biodiversity with immediate effect. The major problem in biodiversity studies in lichens and butterflies across India is the identification of lichen and butterfly varieties.

To identify lichens rapidly without following the conventional methods such as morphological, anatomical, biochemical, and molecular techniques, there is no easy reliable and reproducible protocol made available for lichenologists (Hamuda et al., 2016). Similarly, easy, reliable conventional methods are not available to identify butterflies using the pattern of wings and their tiny scales. Hence, it is proposed to develop a simple protocol that includes IT-based image processing techniques to identify lichen and butterfly species. Similarly, butterflies can be identified rapidly using various data like color and size including shape and wings with tiny scales using image processing techniques with cent percent accuracy without any repetition (Srygley and Thomas, 2002). The major outcome is to reduce the skilled workforce and time consumption for the identification of lichen and butterfly species which will be made accessible for the public domain through cloud computing technology. Lichen and butterflies are subjected to identify the genus and species and capture the images subsequently stored in the database using SQL and ASP.NET servers followed by image pre-processing, segmentation, feature extraction, and extrapolation performed using MATLAB®. Further identification may be performed by developing a lichen finder algorithm (LFA) using an ANN, which is an efficient soft computing technique. The technology for the identification of lichen and butterfly species developed may be made available in the public domain through cloud computing methods.

22.3.4 IMAGE PROCESSING TECHNIQUES IN CLOUD COMPUTING

To identify plant and insect samples rapidly, an image processing technique is essential with limited numbers of skilled manpower and large numbers of specimens. Digital image recognition is an important process normally used to analyze the content of digital images in general such a way that image objects may be identified quickly from known digital patterns in particular (Kulkarni, 1994). Image recognition is normally used to identify the unknown samples in which how abstract patterns of sample images are matched or classified into known categories based on the percentage of expression. According to Fu (1996) pattern matching process between known and unknown digital images is being achieved using either the decision-theoretic approach or the syntactic approach. Among these approaches, the decision-theoretic approach is accomplished to identify the unknown images by statistical methods in which a limited set of characteristic measurements or characteristic features are widely used so that classification of digital images is simply carried out using some easy, reliable statistical models.

Most of the statistical models generally feed the numerical inputs during the pattern matching process and perform the recognition process of unknown images by assigning the characteristic features. Further they are working based on the numerical measurements of the features, the test pattern of visual recognizing process accordingly into a finite set of pattern classes (Fu, 1996). The syntactic approach or decision-theoretic approach of a pattern matching process uses a tree-like pattern (or hierarchical pattern) in which description language as input image of unknown samples showing the pattern recognition process is observed by performing a grammar syntax analysis as one of the statistical models. This method is functioning purely based on the number of characteristic measurements of input image (Hale and Mason, 2008).

Computer pattern recognition of input digital images is an automated process to execute the processes such as machine recognition, description and classification of test patterns based on the number of characteristic measurements of numerical inputs that are converted into known pattern classes and their features (Chellappa et al., 1995).

Since it is an automated pattern recognition process, many benefits are enumerated to perform visual recognition of input images implemented in many IT-based techniques and real-life applications. In this automated pattern recognition, the various approaches and methods such as statistical approaches, template-matching process, syntactic analyzers, and artificial neural networks are normally used. Among these four widely used approaches, ANNs are now extensively used in image processing techniques, especially in biotechnology and biomedical researches in which ANN is used as a classification tool (Smach et al., 2006). In biomedical research, ANN is commonly applied to x-ray image segmentation, image classification, image segregation, enzyme and protein structure prediction, and nucleic acids and protein sequencing studies (Antowiak and Chalasinska, 2003).

Most lichenologists have identified and classified lichen samples into three main lichen growth forms such as crustose, foliose, and fruticose. In general, lichen are identified by following conventional methods such as morphological, anatomical, biochemical, physiological, and molecular biological techniques. The conventional methods of lichen classification and identification relies on the human expert with skilled manpower and time-consuming process. In recent days, lichens are identified using the latest techniques like image processing and fingerprinting techniques. These methods rely on computational biology experts and/or biotechnologists with an image recognition or classification system which can automate the degree of recognition process towards rapid identification. The advantage of using image processing technique is to identify the unknown lichen samples rapidly with cent percent accuracy. Since it is an automation process working based on lichen input images applying ANN, good image quality, variable features, sizes, and shapes with high resolution of various degrees of digital images are needed (Belongies et al., 2002).

Nowadays it has become a trend throughout the world to authenticate the identity of lichen *taxa* by following information technology. The method solves taxonomic problems and helps in understanding the evolution of a taxa, including identification. In the current decade most of the lichen monographic and floristic studies have been compiled for North America in the form of floras, checklists, and identification keys, which gives a fair idea regarding the lichen wealth in their country. However, for South and Central America, there are not many compiled floras but significant lichenological studies are available in scattered literature using image processing techniques (Lucking, 2008).

22.4 METHODOLOGY

Lichen species and their digital images were collected from different agroclimatic conditions of Western Ghats covering Nilgiris, Palani Hills, Silent Valley National Park, Kodaikanal, and Chikamagalur areas of southern part of India using standard techniques. The digital images of lichens were obtained using digital camera (Canon, Inc. Japan). The Awasthi's lichen identification manual was followed for matching the identification characters of the lichen samples under morphological, anatomical, and biochemical investigations (Awasthi, 2007). The lichen and butterfly images were captured in three views, such as front, close-up, and full. These images are stored as a data set. The collected images were subjected to pre-processing to minimize undesired distortions or to enhance the quality of images for further processing. The images were pre-processed by resizing (resize the images), conversion (intensity information), and enhancement (image lighter or darker). The present pre-processing study is based on domain enhancement techniques such as spatial domain enhancement techniques which includes morphological operation, Gaussian filter, unsharp masking, and adaptive filter methods (Brindha et al., 2015). Frequency domain enhancement techniques, which include Wavelet transform technique, were used for the processing of images (Sheikh and Raghad, 2016). MATLAB® R2010b software was used for analyzing the digital data of lichens and butterflies as per the method of Gomez and Gomez (1984).

The classification of lichen and butterfly images was done using a Support Vector Machine (SVM) classifier in which the selected features such as contrast, correlation, energy, homogeneity, mean, standard deviation, entropy, root mean square, variance, smoothness, kurtosis, and skewness are extracted from the image and used as input. The features of input sample images were used as a training data set in SVM classifier. In this method, the features of input sample image are compared with training data set to find out the species name of input lichen and butterfly images (Le Hoang et al., 2012). Structured Query Language (SQL) was used for managing image held in a Relational Data Base Management System (RDBMS) and for the creation of lichen and butterfly images database. Active Server Pages (ASP) was used to develop and run dynamic, interactive web server applications for lichen and butterfly images database. A computational tool was then created to store and archive lichen and butterfly images through SQL Server 2000 as front end and ASP.NET as back end (Belongies et al., 2002). ANN was used for the image segmentation based on the texture and non-texture shapes from the digital images of lichens and butterflies. The ANN implementation was completed by training the lichen data set and testing the unknown lichen and butterfly images with the trained data set for recognition. A total of 1,500 images were taken for the present study, from which 130 x 130 pixels of lichen and butterfly images were segmented using lichen/butterfly finder algorithm for further scanning. Lichen and butterfly images from top to bottom and left to right from the above scanning, opted shapes selected and trained in ANN as an input while scanning; sub-images were extracted subsequently and compared with ideal shapes from the data set (Smach et al., 2006).

The feature of lichens such as type of lichen growth forms (crustose, foliose, and fruticose), color, size, nature of thallus, the emergence of fruiting bodies on thallus, outer layer of lichens, and presence of rhizoids were extracted using the following formula. Similarly, the type of butterflies, color, head, legs, abdomen, the pattern of wings and veins, size and arrangement of antenna, and thorax were extracted using the following formula proposed by Arun et al. (2013) with slight modifications:

$$P(xi) = k/N \qquad (22.1)$$

where $P(xi)$ is defined as the probability of occurrence of gray levels, k is the number of pixels with gray-level contrast, N is the total number of pixels in various regions of lichens and butterflies. The number of features were extracted based on the number of samples collected in each species of lichen and butterfly images. The variance between lichen and butterfly species ($\mu 1$) was referred to as the measure of gray-level contrast used to describe the descriptors of relative smoothness of lichen thallus and butterfly morphology images with values:

$$\mu 1 = \sum_{i=0}^{L-1}(xi - \mu 0) \ P(xi) \qquad (22.2)$$

where $\mu 1$ is the mean of lichen and butterfly samples, $\mu 0$ is the gray-level contrast mean, Σ standard deviation, L-1 and i=0 are the standard error and critical difference, respectively, between close samplings, and xi and $\mu 0$ are the variations between measurements. The number of image samples closely associated and large deviations between samples were statistically analyzed based on standard deviation and correlation coefficient. The standard error and critical difference between samples were also calculated. The extracted features, feature values, and enhancement values were determined in terms of contrast, energy, homology, and entropy between images.

22.5 OBSERVATIONS

Both the lichen and butterfly images are captured in three views, such as front, close-up, and full. These images are stored as a data set and the digital camera is interfaced to a computer in which digital images are transferred for further analysis. The input images are needed in RGB format in general. For getting the feature extraction, a simple and accurate pre-processing phase without noise error is required for critical analysis of the images. Tested the various filtering techniques and transforms by applying them to the input images and chose the best filter, which removes the noise errors from the input lichen image. Removing noise may reduce the pixel size in the computer, which leads to less storage data. The input images have to be enhanced to obtain better segmentation to get the significant results.

22.5.1 PRE-PROCESSING OF LICHEN IMAGES

The collected lichen images were subjected to pre-processing to minimize undesired distortions or to enhance the quality of images for further processing (Figure 22.1). The detailed methodology is shown in Figure 22.2. The images were pre-processed by resizing (resizing the images), conversion (intensity information), and enhancement (image lighter or darker). The present pre-processing study is based on domain enhancement techniques such as spatial domain enhancement techniques which includes morphological operation, Gaussian filter, un-sharp masking, and adaptive filters (Brindha et al., 2015). Frequency domain enhancement techniques and wavelet transform techniques were used (Sheikh and Raghad, 2016).

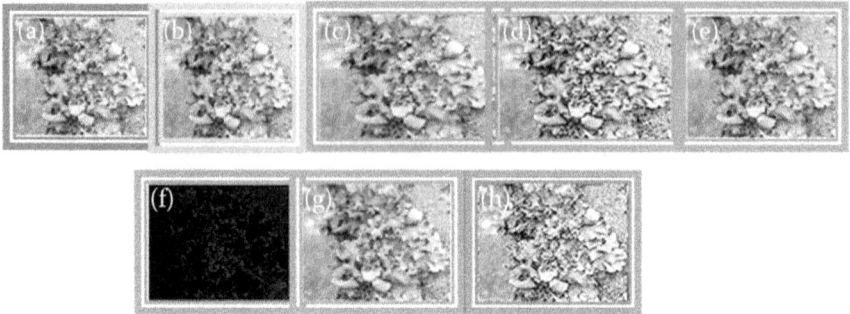

FIGURE 22.1 Pre-processing of collected lichen images [(a) input image, (b) resized image, (c) extrapolated image, (d) morphological operation, (e) un-sharp masking, (f) adaptive filter, (g) gaussian filter, (h) wavelet transform].

The lichen images are captured in three views, such as front, close-up, and full, and stored as a database for further processing. The collected images are pre-processed in MATLAB using the Image Processing Toolbox. For better quality image, various enhancement techniques were applied on the input lichen image in the pre-processing function and comparative analysis was done on the various enhancement techniques using error measurement parameters like Signal-to-Noise Ratio (SNR), Peak-to-peak Signal-to-Noise Ratio (PSNR), Mean Square Error (MSE), Root Mean Square Error (RMSE), Mean Absolute Error (MAE), Measurement of Enhancement (EME), and Correlation Coefficient.

This process has improved the quality of the input image significantly. The input image was converted from RGB to gray-scale format as per the data conversion process. In digital imaging, the object matching concept is applied to compare two images. This method performs very fast in detecting the similarity by means of an interest point detector even if the scale of the image is rotated and invariant. Based on the degree of image comparison, the state of interest points could be analyzed without affecting the original quality of both the 2D and 3D images. Speed Up Robust Feature (SURF) is a phenomenon of object matching concept, which produces accurate results. This method is more advanced than the Gaussian filter algorithm (which considers only gray information of the images), whereas the SURF method considers both the gray information along with the image edge structure information.

The enhancement techniques revealed that Gaussian filters exhibited highest PSNR value 18.46 and lowest MSE value of 935.13 followed by wavelet transform and morphological operation. The present pre-processing of lichen images showed Gaussian filters were better significant in enhancing image quality and features of lichen thallus. The consequence of lichen image processing Gaussian filter was used to improve the image quality. The data is presented in Table 22.1.

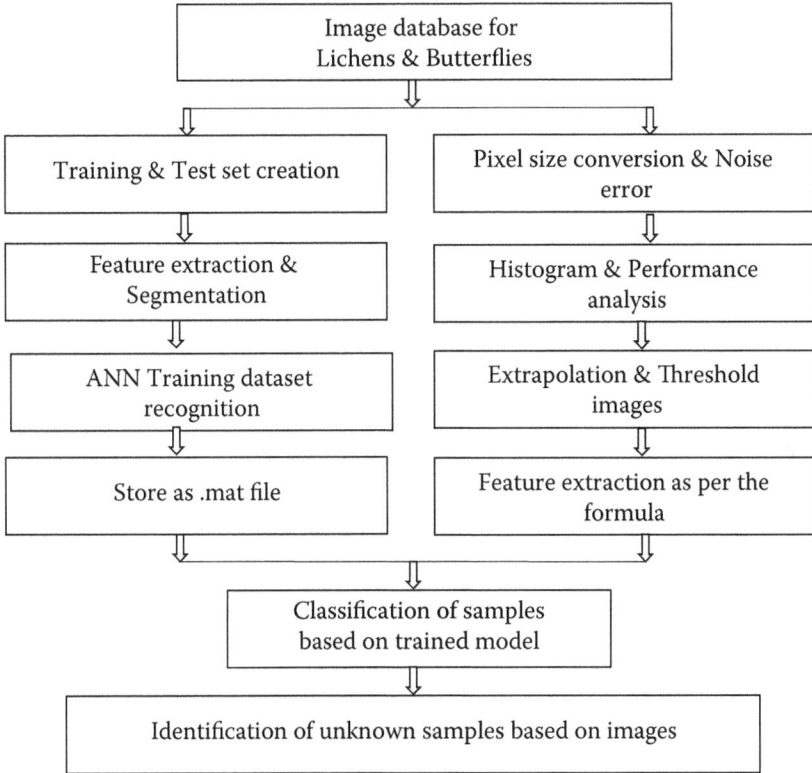

FIGURE 22.2   Classification of results in cloud computing.

22.5.2   SEGMENTATION OF PRE-PROCESSED LICHEN AND BUTTERFLY IMAGES

The lichen and butterfly images were further segmented to study the particular region of interest in lichen thallus and butterfly wings and their tiny scales or to predict important features. Image segmentation was done by using the following methods such as Thresholding (Senthilkumaran and Vaithegi, 2016), Active Contour (Khaldi and Farida, 2012), and K-Means Clustering (Piyush et al., 2013). In the thresholding level, T threshold was set, and segments were converted into two pixel values such as white and black format. During the segmentation process, both lichen and butterfly images were converted into gray-scale images and better segmentation and classification process. Moreover, the intensity of the input images was also greatly improved.

If the input image intensity f(x,y) was less than the threshold limit, then the pixel value of the input image was replaced with black pixel size so that the image clarity was better. A white pixel was replaced if f(x,y) was greater than T. The 2D gray-scale lichen and butterfly images into foreground (object) and background regions

TABLE 22.1

Analysis of Various Enhancement Techniques of Collected Lichen Images

Parameters	Enhancement Techniques				
	Morphological Operation	Un-sharp Masking	Adaptive Filter	Gaussian Filter	Wavelet Transform
PSNR	18.08607	18.07415	16.3797	**18.45608**	18.08307
SNR	−6.29727	−6.14960	−12.61189	−5.67425	−6.25833
RMSE	31.91071	31,95455	38.83755	30.57989	31.92172
MSE	1018.29330	1021.093	1508.355	**935.12955**	1018.9965
EME	4.72615	4.28513	0	6.29239	4.42760
Correlation coefficient	65535.00	57155.89	23234.85	55268.16	58891.22
MAE	6.28961	6.59203	6.38513	6.36874	6.19708

using a mask in the active contour method were applied. The basic K-means clustering was developed for lichen and butterfly images by the following steps:

1. Selection of K cluster center, degree of images, either randomly or based on image input heuristic method.
2. Assign each high-resolution pixel size in the input image to the K cluster that minimizes the space between the pixel size and the cluster center for good clarity.
3. Re-compute the cluster center of better clarity by averaging all of the pixel sizes in the selection of K clusters.
4. Repeat steps 2 and 3 until convergence and better clarity of input digital images is attained clearly.

The quality of the solution towards improving pixels depends on the initial set of clusters and the value of K on every image of lichens, which is useful for better clarity of the input images. It was purely based on the working principles of thresholding, active contour, and K-means clustering process (Khaldi and Farida, 2012; Senthilkumaran and Vaithegi, 2016).

The Region of Interest (ROI) in the input image was segmented from the input image using the thresholding, K-means clustering algorithm, and active contour method. K-means clustering revealed better segmentation for feature extraction than the other two methods tested in the present study. It showed the lichen thallus with all regions of interest, whereas thresholding exhibited the least characteristic feature of lichen thallus with other plants (background details) in the images. The contour of lichen thallus contains less detail in morphological and anatomical features. Then the features were extracted from the ROI using region props for SVM classifier for further analysis. Figure 22.3 shows the segmented image from the input lichen image using thresholding, active contour, and K-means clustering methods, respectively.

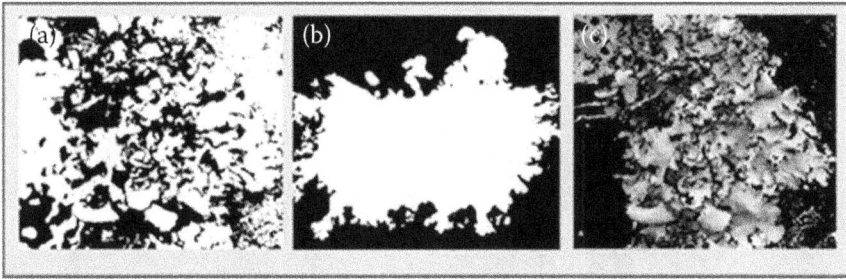

FIGURE 22.3 Segmentation of region of interest by various method [(a) thresholding, (b) active contour, (c) k-means clustering].

22.5.3 CLASSIFICATION AND PREDICTION OF LICHEN AND BUTTERFLY SPECIES

The classification and group of lichen and butterfly digital images have attempted using a Support Vector Machine (SVM) Classifier (Le Hoang et al., 2012). SVM is a supervised machine learning algorithm commonly used in all image processing techniques to identify unknown specimens, which can be used normally in both classification and regression challenges. The selected features such as contrast, correlation, energy, homogeneity, mean, standard deviation, entropy, root mean square, variance, smoothness, kurtosis, skewness, and IDM are extracted from the digital image results and used as an input image. The features of input lichen images were used as a training data set in the SVM classifier. In the SVM method, the features of input lichen images have been compared with training data set to find out the species name of input lichen image. The SVM classifier classifies the samples to be used for identification in which each row in TEST using the SVM classifier structure SVMSTRUCT, which created using SVMTRAIN is then applied. During the process, it returns the predicted class level GROUP significantly. TEST must contain the same number of columns as the data of images used to train the classifier in SVMTRAIN in rows. The results on GROUP indicated the group to which each row of TEST and its corresponding column having the images are assigned properly. Figures 22.4 and 22.5 show the step-by-step results obtained from the SVM classifier in various steps such as resized input image, contrast enhanced, thresholding, HSI image, image labeled by cluster index, cluster 1 image, cluster 2 image, cluster 3 image, selected the cluster contain ROI, selected cluster image, and converted gray-scale image of species.

22.5.4 IDENTIFICATION OF LICHEN AND BUTTERFLY IMAGES

Parmotrema lichen species were selected for image processing techniques to identify the name of the species without following the conventional method of the identification process (Figure 7.3). This genus belongs to the family Parmeliaceae, kingdom Fungi, division Ascomycota, class Lecanoromycetes, and order Lecanorales. *Parmotrema* is one of the largest genera of parmelioid core in the family Parmeliaceae in the lichen group (Ponmurugan et al., 2016). Based on the results, the selected lichen species was identified as *Parmotrema tinctorum* (Figure 22.6).

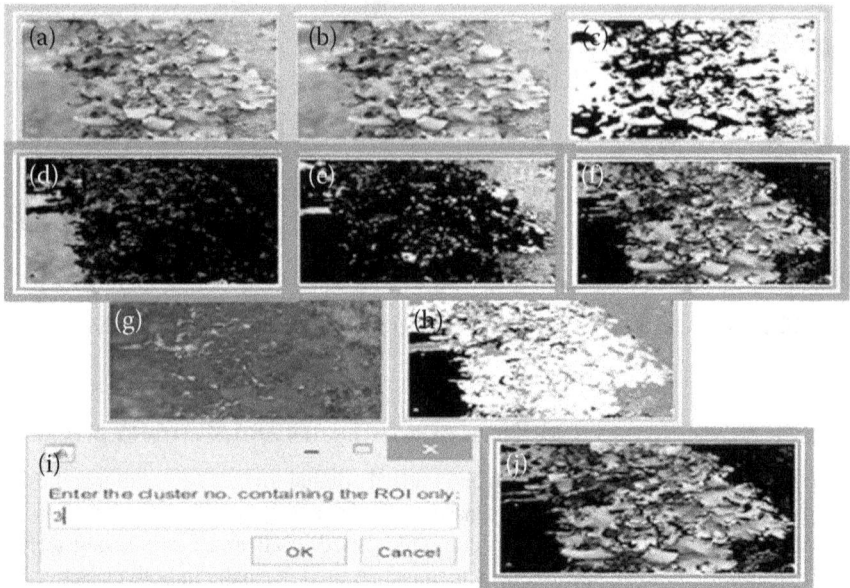

FIGURE 22.4 Classification and prediction of lichen species based on image processing techniques [(a) resized input image, (b) contrast enhanced, (c) thresholding, (d) HSI image, (e) image labeled by cluster index, (f) cluster 1 image, (g) cluster 2 image, (h) cluster 3 image, (i) select the cluster contain ROI, (j) selected cluster image converted grayscale image].

Butterfly species are identified based on wings, coloring patterns, tiny scales, antennae with/without clubbed; long/short with slim/fat abdomen, nature of head, and eye color. The images were taken using a digital camera during flying without disturbing the activity (Figure 7.4). They are widely used as insect model organisms to investigate the impact of habit and their habitat loss and fragmentation, environmental deterioration, and climate change. They are ecosystem indicators of a healthy environment in a particular location. It has been reported that they have numerous environmental benefits like inducing the pollination in higher plants and act as natural pest control, which is an important element of the food chain (Murugan, 2009). Based on the results, the selected butterfly species was identified as *Thymelicus sylvestris* (Figure 22.7).

After identifying selected species of lichen and butterfly using image processing techniques, the selected features and its values extracted from the pre-processed input image are shown in the Tables 22.2 and 22.3. The results indicated a significant difference between extracted features, feature values, and enhancement values of pre-processed input images of lichens and butterflies. It is because of growth habits and species diversity of lichens and butterflies (Ponmurugan, 2018). The analysis further showed that the enhancement values of pre-processed input images were higher than those of extracted features and feature values exhibited in both lichen and butterfly samples. Similarly, correlation coefficient and standard

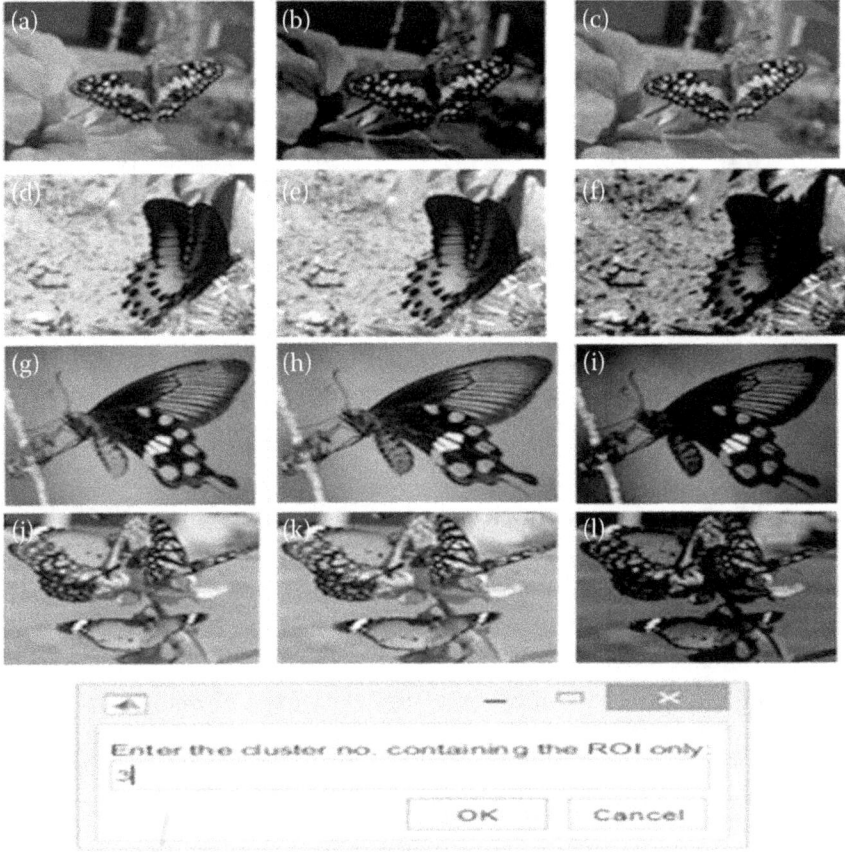

FIGURE 22.5 Classification and prediction of butterfly species on image processing techniques [(a) resized input image, (b) contrast enhanced, (c) thresholding of species 1, (d) resized input image, (e) contrast enhanced, (f) thresholding of species 2, (g) resized input image, (h) contrast enhanced, (i) thresholding of species 3, (j) resized input image, (k) contrast enhanced, (l) thresholding of species 4].

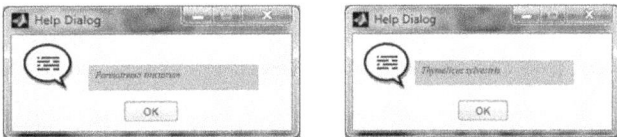

FIGURE 22.6 Results of SVM classifier of lichen *parmotrema tinctorum* and butterfly *thymelicus sylvestris*.

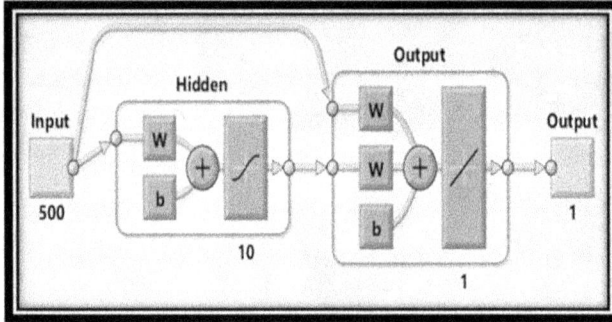

FIGURE 22.7   The cascade-forward model used by ANN.

TABLE 22.2
Extracted Features from Input Lichen Images

Extracted Features	Contrast	Correlation Coefficient	Energy	Homogeneity	Mean	SD	Entropy
Extracted features	4.57	2.561	0.12	0.52	44.23	52.55	3.56
Feature values	2.52	0.755	0.21	0.81	68.12	74.74	5.01
Enhancement values	9.03	5.118	1.07	1.84	5.60	25.23	5.84

TABLE 22.3
Extracted Features from Input Butterfly Images

Extracted Features	Contrast	Correlation Coefficient	Energy	Homogeneity	Mean	SD	Entropy
Extracted features	7.41	3.653	0.53	0.55	32.58	66.34	4.23
Feature values	4.55	2.845	0.24	0.58	42.42	85.65	5.88
Enhancement values	13.87	6.867	2.69	2.71	6.58	36.47	6.63

deviation were significantly varied in varying levels between features of lichen input images. It might be due to the nature of lichen thallus and butterfly sizes and shapes including various color variations (Vaishnavi et al., 2019).

The selected features were normally used for image classification in the SVM classifier, which provides accurate results. The name of the species of input lichen/ butterfly images will be displayed as a result of the SVM classifier. Figure 22.6 shows the resulting message box which contains the species name of input lichen and butterfly images. The SVM classifier classified each row in TEST using the support vector machine classifier structure SVMSTRUCT created using SVMTR-AIN. It returned the predicted class-level GROUP. TEST had the same number of columns as the data used to train the classifier in SVMTRAIN. GROUP indicated the group to which each row of TEST was assigned.

22.5.5 IMPLEMENTATION OF ARTIFICIAL NEURAL NETWORKS (ANNs)

The implementation of ANN consists of two processes in the present investigation such as 1) training and 2) testing process in identifying the lichen and butterfly images through image process techniques. In the image process techniques, ANN is playing an important role in lichen and butterfly images identification through training and testing processes. ANN training is a mathematical model in which a large number of numeric data such as values of extracted features, correlation efficiency, energy, entropy, and homogeneity were entered. These values consisted of several highly interconnected processing elements between two sets and subsequently organized into layers such as geometry and functionality. They normally resemble that of the human brain in terms of analysis and processing of input data. In general, ANN might be observed as enormously parallel distributed processor data that have a natural propensity for storing varying degrees of experiential knowledge upon a particular area of interest. Finally, the ANN process results may be made available in public domain for public use (Baxt, 1995). Among the various ANN processes, the cascade-forward propagation (CFP) network is generally used as the classifier on digital input original image and sub-image to be studied, which is required in this study consists of two layers. The observation revealed the first layer consisted of 145 input elements in accordance with the 500 feature vectors selected from the histogram of oriented gradients (HOG) features of sub-image (Smach et al., 2006). The further observations revealed that the number of neurons in the hidden first or second layers is recorded as 10. The single neuron in the output first/second layer towards the CFP network represents the recognition of species of lichen and butterfly images. The ANN has been continuously trained to adjust the connection weights and biases in order to produce the desired mapping of lichens and butterflies efficiently. In this stage of various processes, the feature vectors are employed as a digital input image to the network, adjusting its variable parameters, degree of weights and biases, to capture the relationship between the input patterns and output results of both lichens and butterflies. In ANN training, the 3 130*130 pixel sub-image features were significantly extracted from the lichen image database, which contains front, close up, and full view of lichen image and stored as a data set. The data set is trained with an artificial neural network to obtain the classification result. In ANN testing, the single 130*130 sub-image and features are being extracted from the unknown input lichen and butterfly images and then obtain the classification result by comparing sub-image features with the trained data set.

The ANN implementation is completed by training the lichen data set and testing the unknown lichen image with trained data set for recognition. Figure 22.7 showed the structure of ANN that we used to classify the lichen image. The structure that we used is based on 500 sub-image feature inputs extracted from 145 input lichen data set. Then, we have used one hidden layer where the hidden layer has 10 neurons. The single output layer gives the classification result.

The performance graph of lichen and butterfly images and error histogram result of ANN training revealed the performance analysis plots error vs. epoch for the training, validation, feature extraction, and test performances of the training records. In training records, several input images of lichen and butterfly were trained continuously in which histogram result of ANN training was obtained. Continuous training is necessary to validate the results without getting any errors which in turn to provide the best test performance. In this view, the input image of various lichen and butterfly species was trained to get the tangible results of output by means of several test performances. Due to continuous test performance, the number of errors were minimized considerably. Both input and output errors reduce after more epochs of the training process, but it might start to increase on the validation data sets as the network starts upon fitting the training data correspondingly. During the training process, a default setup is needed in which the training stops after six to eight consecutive increases in validation data error takes place. The best performance based on the number of validation errors is being considered from the epoch with the lowest validation errors among the training data sets. Error histogram is designed, wherein a histogram of error values was subjected to a continuous ANN training process, validation of output and testing for better performance. It is used to visualize errors between target values and predicted values after training the artificial neural network.

22.5.6 GRAYSCALE SUB-IMAGES OF LICHENS AND BUTTERFLY EXTRACTED FROM INPUT IMAGES

The sub-image extraction is the second step in ANN classification after pre-processing. The sub-images are extracted from pre-processed input image and each sub-image contains 130*130 pixels (i.e. Information) from the pre-processed input image. These sub-images are used to compare with lichen and butterfly image databases for recognition or identification in ANN tool boxes. We have tried to extract 4 130*130 pixel sub-images and 12 130*130 pixel sub-images. Figure 22.8 shows the sub-images extracted from grayscale input image and color input image, respectively. The lichen and butterfly images were extracted from the sub-images of various regions of interest with specified pixels. The sub-images and its orientation or segmented images were stored in the lichen and butterfly database. Likewise, all lichen and butterfly sub-images and parameters will be stored in the lichen and butterfly database. The system will be trained to predict the accurate unknown species using the ANN. Lichen and butterfly sub-images were stored on the basis of grayscale or color-based images.

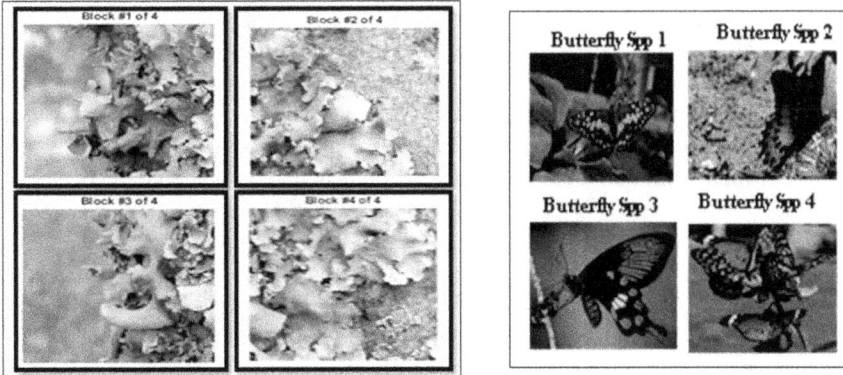

FIGURE 22.8   Grayscale lichen and butterfly sub-images extracted from input images.

22.5.7   CLOUD COMPUTING TECHNIQUES

Cloud computing plays one of the most vital roles in the business conception, because it doesn't require the user to have any PCs or other equipment (Janani et al., 2015). Cloud computing is mainly useful in business for bulk data storage, which is also specified by the allocated space and can be used as a normal PC system helpful for many people in this world. Cloud computing is in two different ways. The first one includes cloud storage, along with the requirements of the applications like operating system, application software, and storage. These are provided by companies like Google, Microsoft, and Amazon etc. These require a huge amount of space. The second one provides Web Interface along with the cloud storage. This requires a data cloud for storage of data sets (Maini and Aggarwal, 2010). In our proposed method, we use the web interface cloud, which incorporates MATLAB code and storage space on the web. The MATLAB code is converted into .dll format which allows interacting with the web interface and generates the result in the cloud computing methods.

Lichen and butterfly species were characterized and then identified based on the morphology, anatomy, and molecular data of DNA and protein sequencing. The present pre-processing of lichen and butterfly images showed Gaussian filters were significant in enhancing image quality and features of selected species. The consequence of lichen and butterfly species image processing Gaussian filter was used to improve image quality.

22.6   CONCLUSION

The lichen and butterfly images were obtained at random in Western Ghats of Tamil Nadu, India for the present study and were subjected to identify them based morphological and anatomical characteristic features. The collected images were pre-processed using MATLAB 2016 and subjected to machine learning technique for the identification from genus to species level. The pre-processing includes resizing, contrast enhancement, and image conversion. The Region of Interest (ROI) was segmented from the input image using K-means clustering algorithm and active contour methods. Then the selected features were classified by using the Support Vector Machine (SVM). The result indicated that 90% accuracy is obtained in image classification using the SVM classifier. The training process in ANN implementation was done and then the testing process which includes sub-image and feature extraction on both color and grayscale image and implementation of lichen/butterfly finder algorithm that compares the features of sub-images with the data set was done. The ANN classification gives 96% accuracy for lichen and butterfly image classification. The comparison of the SVM classifier and ANN classifier was done. The comparison result shows ANN classification is best for lichen and butterfly images and it will be used for further species classification. The ANN process was used to find out the trained images for identification purposes with least time interval and skilled manpower. The developed protocol is deployed in the lichen and butterfly image databases in cloud environments using Amazon web service for public access.

ACKNOWLEDGMENTS

The authors would like to acknowledge DST-SERB, New Delhi for financial support to carry out an Extramural Research project entitled "Development of protocol for identification of Lichens using Image processing techniques in cloud computing." The authors are indebted to Dr. D.K. Upredi, Director (Formerly) and Dr. Sanjeeva Nayaka, Principal Scientist, Lichenology Laboratory, CSIR-National Botanical Research Institute, Lucknow, Uttar Pradesh, India and Dr. G. Ayyappadasan, Assistant Professor, Department of Biotechnology & Dr. P.G. Geetha, Department of Computer Science and Engineering, KSR College of Technology, Tiruchengode, Tamil Nadu, India for allowing us to access their laboratory facilities. The authors are thankful to Prof. Dr. P. Kaliraj, Vice Chancellor and Prof. Dr. T. Devi, Professor and Head, Department of Computer Applications, Bharathiar University, Coimbatore, Tamil Nadu, India for their support in writing this book chapter.

REFERENCES

Antowiak, M., Chalasinska, M.K., 2003. Finger identification by using artificial neural network with optical wavelet preprocessing. Optoelectronics Review 11, 327–337.

Arnal Barbedo, J.G., 2013. Digital image processing techniques for detecting, quantifying and classifying plant diseases. Springer Plus 2, 660–665.

Arun, C.H., Emmanuel, W.R.S., Durairaj, D.C., 2013. Texture feature extraction for identification of medicinal plants and comparison of different classifiers. International Journal of Computer Applications 62, 1–9.

Awasthi, D.D., 2007. Compendium of the macrolichens from India, Nepal and Sri Lanka. Bishen Singh Mahendra Pal Singh, Uttarakhand, India.

Ayyappadasan, G., Madhupreetha, T., Ponmurugan, P., Jeyaprakash, S., 2017. Antibacterial and antioxidant activity of *Parmotrema reticulatum* obtained from Eastern Ghats, Southern India. Biomedical Research 28, 1593–1597.

Baxt, W.G., 1995. Application of artificial neural networks to clinical medicine. The Lancet 346, 1135–1138.

Belongies, S., Malik, K., Jitendra, L., Puzicha, L., 2002. Shape matching and object recognition using shape contexts. IEEE Transactions on Pattern Analysis and Machine Intelligence 24, 121–137.

Brindha, B., Anusuya, P., Karunya, S., 2015. Image enhancement techniques. International Journal of Research in Engineering and Technology 4, 455–459.

Chellappa, R., Wilson, C., Sirohey, S., 1995. Human and machine recognition of faces: A survey. Proceedings of the IEEE 83, 705–740.

Dennis, R.L.H., Shreeve, T.G., Arnold, R., Henry, R., David, B., 2005. Does diet breadth control herbivorous insect distribution size? Life history and resource outlets for specialist butterflies. Journal of Insect Conservation 9, 187–200.

Fu, K.S., 1996. Digital Pattern Recognition. Springer-Verlag, London, UK. 228 pp.

Gomez, K.A., Gomez, A.A., 1984. Statistical Procedure for Agricultural Research, 2nd edn. International Rice Research Institute, Los Banos, The Philippines, pp. 183–190.

Hale, F., Mason, E., 2008. Biology of Lichens and Identification Procedures. Edward Arnold Publishers Ltd, London, UK. 325 pp.

Harpel, D., Cullen, D.A., Ott, S.R., Jiggins, C.D., Walters, J.R., 2015. Pollen feeding proteomics: Salivary proteins of the passion flower butterfly, *Heliconius melpomene*. Insect Biochemistry and Molecular Biology 63, 7–13.

Janani, P., Premaladha, J., Ravichandran, K.S., 2015. Image enhancement techniques: A study. Indian Journal of Science and Technology 8, 1–12.

Hamuda, E., Glavin, M., Jones, E., 2016. A survey of image processing techniques for plant extraction and segmentation in the field. Computers and Electronics in Agriculture 125, 184–199.

Kalidoss, R., Ayyappadasan, G., Gnanamangai, B.M., Ponmurugan, P., 2020. Antibacterial activity of lichen *Parmotrema* spp. International Journal of Pharmaceutical Biological Sciences 8, 7–11.

Kalidoss, R., Poornima, S., Ponmurugan, P., 2020. Anti-microbial and antiproliferative activities of depside compound isolated from the mycobiont culture of *Parmotrema austrosinense* (Zahlbr.) Hale. Journal of Pure and Applied Microbiology 14, 2525–2541.

Khaldi, A., Farida, M.H., 2012. An active contour for range image segmentation. Signal & Image Processing: International Journal of Computing 3, 17–29.

Kulkarni, A.D., 1994. Artificial Neural Networks for Image Understanding. International Thomson Publishers, New York, US, 421 pp.

Le Hoang, T., Hai, T.S., Thuy, N.T., 2012. Image classification using support vector machine and artificial neural network. International Journal of Information Technology and Computer Science 5, 32–38.

Lucking, R., 2008. Foliicolous Lichenized Fungi. New York Botanical Garden Press, Bronx, New York, US, 741 pp.

Maini, R., Aggarwal, H., 2010. A comprehensive review of image enhancement techniques. Journal of Computing 2, 8–13.

Mariraj, M., Kalidoss, R., Vinayaka, K.S., Nayaka, S., Ponmurugan, P., 2020. *Usnea dasaea*, a further new addition to the Lichen Flora of Tamil Nadu State, India. Current Botany 11, 138–141.

Murugan, K., 2009. Biodiversity conservation of butterflies in the Western Ghats, Southern India. In: Victor, R. & Robinson, M.D. (eds) Proceedings of the International Conference on Mountains of the World, Ecology, Conservation and Sustainable Development. Sultan Qaboos University, Oman, pp. 74–77.

Narendran, T.C., 2001. Taxonomic entomology research and education in India. Current Science 81, 445–447.

Piyush, M., Shah, B.N., Vandana, S., 2013. Image segmentation using K-mean clustering for finding tumor in medical application. International Journal of Computer Trends and Technology 4, 1239–1242.

Ponmurugan, P., 2018. Biotechnology Techniques in Biodiversity Conservation. New Age International, New Delhi, India, 222 pp.

Ponmurugan, P., Ayyappadasan, G., Verma, R.S., Nayaka, S., 2016. Survey, distribution pattern and elemental composition of lichens in Yercaud hills of Eastern Ghats in southern India. Journal of Environmental Biology 37, 407–412.

Senthilkumaran, N., Vaithegi, S., 2016. Image segmentation by using thresholding techniques for medical images. Computer Science & Engineering International Journal 6, 1–13.

Sheikh, T., Raghad, R., 2016. A comparative study of various image filtering techniques for removing various noisy pixels in aerial image. International Journal of Signal Processing 9, 113–124.

Shrestha, G., El-Naggar, A.M., St. Clair, L.L., O'Neill, K.L., 2015. Anticancer activities of selected species of North American lichen extracts. Phototherapy Research 29, 100–107.

Smach, F., Atri, M., Mitéran, J., Abid, M., 2006. Design of a neural networks classifier for face detection. Journal of Computer Science 2, 257–260.

Srygley, R.B., Thomas, A.L.R., 2002. Aerodynamics of insect flight: Flow visualisations with free flying butterflies reveal a variety of unconventional lift-generating mechanisms. Nature 420, 660–664.

Tanas, S., Odabasoglu, F., Halici, Z., Cakir, A., Aygun, H., Aslan, A., Suleyman, H., 2010. Evaluation of anti-inflammatory and antioxidant activities of *Peltigera rufescens* lichen species in acute and chronic inflammation models. Journal of Natural Medicine 64, 42–45.

Vaishnavi, R., Jamuna, S., Usha, C.S., 2019. A survey paper on identification of diseased leaves in plants with the implementation of IOT and image processing. International Journal of Computer Engineering and Sciences Research 1, 25–29.

Vartia, K.O., 1973. Antibiotics in lichens. In: Ahmadjian, V., & Hale, M.E. (eds) The Lichens. Academic Press, New York, US, 561 pp.

Vivian, M., Françoise, C.M., Daren, B., Shannon, S., Gary, D., Julian, D., 2001. Taxonomic status: Present and future. Trends in Biotechnology 19, 349–355.

Vukusic, P., Sambles, J.R., Ghiradella, H., 2000. Optical classification of microstructure in Butterfly wing-scales. Photonics Science News 6, 61–66.

Yago, M., Yoshitake, H., Ohshima, Y., Katsuyama, R., Sivaramakrishnan, S., Murugan, K., Ito, M., 2010. Butterflies collected from Coimbatore, Tamil Nadu, South India with comment on its conservation significance. Butterflies 54, 45–53.

23 Artificial Neural Network for Decision Making

K.M. Sakthivel[1] and C.S. Rajitha[2]

[1]Associate Professor, Department of Statistics, Bharathiar University, Coimbatore, India

[2]Assistant Professor, Department of Mathematics, Amrita School of Engineering, Amrita Vishwa Vidyapeetham, Coimbatore, India

CONTENTS

OBJECTIVES

This chapter starts with a clear-cut presentation of ANN (artificial neural network) and progresses with different components and structure of ANN along with a detailed explanation. After that it provides an overview of the learning procedure of ANN with different learning algorithms and discusses ANN applications in various fields. This chapter also provides a short discussion on the performance of ANN for count modeling and ends with a comparison study of ANN with eminently used count models like zero-inflated Poisson (ZIP) and Hurdle models to model count data.

DOI: 10.1201/9781003175865-23

23.1 INTRODUCTION

ANNs are generally referred to as a neural network (NN) designed in the similar manner as in the processing of information in the human brain. Since dealing out of the information in the brain is like an extremely multifaceted, nonlinear analogous computer, computations made by the brain are completely different from the typical digital computer. The human brain is comprised of very simple and densely parallel several nerve cells and can learn. Proximity to effectively working like the human brain is the encouraging thing in studying Artificial Neural Networks (ANNs) (Haykin, 1999).

Figure 23.1 shows how our brain processes information. There are billions of cells called neurons in our brain, which help information development in the pattern of electric signals. Exterior motivation arrives through the neuron's dendrites, developed in the neuron cell body, transformed to output, and transited the axon to the subsequent neuron. The next neuron can prefer to agree on it or decline it, depending on the power of the signal. The following steps help to understand in what way our brain processes information:

Step 1: Exterior signal received by dendrites
Step 2: Exterior signal processes in the neuron cell body
Step 3: Processes signal transformed into an output signal and transferred through the axon
Step 4: Output signal received by the dendrites of the subsequent neuron through the synapse

It is acknowledged and wide-ranging of modern brain study proposals that the brain of human beings is further convoluted as several of its cognitive tasks are still mysterious. The following are the major features measured and explained as universal tasks in actual and artificial networks:

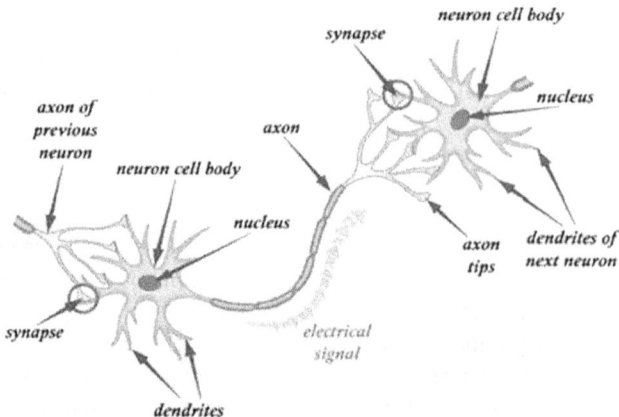

FIGURE 23.1 A biological neuron.

- Generalization
- Associative storage of information
- Learning and adaptation
- Spatiotemporal information processing
- Robustness

It is not required to program a neural network in an explicit manner. It can learn from training samples or through support. The ability of the learning procedure is that the network can generalize and associate the data. After effective training of a neural network, we can get sensible results for identical problems of a similar category that were not trained explicitly. This successively produces results in a high degree of accuracy besides piercing input data.

To attain a better performance through learning process, ANN uses a monolithic interdependence of parallel computational units usually referred to as the processing units or neurons (Ibiwoye et al., 2012). An artificial neuron is an electric imitation of an organic neuron; it obtains stimulus from neighboring cells, or as of its surroundings, and produces a customized nerve signal (Ajibola et al., 2011).

"According to Haykin (1999), a neural network is characterized as a massively parallel dispersed processor or computer including simple computational units, which has a natural tendency for keeping experimental knowledge and making it accessible for use. It reminds you of the brain in two ways:

1. *During the learning process, the network attains the necessary knowledge from its surroundings.*
2. *For storing the knowledge attained by learning process, the interneuron connection strength, also called synaptic weights are used."*

The learning algorithm is the procedure used for performing the learning process. The role of the learning algorithm is to qualify the synaptic weights (SW) of the network in a well-ordered manner to arrive at a trusted designing target. Association networks, neuro computers, parallel dispersed processors, etc. are the other names of NNs in the literature.

To compose matter clearer, let's realize ANN using a simple example: A bank wishes to measure whether to agree a loan request to a customer (client), so it needs to forecast whether a client is to be expected to fail to pay on the loan. The data in Table 23.1 can be used to forecast whether a client is expected to fail to pay the loan. The model generated will take the values for the customer age, customer debit ratio and monthly income and map them to "Yes" or "No."

So, we need to forecast the last column (default prediction). A forecast nearer to 1 points out that the client has added probability to nonpayment. Overall, a simple ANN structural design for the above instance might be like the subsequent Figure 23.2. The ANN in Figure 23.2 receives three inputs, X_1, X_2 and X_3, and produces a single output, O_3. The ANN calculates the output value from the input values as follows. First, the input values are taken from the attributes of the training example, as it is inputted to the ANN. These values are then weighted and fed into the next set of nodes, which in this example are H1 and H2. A nonlinear activation function is then

TABLE 23.1

Prediction of Nonpayment

Customer ID	Customer Age	Debit Ratio (% of Income)	Monthly Income ($)	Defaulting Debtor Yes: 1, No: 0	Prediction of Nonpayment
1	45	0.80	9,120	1	0.76
2	40	0.12	2,000	1	0.66
3	38	0.08	3,042	0	0.34
4	25	0.03	3,300	0	0.55
5	49	0.02	63,588	0	0.15
6	74	0.37	3,500	0	0.72

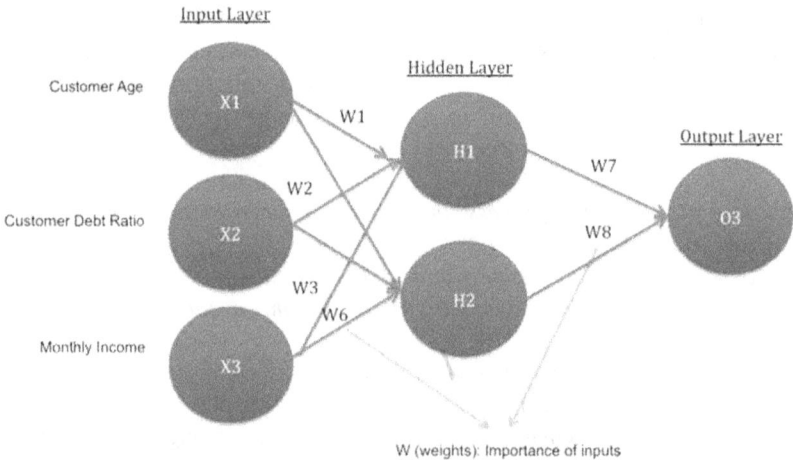

FIGURE 23.2 ANN structure.

utilized to this weighted sum and then the resultant value is passed to the succeeding layer, where this procedure is replicated, until the last value(s) are output. The ANN learns by gradually reviewing its weights so that all through the training period, the estimated output value moves nearer to the experimental value. The most popular algorithm for adapting the weights is the backpropagation algorithm (Rumelhart et al., 1986). As a result of the nature of ANN learning, the entire training set is applied repetitively, where each application is mentioned as an epoch.

23.2 COMPONENTS OF ANN

According to Haykin (2009), ANN forms a directed graph by connecting the artificial neurons, the basic processing components of the network. The three basic components of a NN are the fundamental computing elements, known as neurons or nodes; the network structural design which describes the association among computing units or neurons; and the training rule accustomed to locate the weights which modify the strength of the input for performing a particular task.

The fundamental building block of a NN is the neuron, which is an information processing unit. Layers of units are used for constructing ANNs; therefore it is termed multi-layer ANNs. The first layer is called the input layer to accept external information; they are considered independent variables as per statistical literature. The final layer is the output layer, which generates the model solution. In statistical terminology, these units are called the response or dependent variable. The layers connecting input and output layers are named hidden layers. Agatonovic Kustrins and Beresford (2000) described that a NN's behavior is influenced using its neurons' transfer functions, through the learning rule, and with the structural design itself. The key elements of the neuronic model are:

1. **Synapses, also known as connecting links**, are used for operating neurons by receiving signals from other neurons. A weight or strength is used for characterizing a synapse called SW. Precisely, multiplying each unit x_j at the input layer of synapse j associated to neuron k with SWw_{kj}. Negative and positive values can be used as the weight of an artificial neuron.
2. **An adder, or LC**, is used to find the total of the input signals (IS). The respective synapses weigh the IS of the neuronal model.
3. **Activation function or transfer function**: The output amplitude is limited by using this function.

According to Stergious and Siganos (2007), the performance of an ANN depends on both the weights and transfer function (activation function) that is determined for the units. The essential part of ANN is finding out or learning the weights that reproduce the wanted output for a given series of inputs. Backpropagation algorithm is one of the generally adopted ways of finding and training the weights.

A general model of ANN might be like Figure 23.3. The normalized magnitude range of neuronal output in general lies between [0, 1] or [-1, 1]. b_k denote an externally applied bias of the neural modal. The bias b_k has the impression of rising or declining the net input of the transfer function; relying upon either is positive or negative. Mathematically, a neuron k can also be summarized by the subsequent equations:

$$u_k = \sum_{j=1}^{m} w_{kj} x_j$$
$$y_k = \phi(u_k + b_k)$$

where $x_1, x_2, \ldots, x_m$ denote the IS; SWs of neuron k are characterized by $w_{k1}, w_{k2}, \ldots, w_{km}$; u_k is the linear combiner (LC) output due to the IS; $b_k = w_{k0}$ is the externally applied bias; $\phi(.)$ denote the activation function; output signal of the neuron is denoted by y_k. To make use of the bias b_k, the affine transformation is used to the output u_k of the LC:

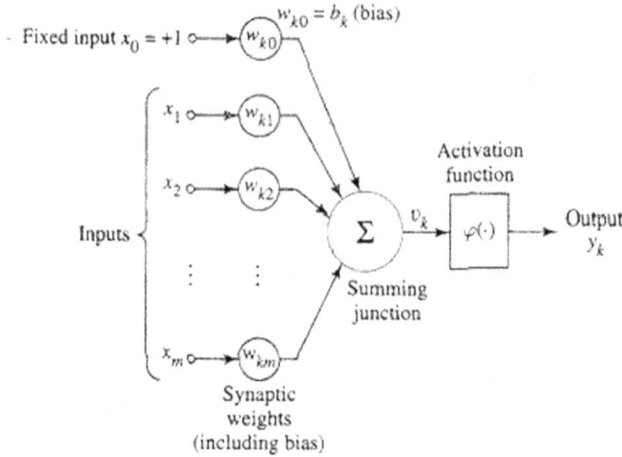

FIGURE 23.3 A general model of ANN.

$$v_k = u_k + b_k$$

v_k is called the induced local field (ILF). The association between the LC output u_k and activation function potential v_k or the ILF of neuron k modified on either the bias b_k is positive or negative. The bias b_k denotes an externally applied bias of artificial neuron k. We may combine the above three equations as follows:

$$v_k = \sum_{j=1}^{m} W_{kj} x_j$$
$$y_k = \phi(v_k)$$

A variety of transfer (activation) functions are available, including threshold function, sigmoid function, and piecewise linear function, of which sigmoid function is the most frequently used function. It is the logistic function:

$$\phi(v) = \frac{1}{1 + \exp(-av)}$$

where a denotes slope parameter of the sigmoid function. Several possibilities of utilizing transfer functions of various types in neural models are given in Duch and Jankowski (2001).

23.3 STRUCTURE WITH EXPLANATION

The structure of the network refers to the arrangement of the units and the types of connections permitted. The network consists of a set of neurons which can generally label with positive integers. The neurons are associated in the sense that the output of one unit will serve as a component of the input to another. For every network, there is a network associated with each connection. Coordination of the computing units and the variety of connections allowed by the network are mentioned by the network architecture.

23.3.1 NETWORK ARCHITECTURES

The two commonly used types of networks are feed-forward networks (FFN) and recurrent networks (RNs). If the flow of information within the network is only in the forward direction and the behavior of the network does not depend on the past, then it is called FFN. Recurrent neural networks include at least one feedback connection.

23.3.2 FEEDFORWARD NEURAL NETWORKS

It is a layered-type neural network. In 1950s Rosenblatt commenced the layered feed-forward network referred to as single-layer perceptron since it has only one layer. All the layers and nodes are connected in a feed-forward manner for a perceptron. But it is only suitable for solving linearly separable problems. Minsky and Papert (1969) provided the mathematical restrictions of a distinct layer network in their famous book, *Perceptrons*. Hence, to overcome the limitations of the single-layered feed-forward network, a multi-layer feed-forward network with one or more hidden layers referred to as multi-layer perceptron has been developed. In this network computation, nodes or neurons of the hidden layer are called unseen units or hidden neurons and it can be trained using backpropagation algorithm (BPA). And multi-layer feed-forward network (MLFFN) is the generally used type of NN used in statistical applications. In the MLFFN, units are ordered in a series of layers. This is one of the network types most often used in statistical applications.

23.3.3 BACKPROPAGATION TRAINING ALGORITHM

BPA was first introduced by Werbos (1974). But his work stayed without getting much attention from the scientific community. Parker (1985) worked on this technique and published his findings. After some time, this technique was again rediscovered by Rumelhart et al. (1986), which led to the backpropagation technique to become an outstanding supporter of neuro computing. This technique is the most popular for network modeling and maintains superior performance among all the existing models.

For finding the discrepancy between real and required network outputs, cost function (equal to the mean squared error) is used in the backpropagation algorithm and this algorithm employs a gradient descent procedure to reduce the cost function. Gradient descent technique is a computational method trying to find the accurate weight values employed with the backpropagation training algorithm. The algorithm proposed by Rumelhart et al. (1986) contains the demonstration of a set of pairs of output and input outlines. At first, the input vector is used to produce actual network output or its own output and then compares the two outputs, actual and the desired output (target vector). There is no need to train the data if the difference among the real and the required output is zero; otherwise change the network weights for dropping the difference between these two outputs.

23.4 TYPES OF LEARNING

The practice of adjusting parameters of NN to get better performance is normally called learning. Quite a few components are required for learning. Primary, as the modification of network parameters, the functioning should get better. Consequently, the description of a performance appraisal is necessary and the regulations for varying the parameters have to be defined. Third, this practice of network training must be completed using well-known (historical) data. However, until now the learning algorithms are applied and arranged into three groups.

23.4.1 SUPERVISED LEARNING (SL)

If the performance function is derived from the description of an error gauge, it is called SL. Usually the error is specified as the variation of the output of the ANN and a predefined peripheral required indication. In industrial purposes where the required functioning is identified, SL paradigms be converted into extremely significant. The training illustrations be composed of input vectors x and the required output vectors y and training is carried out up to the NN "be trained" to connect every input vector x to its consequent output vector y (estimated a function $y = f(x)$). It converts the illustration in its interior arrangement.

For the category of SL, three essential judgments are required to be made: an alternative to the error measure, how the error is transmitted throughout the network, and what restriction (stationary or crosswise time) one entails on the network output. The primary problem is associated with the formula (the cost function) that calculates the error. The next feature is connected to systems that change the network parameters in a mechanized style. At this point, we will notice that gradient descent learning is the primary of frequent learning in SL methods. The third feature is connected with how we restrict the network output against the required signal. One can point out merely the behavior at the finishing time called fixed point learning (FPL); i.e. we do not confine the values that the output gets on with the required behavior. Or, we can confine the intermediary values and is called trajectory learning (TL). Note that a FFN, as it is an immediate mapper (the reaction is attained in recent step), can merely be taught by FPL. On the other hand, RNs can be trained by indicating either the last instance behavior (FPL) or the behavior next to a path (TL). Learning necessitates the requirement of a data set for network training. This is usually entitled as the train set. Performance of the learning should be assured next to a mutually exclusive set of data, named as the test set. It is of basic significance to select a suitable training set size, and to offer representative exposure of all potential circumstances. Throughout learning, the network is directed to find out the most excellent mapping among the input data and the required concert. If the data employed in the training set is not a mediator of the input data class, we can anticipate an unfortunate presentation with the test set. Although functioning can be perform outstandingly with the training set. There are essentially three convenient characteristics connected to learning: 1. Variable selection set and size of the training data set, 2. the choice of training algorithm and algorithmic parameters, and 3. what time to discontinue the learning to stop overdoing it. Regrettably, there are no "formulas" to choose these parameters. Merely a number of common policies can be appropriate and a bunch of testing is essential. By the way, the accessibility of rapid replication environment and comprehensive questioning abilities are a specific advantage.

23.4.2 Unsupervised Learning (UL)

This category of learning transforms the network weights in relation to various predefined internal rules of interface (unsupervised learning). As a result there is no "outside teacher." This is the motive of calling UL as self-organization. Self-organization may be extremely suitable for attribute detection (characteristic extraction) in multifarious signals with redundancy. Only input vectors x are issued and the NN learns a few internal characteristics of the entire set of all the input vectors offered to it. Modern unsupervised algorithms are further divided into two (i) noncompetitive and (ii) competitive.

23.4.3 Reinforcement Learning (RL)

It is also stated as a reward penalty learning method. In RL the outside trainer immediately points out the worth (fine or terrible) of the reply. RL is still in a research stage; however, it may cling to the input to online learning. The input vector is described, and the NN is permitted to compute the subsequent output, and if it is good quality, then the active connection weights are improved (rewarded), or else the connection weights associated are reduced (punished).

23.5 APPLICATION

As a result of some outstanding characteristics, ANNs have numerous applications:

i. *Image Processing and Character Recognition*: Given ANNs' capacity to acquire a lot of inputs, treat them to deduce unseen along with composite, nonlinear associations, ANNs are performing a gigantic task in image and character recognition. Character recognition like writing style, has plenty of implementations in fraud detection (e.g., bank fraud) and national safety measurements. Image detection is a continually increasing area with extensive demands from face detection in public networks, cancer screening in the medical industry to satellite-based image processing for agronomic and defense service. The study on ANN now has opened the door for deep NNs that provide the support for "deep learning," which has now commenced all the stimulating and reconstructive novelties in artificial intelligence, voice recognition, and programming language – well-known examples being self-driving cars.

ii. ***Forecasting or Prediction***: Prediction is necessary in daily decision making in business (e.g., sales, budgetary appropriations between products, use of the capacity), in financial and fiscal policy, in funding, and the equity market. Frequently, prediction problems are difficult; for instance, forecasting stock prices is a difficult crisis with numerous essential components (some recognized, some hidden). Conventional predictive models throw up restrictions with respect to these multifarious, nonlinear relationships. ANNs, implemented in the proper way, will be able to supply persistent substitute, given its capacity to model and pull out hidden characteristics and associations. In addition, contrary to these conventional models, ANN doesn't oblige any constraint on input and remaining distributions. Further research is going on in the field.

It is found that the majority of ANN applications mostly fell off in the class of forecast, in which locating an unexplained connection subsists among a set of input factors and an output is of key attention. The training process of ANN model results in ascertains the underlying connection between the variables with existing data. The foremost drawback is that ANN models do not illustrate any substantial interior system that monitors the processes. On the other hand, the application of ANN model has been remaining urged in the majority of the circumstances because of the precise guess or prediction compared to conceptual models. In statistical terms, the ANN output estimates the mean of the fundamental objective trained on the NN model input vector; though ANN predictions express no information concerning the sampling errors and the prediction accurateness. The restricted recognition of the ANN model applications can be probably endorsed to the complexity noticed in conveying self-confidence interval (or prediction interval) to the output, which may develop the consistency and reliability of the predictions. Consequently an inquiry into computing the improbability connected with the ANN model predictions is basically required. Modern studies show that modeling count data using ANN offers comparatively superior performance against traditional statistical models such as GLM, hurdle models, zero-inflated models, etc. But all these approaches used for modeling the count data, including the zero-inflated count models are dependent on a set of rigorous assumption and conditions such as linearity, independence, normality, etc. But, actually for modeling count data, it may not be possible to meet an optimal situation to satisfy all of these assumptions. We can use NNs as a substitute to all these traditional methods and have attained remarkable reputation in the current years, especially in prediction, estimation, classification, and forecasting due to some specific properties such as nonlinearity, nonparametric nature, and adaptive learning properties.

Previously we have discussed the number of eminent ones, but they have extensive applications through various distinct areas in medical science, defense, banking/finance and government, farming, and security. And a number of existing applications of ANN in general are

- *Function estimate, when a set of data is presented*
- *Pattern organization*

- *Data clustering, classification, and conceptualization*
- *Learning statistical parameters*
- *Cumulating knowledge through training*
- *"Acquiring" information through scrutiny of the connection weights*
- *Introducing information in a NN structure for the intention of approximate reasoning*

23.5.1 PERFORMANCE ANALYSIS USING REAL DATA

The superiority of ANN can be proved with the help of an example. For that consideration, a car insurance data set is available in the *Insurance Data* package in R software. The data set comprises a claim file with 120,000 records. It is mandatory to analyze the claim numbers, which is influenced by the age of driver, the value of the vehicle, and duration. The frequency allotment of the claim count is specified in Table 23.2; types of variables (independent and dependent variables) are given in Table 23.3.

A frequency plot of claim counts is presented in Figure 23.4. It is seen that the zero number claim is too large in the data (i.e., 86%). The index of dispersion (ID) is 3.516. It clearly shows the overdispersion of the data.

The study is conducted for 10 percentage to cent percentage of the data. Two diverse ratios for training and testing as 70%:30%, and 80%:20% have been considered, and the mean squared error (MSE) and relative efficiency (RE) for ZIP, Hurdle, and ANN models have been computed. For ANN model making, we used BPA because it exposes reliable and quick approximation with two hidden layers. The result of this analysis is provided in Table 23.4. Table 23.5 shows the mean relative efficiency for ZIP, Hurdle, and ANN models.

23.5.2 RESULTS AND DISCUSSION

23.5.2.1 Results

The performance of various models is measured based on normalized MSE and relative efficiency. Table 23.4 shows that ANN provides superior performance compared to the other two models for 75% of the experiments. The normalized MSE of ANN is comparatively less in contrast to the other two conventional models. As evaluating the mean RE from Table 23.5, ANN presents superior results against ZIP and Hurdle models for this insurance count data.

Figure 23.5 offers RE of all three models with the relevant inflation rate. It is seen that ANN performs better than ZIP for a modest rate of inflation, and also, it is always superior or close to the Hurdle model for different rates of inflation.

23.5.2.2 Discussion

As shown in Figure 23.5, ANN, ZIP, and Hurdle models can predict claim counts well, and close to real number of claims, but the ability of ANN model in contrast of ZIP and Hurdle Poisson regression model is advanced and closer to real claim counts.

TABLE 23.2
Frequency of Claim Counts

Claim Frequency	Count	Percentage	Claim Frequency	Count	Percentage	Claim Frequency	Count	Percentage
0	102,870	85.725	12	19	0.016	25	4	0.0033
1	11,872	9.8933	13	20	0.017	26	1	0.00083
2	2,995	2.496	14	8	0.007	27	2	0.0017
3	1,029	0.8575	15	6	0.005	29	1	0.00083
4	457	0.38	16	8	0.007	30	1	0.00083
5	260	0.2167	17	6	0.005	32	1	0.00083
6	140	0.1167	18	4	0.0033	33	1	0.00083
7	96	0.08	19	3	0.0025	36	1	0.00083
8	63	0.053	20	6	0.005	37	1	0.00083
9	51	0.04	21	4	0.0033	38	1	0.00083
10	35	0.03	22	3	0.0025	43	1	0.00083
11	25	0.021	23	5	0.0042			

TABLE 23.3

Type of Variables

Independent Variables (Input Variables)	Dependent Variable (Target Variable)
1. Driver's age category	Number of claims
2. Vehicle value	
3. Period	

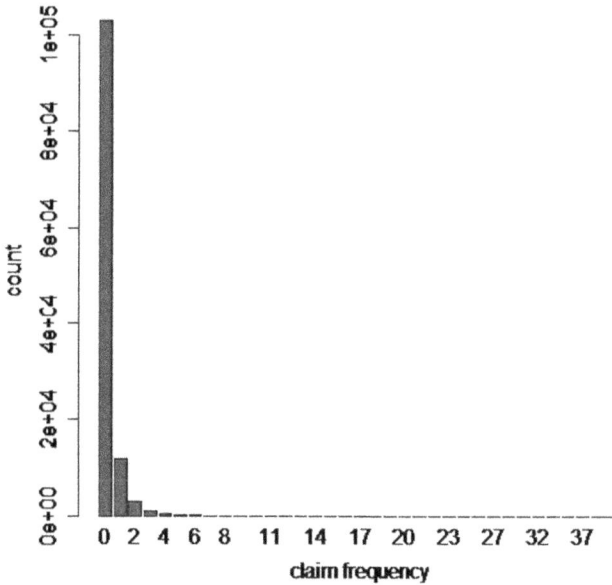

FIGURE 23.4   Frequency of claim counts.

As shown in Table 23.4, statistical analysis of the data revealed that ANN has less normalized MSE compared to ZIP and Hurdle regression models stating high certainty of ANN. There are many metrics available for determining model performance for regression problems, but one of the most frequently used metric is *MSE*. The error in this occasion is the dissimilarity in value concerning a given model prediction and its actual value for an out-of-sample observation. Thus, the MSE is the average of all of the squared errors through all new observations, which is the same as accumulating all of the squared errors (*sum of squares*) and dividing by the number of observations.

To compare the prediction ability of models, one can look at the relative efficiency (ratio of MSE). The relative efficiency indicates how much more efficient ANN is as compared with ZIP and Hurdle regression models. The relative efficiency of ANN vs ZIP and ANN vs Hurdle models is smaller than one indicates that

TABLE 23.4
Summary of the Results

Sl No.	Sample Size (n)	Train:Test	MSE of Models			Relative Efficiency			Model with least MSE value
			ZIP	Hurdle	ANN	ANN/Hurdle	ANN/ZIP	Hurdle/ZIP	
1	12000	80:20	0.6761	0.6771	0.6762	0.09986	1.00015	10.0154	ZIP
	12000	70:30	0.9949	0.9949	0.9932	0.99827	0.99834	1.00007	NN
2	24000	80:20	1.1322	5.6629	1.1302	0.19958	0.99823	5.00168	NN
	24000	70:30	0.9963	0.9963	0.9948	0.99851	0.9985	0.99999	NN
3	36000	80:20	0.6534	0.6534	0.6534	1	0.99999	0.99999	NN
	36000	70:30	0.7512	0.7512	0.7505	0.99896	0.99895	0.99998	NN
4	48000	80:20	1.1386	1.1386	1.1385	0.99989	0.99991	1.00002	NN
	48000	70:30	0.7919	0.7919	0.7925	1.00081	1.00082	1.00001	ZIP
5	60000	80:20	0.8312	0.8312	0.8316	1.00055	1.00055	1	Hurdle
	60000	70:30	0.8326	0.8326	0.8316	0.99877	0.99876	0.99999	NN
6	72000	80:20	0.8312	0.8312	0.8316	1.00052	1.00055	1.00004	ZIP
	72000	70:30	0.7843	0.7843	0.7850	1.00089	1.00089	1	ZIP
7	84000	80:20	0.9039	0.9039	0.9032	0.99919	0.99918	0.99999	NN
	84000	70:30	0.9267	0.9268	0.9262	0.99938	0.99938	1	NN
8	96000	80:20	0.8566	0.8566	0.8565	0.99988	0.99991	1.00002	NN
	96000	70:30	0.8405	0.8405	0.8403	0.99985	0.99983	0.99999	NN
9	108000	80:20	0.8874	0.8873	0.8869	0.9995	0.99944	0.99993	NN
	108000	70:30	0.8441	0.8441	0.8440	0.99996	0.99995	0.99999	NN
10	120000	80:20	0.7321	0.7321	0.7320	0.9998	0.99980	1	NN
	120000	70:30	0.7488	0.7488	0.7487	0.99988	0.99986	0.99999	NN

TABLE 23.5
Avarage MSE and RE

MSE			RE	
ANN	**Hurdle**	**ZIP**	**ANN/Hurdle**	**ANN/ZIP**
0.8573	1.3889	0.8576	0.91470	0.99965

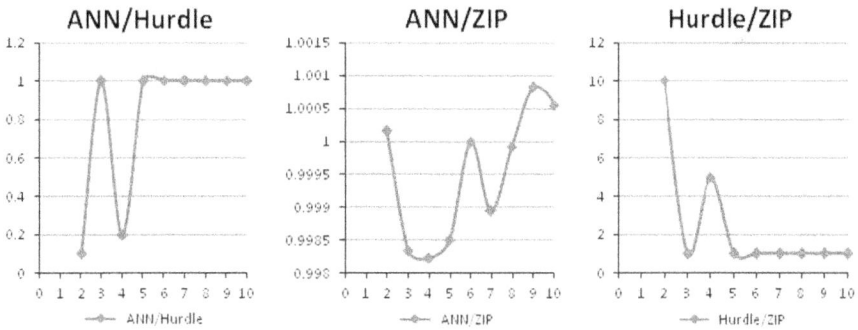

FIGURE 23.5   RE of ANN, hurdle, and ZIP.

ANN is the preferable model. Data presented in Tables 23.4 and 23.5 indicates that ANN can predict claim counts very close to the actual claim counts than ZIP and Hurdle models.

To avoid overfitting ANN, two various ratios for training and testing have been considered for analyzing the insurance data. In the first case, 70% of the data were used as the training set and 30% of the data as testing set. In the second case, 80% of the data were used as the training set and 20% of the data as testing set. Output resulted from predicted data and actual data showed that claim counts predicted with ANN are very close to the actual number of claims in terms of normalized MSE and relative efficiency.

23.6   CONCLUSION

We considered the zero-inflated Poisson regression model, Hurdle Poisson regression model, and ANN to model an overdispersed count data. We compared the suitability of these three models via an actual data study for different inflation rates and different sample sizes. The accuracy of these three models are compared in terms of MSE and RE. Our results demonstrated that for prediction of claim counts, ANN is invariably better and more accurate than Hurdle and zero-inflated Poisson regression models due to the lesser MSE value compared to ZIP and Hurdle regression models for overdispersed count data. While comparing the average relative efficiency, ANN performs better than ZIP and Hurdle models for this particular overdispersed count data. Even though all three models can remarkably predict the claim counts very close to the actual claim counts, the performance of ANNs for prediction of claim counts applying driver's age category, vehicle value, and period as input variables was greater and more accurate. Therefore it could be concluded that it is possible to apply ANNs in place of conventional procedures for the prediction of claim counts.

REFERENCES

Agatonovic Kustrins, S., Beresford, R., 2000. Basic concepts of artificial neural network (ANN) modeling and its application in pharmaceutical research, Journal of Pharmaceutical Biomedical Analysis, 22(5), pp. 717–727.

Ajibola, O.O.E., Olunloyo, V.O.S., Ibidapo-Obe, O., 2011. Artificial neural network simulation of arm gait in Huntington's disease patient, International Journal of Biomechatronics and Biomedical Robotics, 1(3), pp. 133–140.

Duch, W., Jankowski, N., 2001. Transfer functions: Hidden possibilities for better neural networks. Conference: ESANN 2001, 9th European Symposium on Artificial Neural Networks, Bruges, Belgium, April 25–27, 2001, Proceedings, 81–94.

Haykin, S., 1999. Neural Networks: A Comprehensive Foundation, 2nd edn. Prentice Hall, Upper Saddle River, USA.

Haykin, S.S., 2009. Neural Networks and Learning Machines. Pearson, Upper Saddle River, N.J.

Ibiwoye, A., Ajibola, O.O.E., Sogunro, A.B., 2012. Artificial neural network model for predicting insurance insolvency, International Journal of Management and Business, 2(1), pp. 59–68.

Minsky, M., Papert, S., 1969. Perceptrons. MIT Press, Oxford, England.

Parker, D., 1985. Learning-logic, Technical Report TR-47, Center for Computational Research in Economics and Management Science, MIT.

Rumelhart, D., McClelland, J., Williams, R., 1986. Parallel Recognition in Modern Computers Processing: Explorations in the Microstructure of Cognition, Vol. 1, MIT Press Foundations, Cambridge, MA.

Stergious, C., Siganos, D., 2007. Neural Networks. Available: www.Doc.k.ac.uk/and/surprise96/journal/Vol4/cs11/report.html

Werbos, P.J., 1974. Beyond Regression: New Tools for Prediction and Analysis in the Behavioral Sciences, Ph.D. Thesis, Harvard University, Cambridge, MA.

Index

Note: *Italicized* page numbers refer to figures, **bold** page numbers refer to tables

For Product Safety Concerns and Information please contact our EU
representative GPSR@taylorandfrancis.com
Taylor & Francis Verlag GmbH, Kaufingerstraße 24, 80331 München, Germany

www.ingramcontent.com/pod-product-compliance
Lightning Source LLC
Chambersburg PA
CBHW060422220326
41598CB00021BA/2264